400 More
Self Assessment
Picture Tests in
Clinical Medicine

400 More Self Assessment Picture Tests in Clinical Medicine

Year Book Medical Publishers, Inc.

This book is copyrighted in England and may not be
reproduced by any means in whole or part.
Distributed in North America, Canada, Hawaii and
Puerto Rico by Year Book Medical Publishers, Inc.
by arrangement with Wolfe Medical Publications Ltd.

Copyright © Wolfe Medical Publications Ltd, 1988
Printed by South Sea International Press Ltd, Hong Kong
ISBN 0-8151-9393-9

Library of Congress Cataloging-in-Publication Data

400 more self assessment picture tests in clinical medicine.
    p. cm.
  ISBN 0-8151-9393-9
  1. Diagnosis—Atlases. 2. Diagnosis—Examinations, questions,
etc. I. Title: Four hundred more self-assessment picture tests in
clinical medicine.
  [DNLM: 1. Diagnosis—atlases. 2. Diagnosis—problems. WB 18
Z95]
RC71.3.A169 1988
616.07'5—dc19
DNLM/DLC
for Library of Congress

Preface

400 More Self Assessment Picture Tests in Clinical Medicine is published in response to the enormous popularity with which the first volume, *400 Self Assessment Picture Tests in Clinical Medicine*, has been received by medical students and hospital doctors the world over.

Wolfe Medical Atlases represent a source of well over 80,000 colour diagnostic pictures. Since the sharpening of diagnostic skills depends so much upon the recognition of physical and clinical conditions, this second volume, like the first volume, comprises questions and photographs which have been specially set and selected by our own authors. The photographs have been gathered from existing atlases; the questions are completely new and original.

The questions are deliberately varied: some are apparently easy but actually present interesting differential problems. Others appear difficult in some respects but have a very straightforward answer. Others again are a mixture to tease out the many points an aggressive interrogator may want you to recognize.

This second volume will be of value not only to doctors working for higher qualifications and to students, but also to experienced clinicians who enjoy testing their knowledge.

The book source of each picture is traceable through the answers commencing on page 222. To have listed the sources with the questions would have made them easier, which is not the intention of the book!

Acknowledgements

The pictures, questions and answers in this book have kindly been provided by the following authors of many of the Colour Atlas series. The titles are listed on page 7.

Dr Michael Baraitser
Mr Michael A. Bedford
Dr A. Besson
Dr A.C. Boyle
Professor J.C. Brocklehurst
Mr T.R. Bull
Dr Rino Cerio
Dr D.R. Davies
Dr M. Dynski-Klein
Dr R.T.D. Emond
Dr D.C. Evered
Dr Geoffrey Farrer-Brown
Mr R.J. Flemans
Professor H.M. Gilles
Mr James Gow
Professor N.F.C. Gowing
Professor Reginald Hall
Professor F.G.J. Hayhoe
Dr S.M. Herber
Dr Wiliam Jackson
Dr Asif Kamal
Professor Lipmann Kessel
Miss Erna E. Kritzinger
Dr Jack M. Lancer
Mr R.W. Lloyd-Davies
Dr Donald S. McLaren
Dr Joseph B. Michelson
Mr K.L.G. Mills
Professor R.D.G. Milner
Dr Malcolm Parsons
Dr Victor Parsons
Mr M. Robson Parsons
Professor W. Peters
Professor F. Saegesser
Professor Lewis Spitz
Dr G.M. Steiner
Professor V.R. Tindall
Dr W.R. Tyldesley
Mr Roger Watkins
Dr G. Williams
Dr J.G.P. Williams
Dr Robin Winter
Professor R.B. Zachary

Most of the illustrations used in this book have appeared in the following colour Atlases. The code in bold type following each title is repeated by the side of the answer and thus the source of the illustration may readily be identified. Example: **gem**—the illustrations come from **A Colour Atlas of Geriatric Medicine.**

A Colour Atlas of Accidents and Emergencies **ae**
A Colour Atlas of Allergy **al**
A Colour Atlas of Bone Disease **bd**
A Colour Atlas of Cardiac Pathology **cpa**
A Colour Atlas of Chest Trauma Volume One **chtr 1**
A Colour Atlas of Chest Trauma Volume Two **chtr 2**
A Colour Atlas of Clinical Genetics **cg**
A Colour Atlas of Clinical Gynaecology **clgy**
A Colour Atlas of Clinical Neurology **cln**
A Colour Atlas of Clinical Orthopaedics **co**
A Colour Atlas of Endocrinology **end**
A Colour Atlas of ENT Diagnosis **ent**
A Colour Atlas of the Eye and Systemic Diseases **esd**
A Colour Atlas of Fibreoptic Endoscopy of the Upper Respiratory Tract **feurt**
A Colour Atlas of Geriatric Medicine **gem**

A Colour Atlas of Haematological Cytology **hacy**
A Colour Atlas of Infectious Diseases **id**
A Colour Atlas of Injury in Sport **is**
A Colour Atlas of the Newborn **nb**
A Colour Atlas of Nutritional Disorders **nd**
A Colour Atlas of Ocular Tumours **ot**
A Colour Atlas of Ophthalmological Diagnosis **od**
A Colour Atlas of Oral Medicine **om**
A Colour Atlas of Paediatrics **pd**
A Colour Atlas of Paediatric Surgical Diagnosis **psd**
A Colour Atlas of Renal Diseases **rd**
A Colour Atlas of Rheumatology **rh**
A Colour Atlas of Stroke **st**
A Colour Atlas of Tropical Medicine and Parasitology **tmp**
A Colour Atlas of Tumour Histopathology **th**
A Colour Atlas of Urology **ur**
A Colour Atlas of Uveitis Diagnosis **ud**

1 Patches of calcific material are deposited in the skin of the hands. What is the diagnosis?

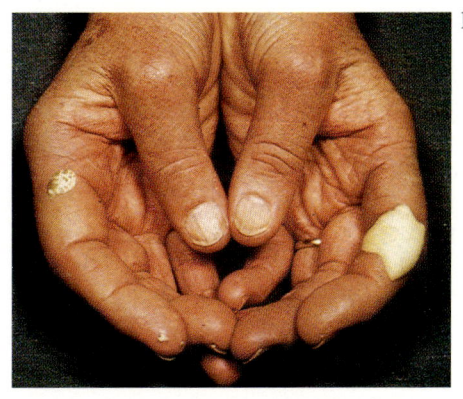

2 This patient, aged 17, complained of lower abdominal pain, occurring at intervals of approximately four weeks on and off for two to three years. On questioning, she had never menstruated.

a) What is the diagnosis?
b) What is the treatment and what are the risks of treatment?

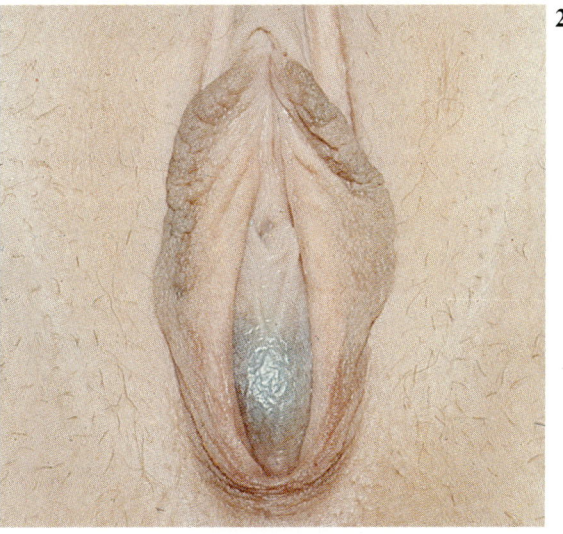

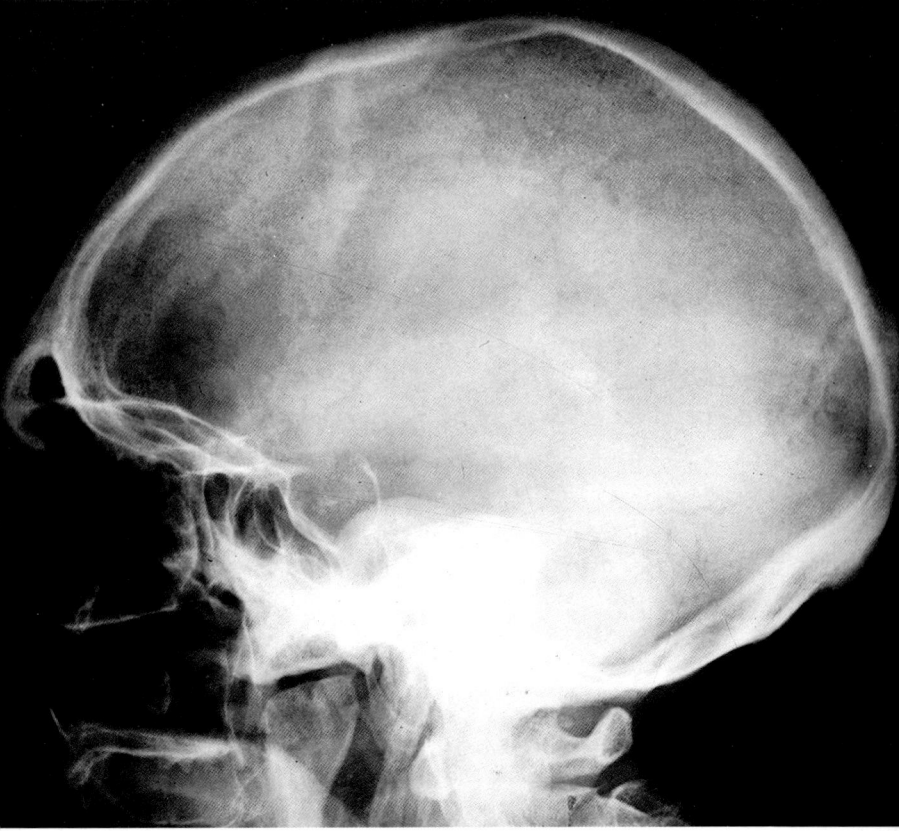

3 The patient with this abnormal X-ray of the skull will probably have:

a) Amaurosis fugax,
b) Hypertension,
c) Increased sweating,
d) Glycosuria,
e) Obesity.

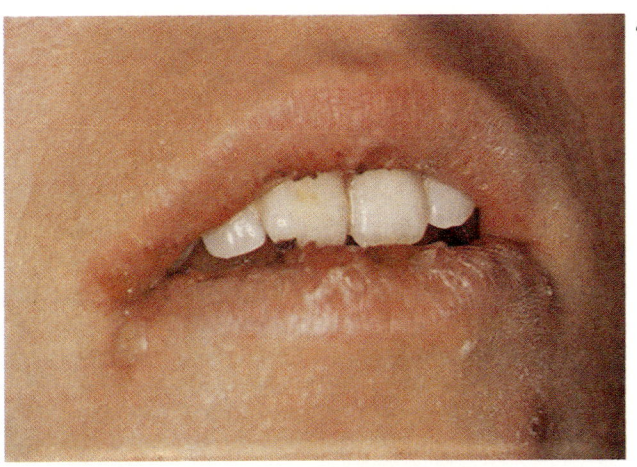

4 This is a common infective condition affecting the mouth.

   a) What is the most likely infective agent?
   b) What is an important differential diagnosis?
   c) What is a possible sequel of this infection?

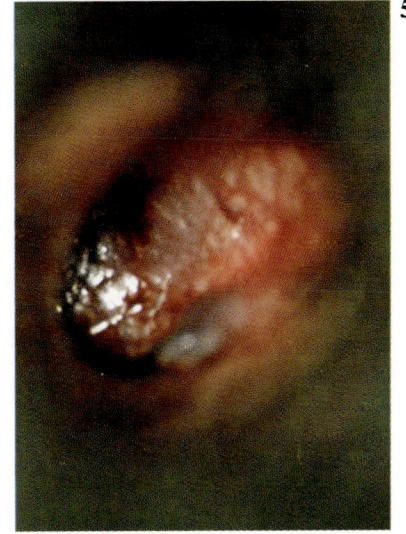

5 An episode of ear ache followed by bleeding without trauma is likely to be due to:

   a) Ramsey–Hunt syndrome?
   b) Bullous myringitis?
   c) Ménière's disease?
   d) An aural neoplasm?

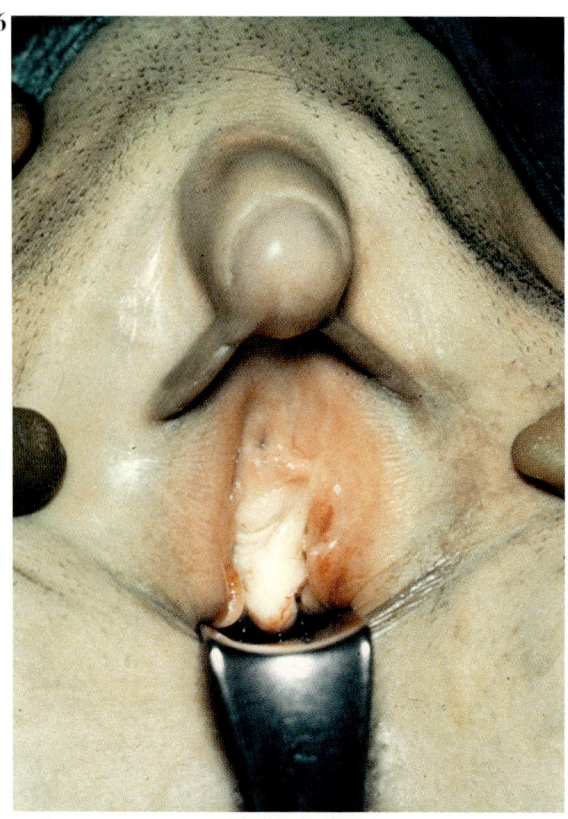

6 This patient had amenorrhoea and signs of virilism.

a) What is the most likely diagnosis and what is the cause?
b) Can it be diagnosed antenatally?
c) With appropriate treatment is the patient likely to be fertile?

7 a) What is this condition?
b) How does it present?
c) What new development in treatment offers rapid relief and return to normal activity?

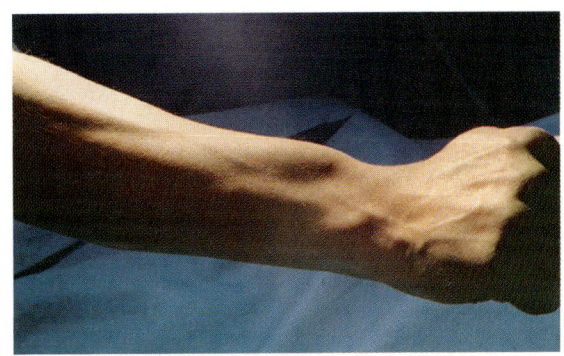

8 A bone marrow smear. Identify the cells shown.

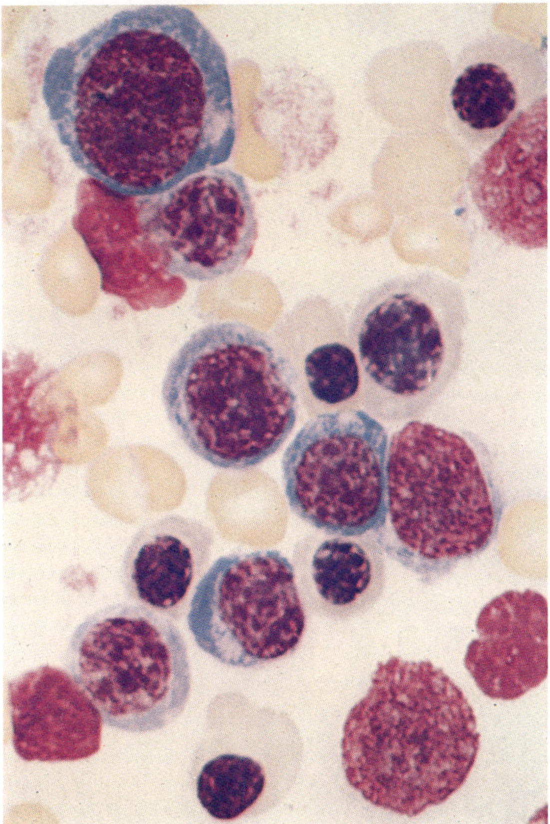

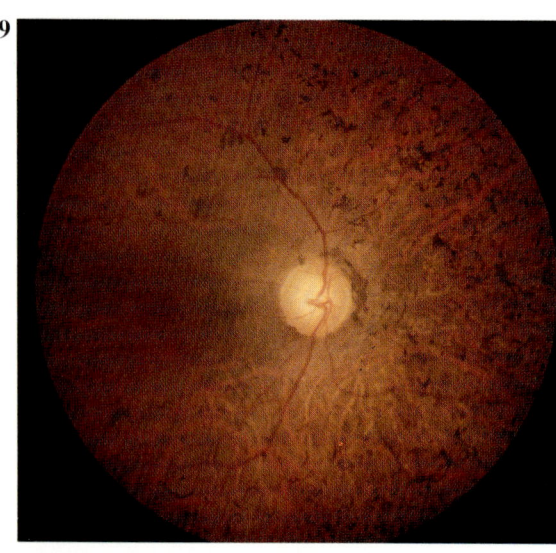

9 a) Name the abnormality and describe the appearance of the fundus.
b) In which syndrome is this ocular abnormality associated with obesity, mental retardation and hypogonadism?
c) What abnormality of the hands is an additional feature of the syndrome?

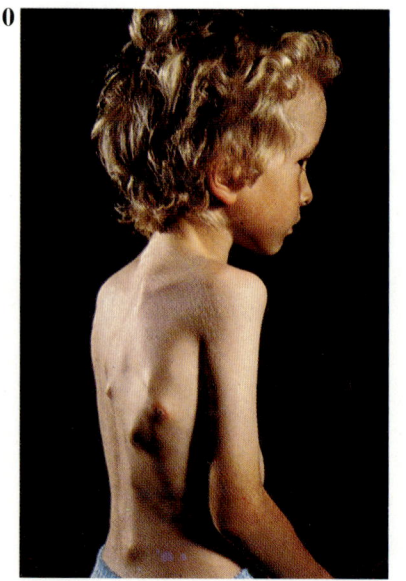

10 There are dense, painful plaques of bony material visible and palpable on this child's back. What is the diagnosis?

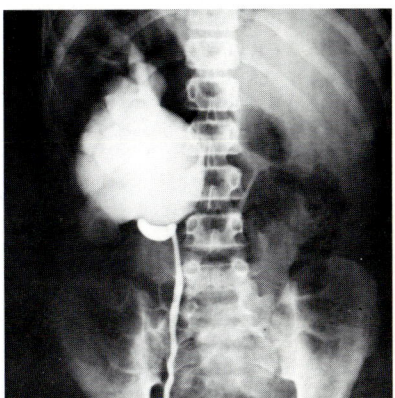

11 Right ureterogram on a patient presenting with fluid induced right loin pain.

  a) What is the abnormality?
  b) What is the probable cause?

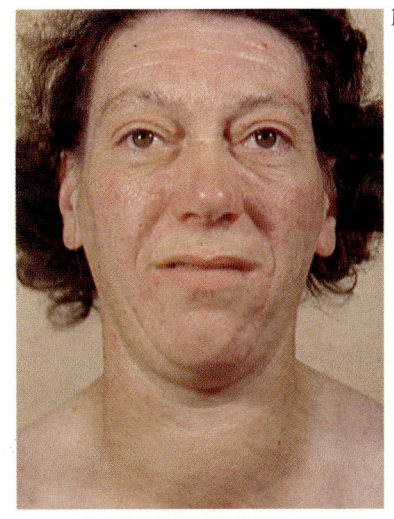

12 a) What is the likely diagnosis in this patient?
  b) List the clinical features shown.
  c) List three major complications of this disorder.
  d) How should the diagnosis be confirmed?

13 An elderly man was referred for examination after a brief period of 'confusion'. The only abnormality found was his inability to draw clocks, for example.

  a) What is this called?
  b) Where is the lesion?
  c) Which other signs in this category are sometimes produced by a lesion at this site?

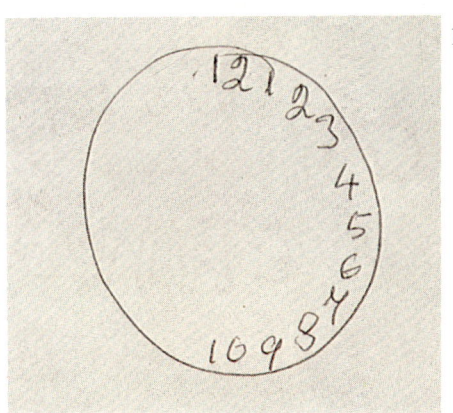

14 This patient with rheumatoid arthritis developed a sudden painful swelling of the left calf. What is the likely diagnosis?

15 Eversion of the lower lid demonstrates a pinkish-yellow lesion on the surface of the bulbar conjunctiva. Which disease is suggested by this clinical sign?

   a) Sarcoidosis?
   b) Conjunctival lymphoma?
   c) Retained foreign body?
   d) Papillae from allergy?

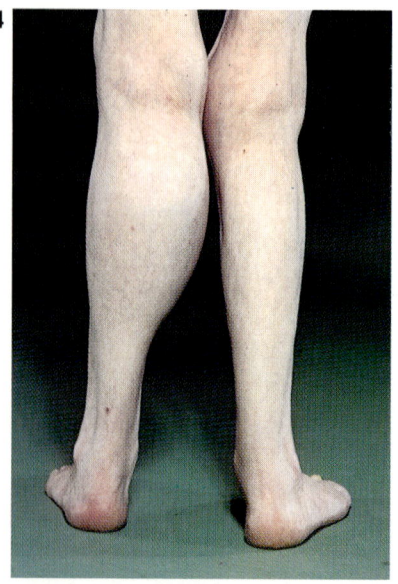

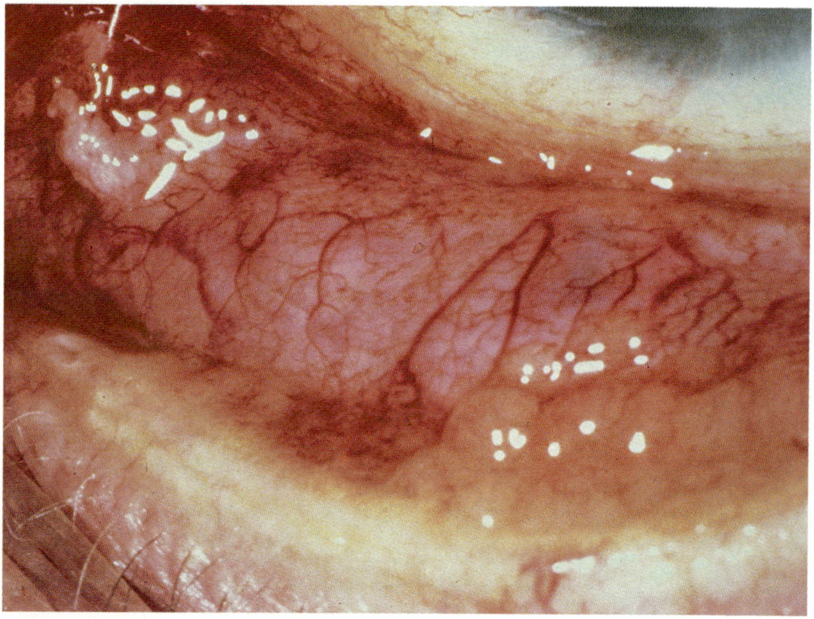

16 This patient may have a history of:

a) Hypothyroidism.
b) Polycythaemia.
c) Hyperadreno-corticism.
d) Pellagra.
e) Chronic corticosteroid ingestion.

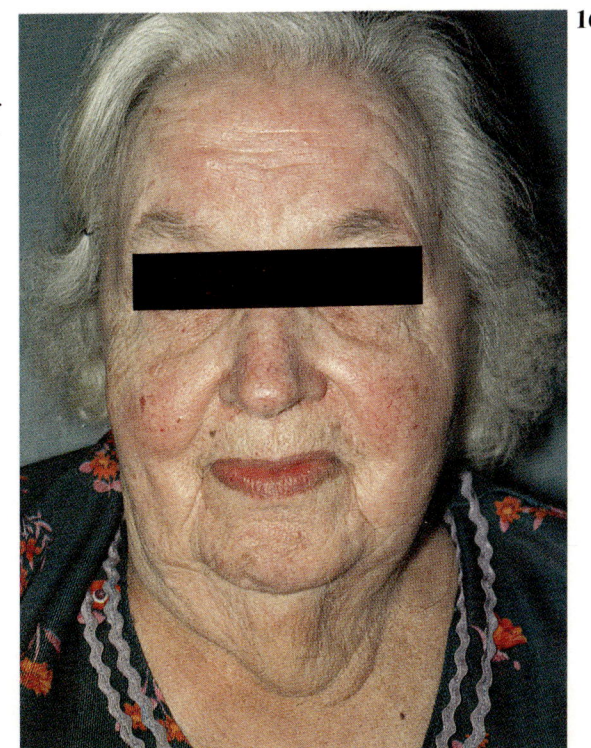

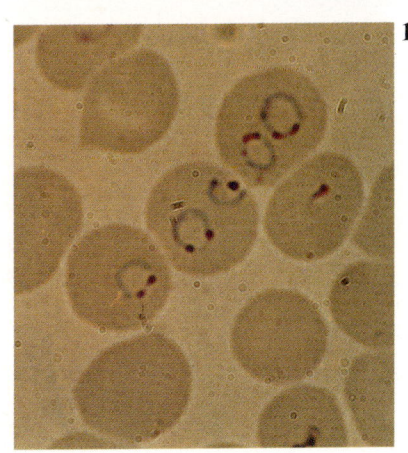

17 What is this parasite found in human blood?

18 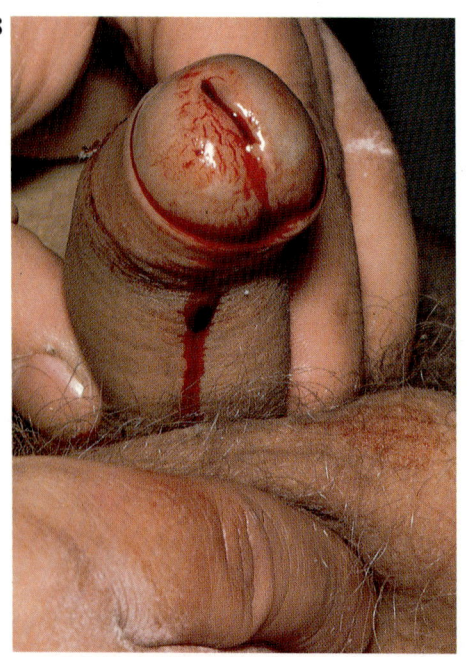 This man was involved in a road traffic accident. His immediate urinary tract investigation should be:

a) Urethral catheterization and cystography to check the integrity of the bladder.
b) Intravenous pyelography to check the integrity of the kidney.
c) Ascending cystourethrogram to check the integrity of the urethra and bladder.

19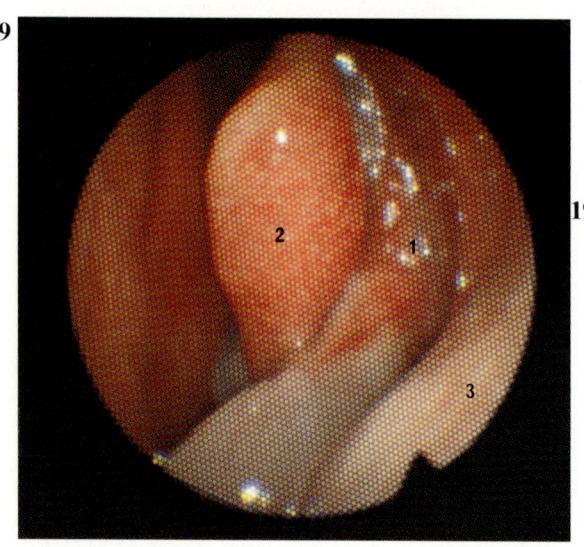

19 a) What is the swelling (1) which is arising between the middle (2) and the inferior (3) turbinates within the nasal cavity?
b) What childhood disease is associated with this swelling?

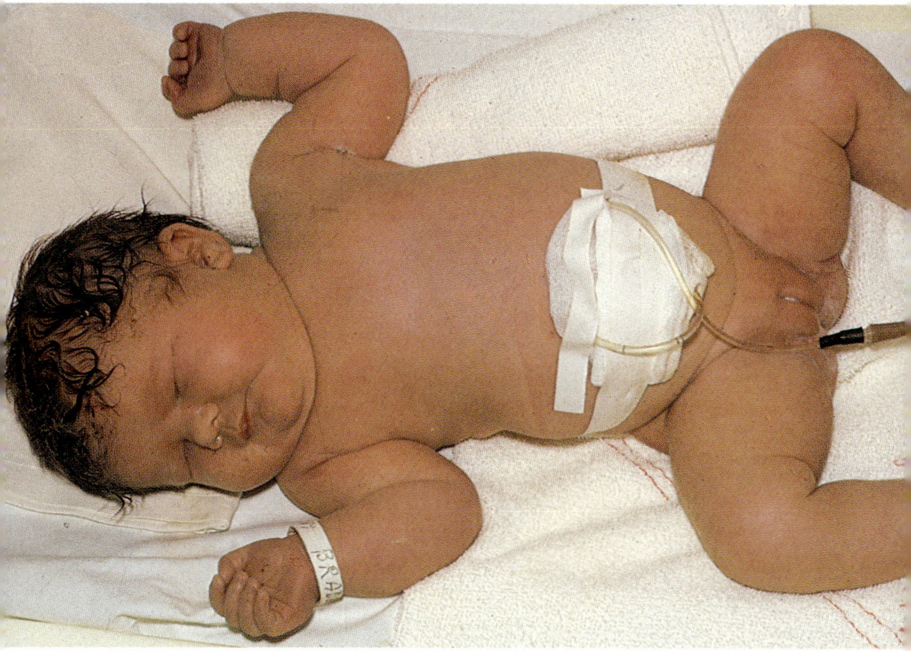

20 This is the infant of a diabetic mother. Which complication is *not* associated with these infants?

a) Hyaline membrane disease.
b) Post-maturity.
c) Hypoglycaemia.
d) Jaundice.
e) Increased incidence of cleft palate.

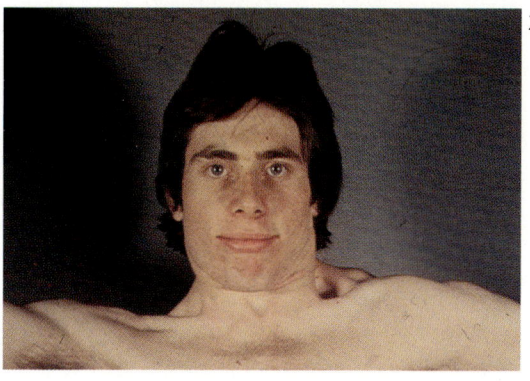

21 What is the name of this characteristic facial appearance, and with what condition is it associated?

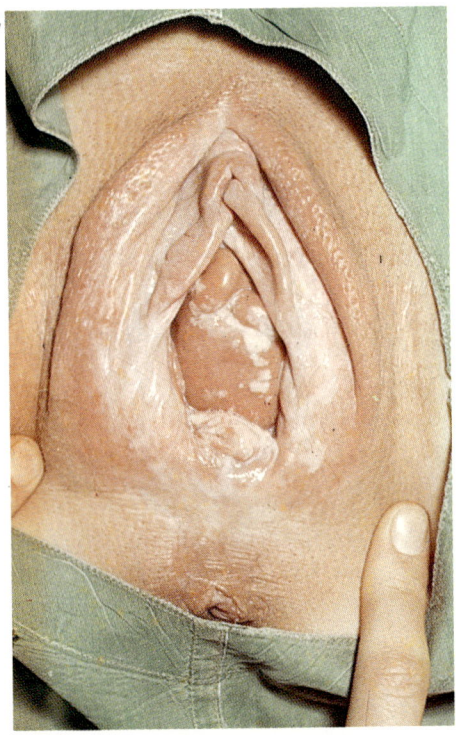

22 This patient complained of pruritus vulva and vaginal discharge.
   a) What is the likely diagnosis and what is the treatment?
   b) Under what circumstance may this type of infection occur?

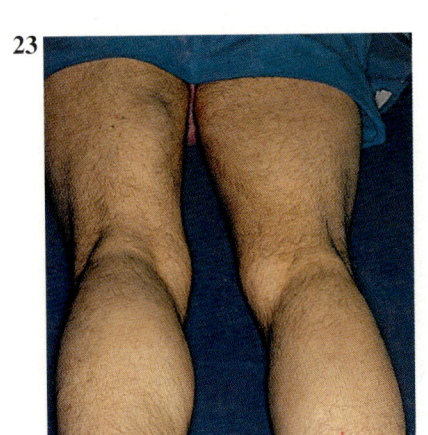

23 This patient presented in clinic with a history of a twisting injury of the knee and inability fully to extend it. Why is it important to examine such patients in prone as well as supine lying?

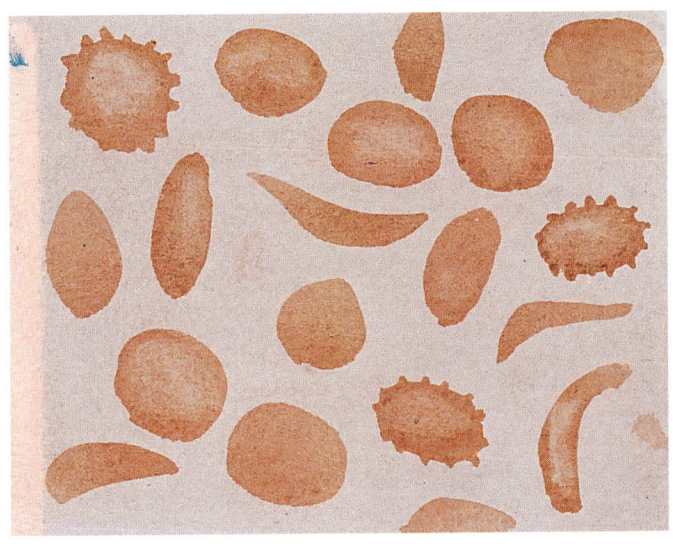

24 This is a blood film taken from a young patient with long-standing history of anaemia, joint pain and minor strokes. It shows:

a) Target cells?
b) Hereditary elliptocytosis?
c) Sickle-cell anaemia?
d) Multiple myeloma?
e) Malarial parasites?

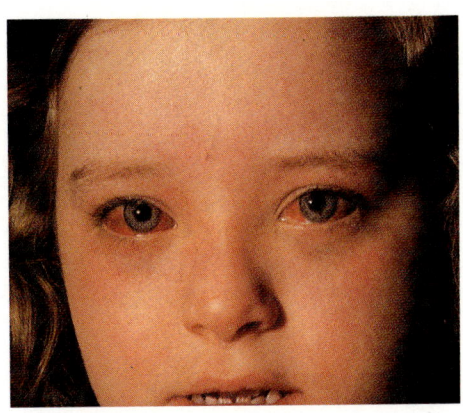

25 This girl was involved in a motor-car accident.

a) What injury was sustained?
b) What is characteristic about the physical sign?
c) How could the injury have possibly been prevented?

26

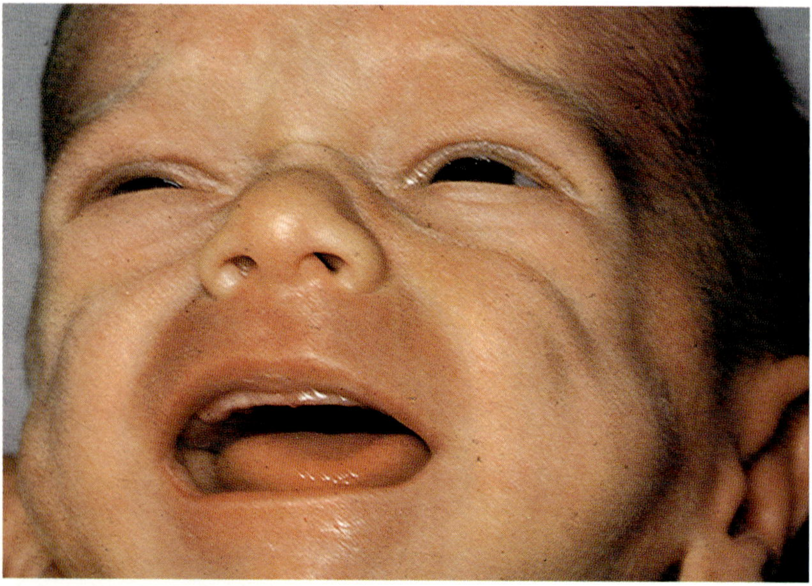

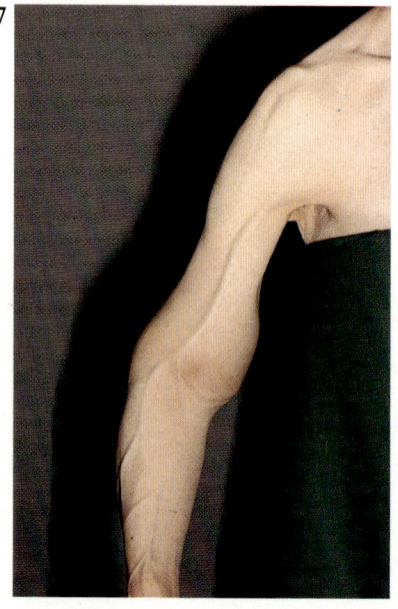

26 What is the rounded swelling on the baby's cheeks?

27 A large painful swelling has appeared in the lower arm of a patient suffering from Paget's disease—note the increased vascularity. What is the likely diagnosis?

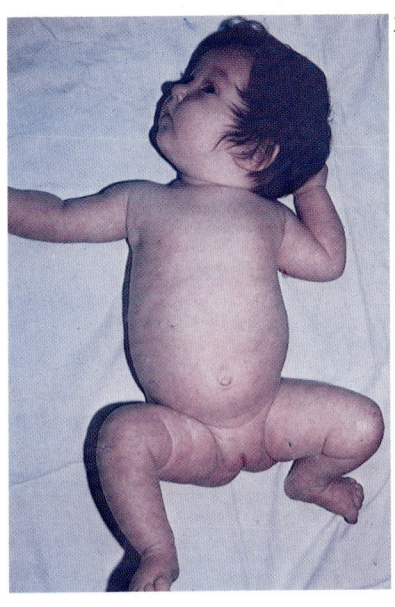

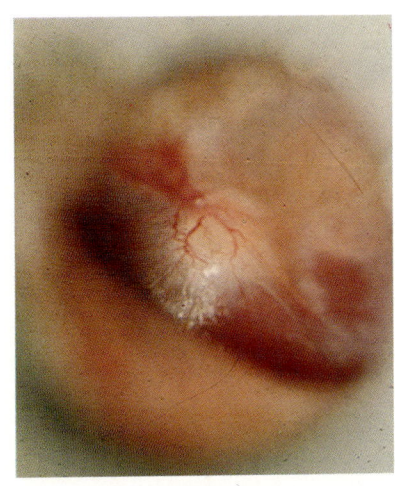

28 What is the name of the baby's peculiar posture?

29 A complaint of pulsating tinnitus without earache with this red tympanic membrane is likely to be due to:

a) A variant of otitis media?
b) 'Glue' ear?
c) A high jugular bulb?
d) A glomus jugulare tumour?

30 Photomicrograph of a rectal biopsy from a mucosal lesion 5-cm in diameter. The patient was a 54-year-old woman. (*H&E* × 90.)

a) What is the lesion?
b) What are the clinical manifestations?

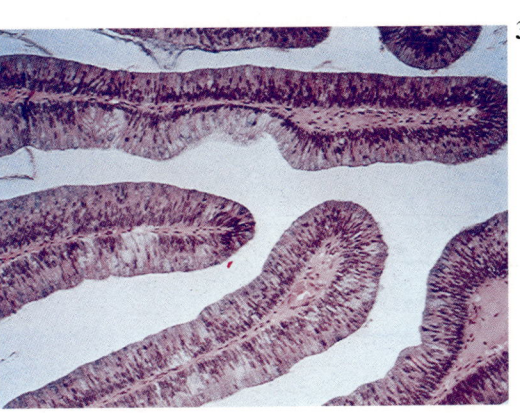

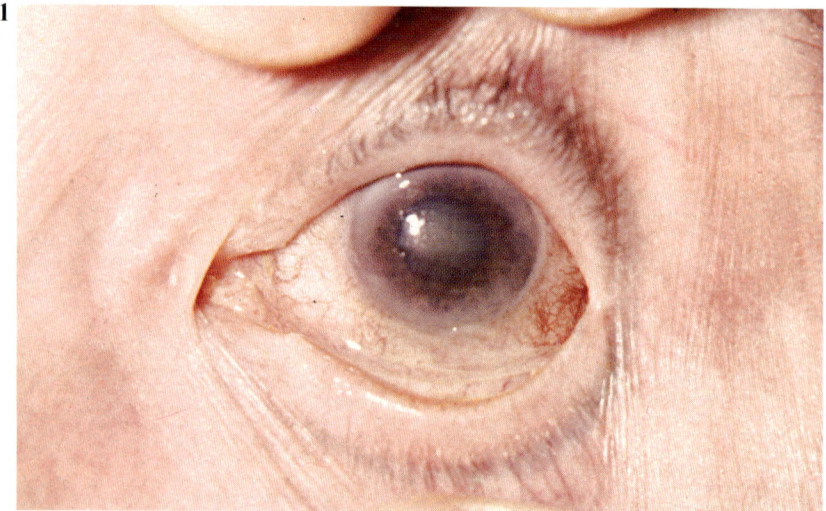

31 The patient complains of a sudden severe pain in his eye, perhaps preceded by haloes around lights. He may be nauseated and even collapse.

a) What are the physical signs and what is the diagnosis?
b) How should it be treated by the general practitioner?

32 a) What names are given to this condition?
b) What organisms are associated with it?

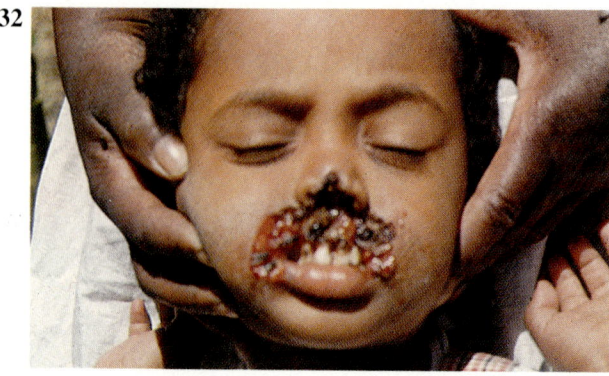

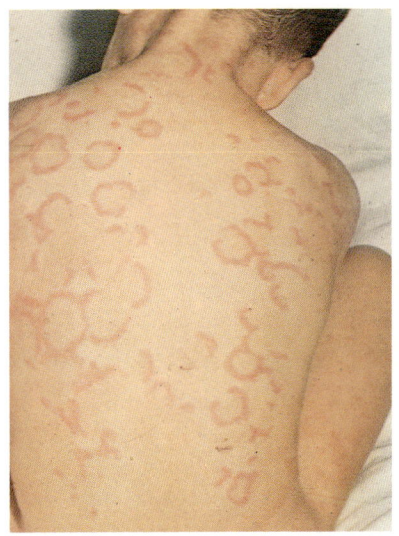

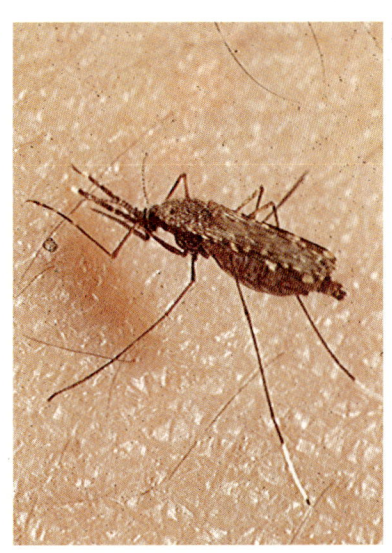

33
 a) What is the name of this erythema?
 b) What is its cause?
 c) With what disease is it associated?

34
 a) What is this insect?
 b) Can it carry any disease to man?

35 A patient admitted from a psychiatric ward.

  a) What is the nature and aetiology of his neurological disorder?
  b) What is the significance of the aetiological diagnosis?
  c) What is the condition with which this disorder is often confused?

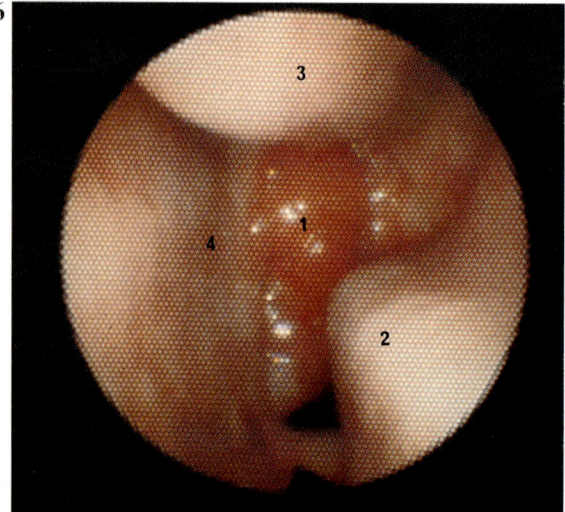

36 This is the nasal cavity of an 8-year-old child whose principle complaints are snoring and nasal obstruction. What abnormality is present?

37 a) What chromosomal abnormality is likely?
b) What physical signs are shown?

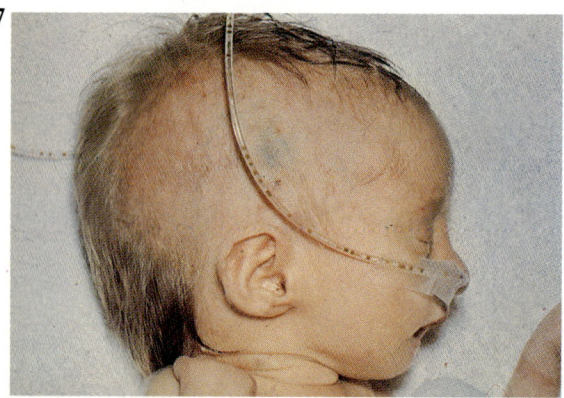

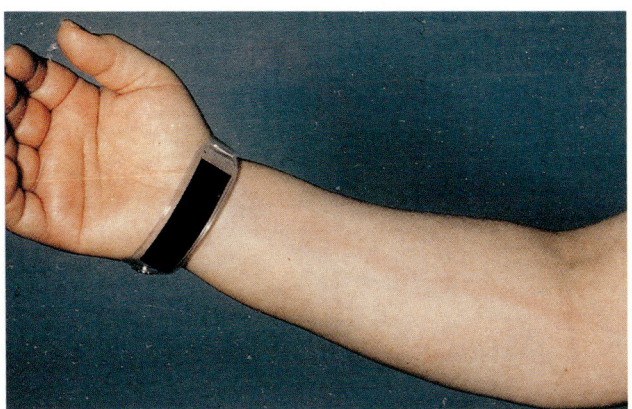

38 Following an infection in his hand, this man developed a tender red linear streak along the anterior aspect of his forearm?

a) What is the condition called?
b) What is the usual causative organism?
c) What associated condition can often be diagnosed by examination of the axilla?

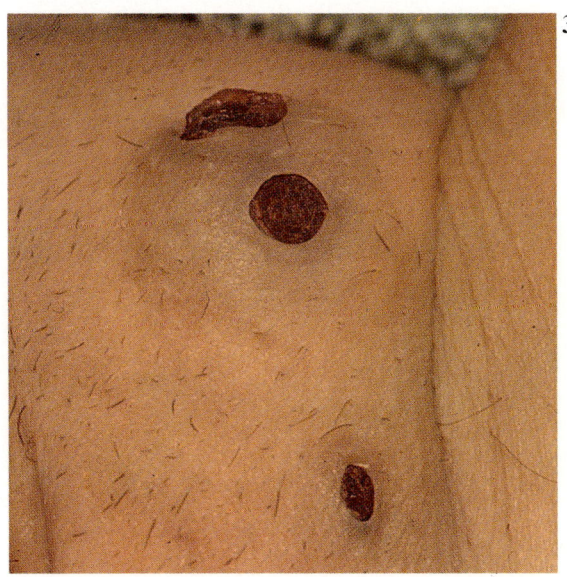

39 a) What is the diagnosis and what other sites may be involved?
b) What is the treatment?

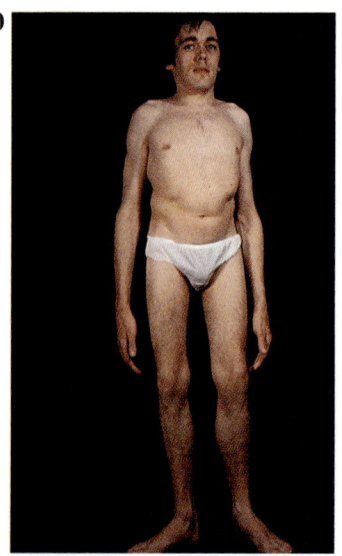 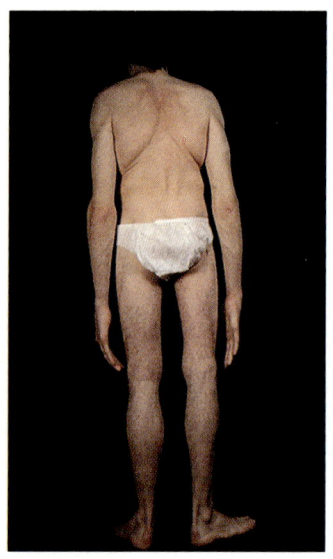

40 This young man has a short trunk and disproportionately long arms. He has a spinal and thoracic deformity. What is the diagnosis?

41 What is the term applied to this unusual form of kwashiorkor?

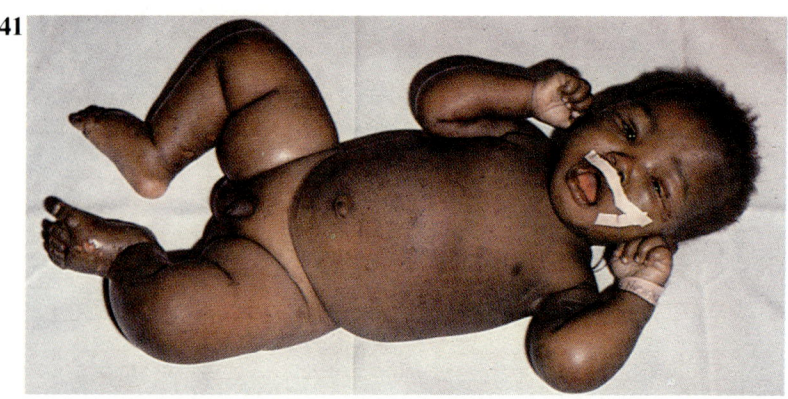

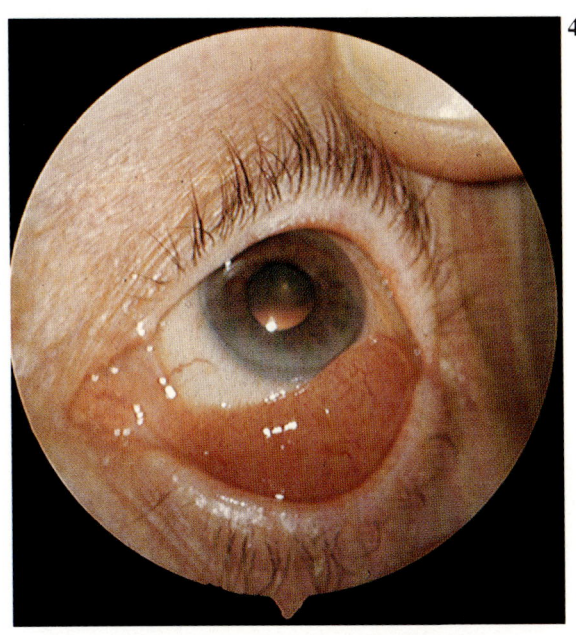

42 The patient complains of a swelling on the outside of the eye.

a) What is the physical sign?
b) What is the likely diagnosis?

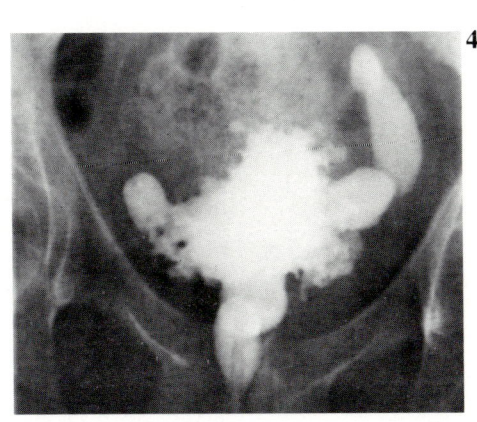

43 a) What abnormalities can be seen in this micturating cystogram?
b) What is the underlying problem?

44

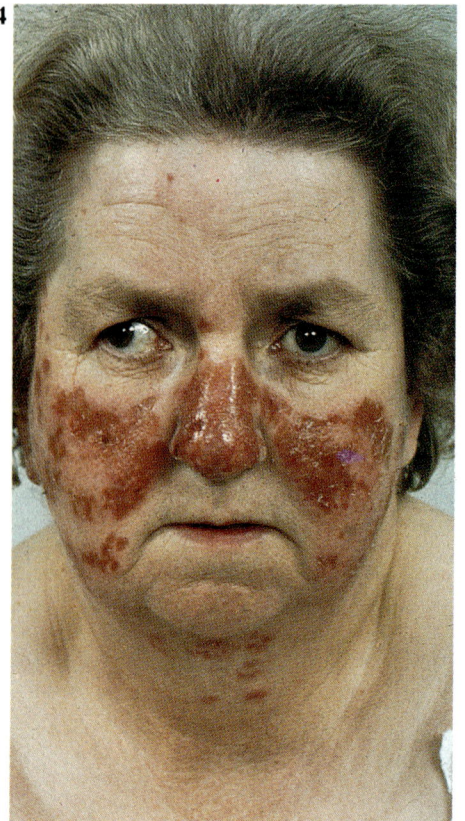

44 This patient is likely to have:

a) Arthropathy?
b) Dementia?
c) Postural hypotension?
d) Proteinuria?
e) Lupus erythematosus?

45

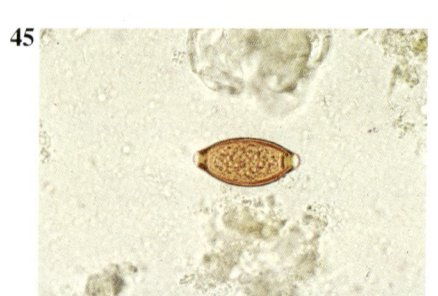

45 A child is brought to the clinic with bloody diarrhoea. Examination of the stool reveals eggs with this characteristic shape. What is the diagnosis?

46 The posterior surface of a heart with nodules scattered in the pericardium. What are the nodules due to?

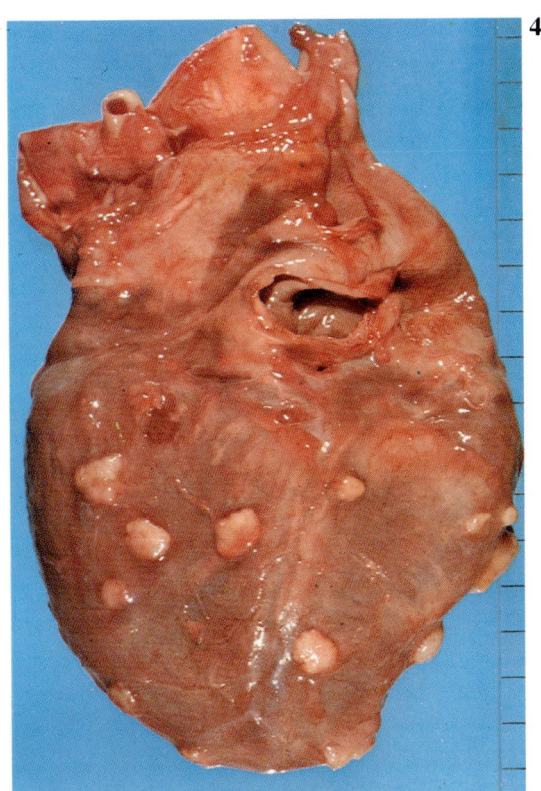

47 The most likely cause of this lesion is:

a) A retained foreign body.
b) Fungal infection.
c) Chronic infection with *Staphylococcus aureus*.

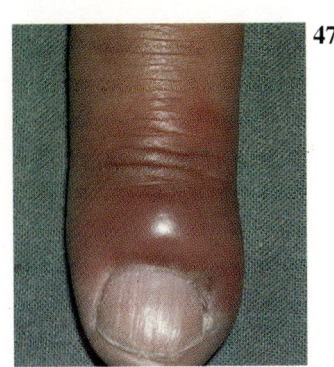

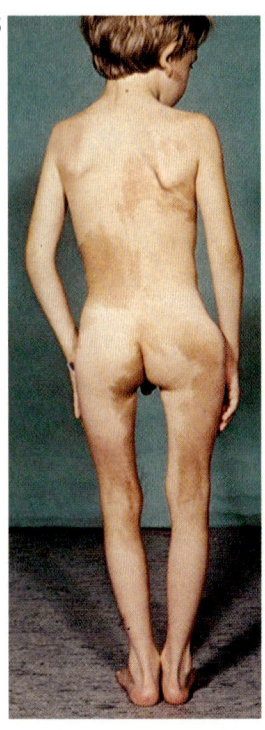
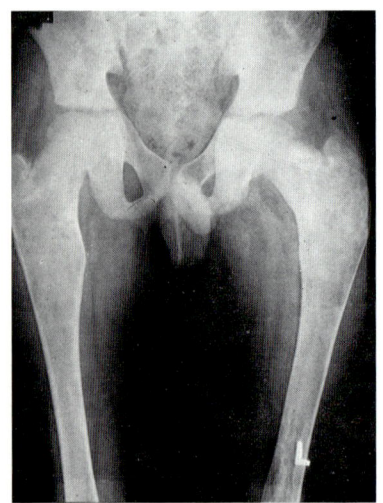

48 This young teenager shows cutaneous pigmentation, and on the X-rays fibrotic areas appear scattered as patches of rarefaction. What is the diagnosis, and with what is it usually associated?

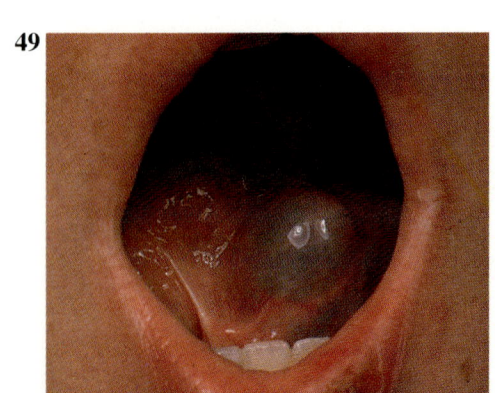

49 Note the bluish swelling in the floor of the mouth.

a) What is the diagnosis?
b) What is the origin?
c) What is the treatment?

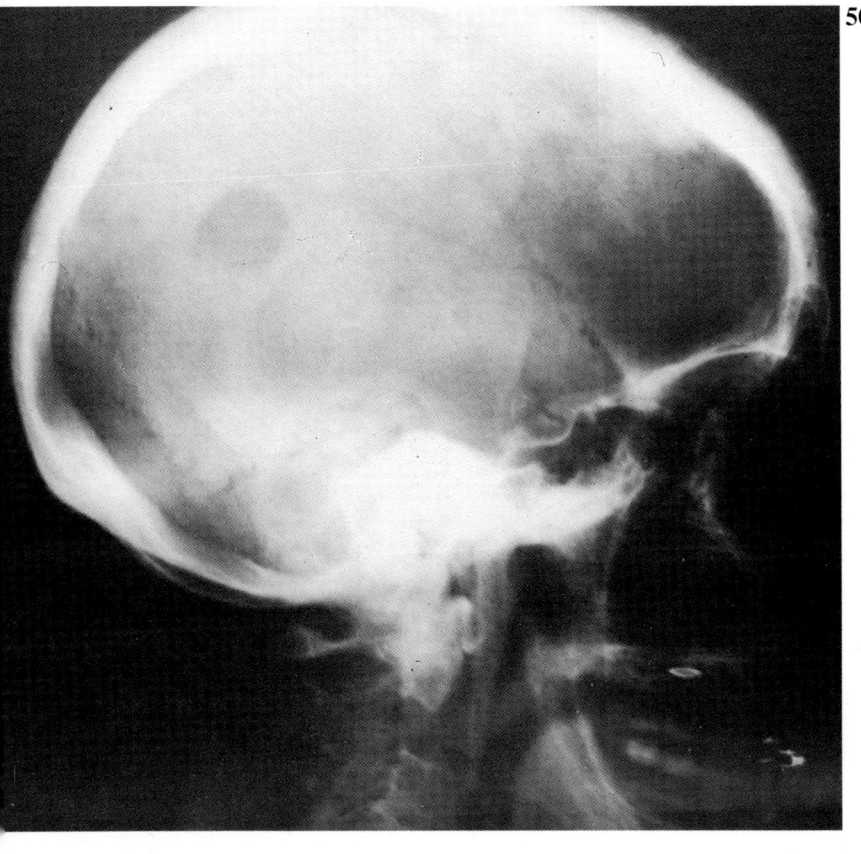

50 This skull X-ray shows:

a) Hyperostosis frontalis interna?
b) Cerebral atrophy?
c) Hydrocephalus?
d) Pick's disease?
e) Osteoporosis circumscripta?

51 a) What is the likely cause of the eruption?
b) How common is it?
c) How can it be prevented?
d) How can it be proved?

52 Heel-to-ear manoeuvre. What is abnormal?

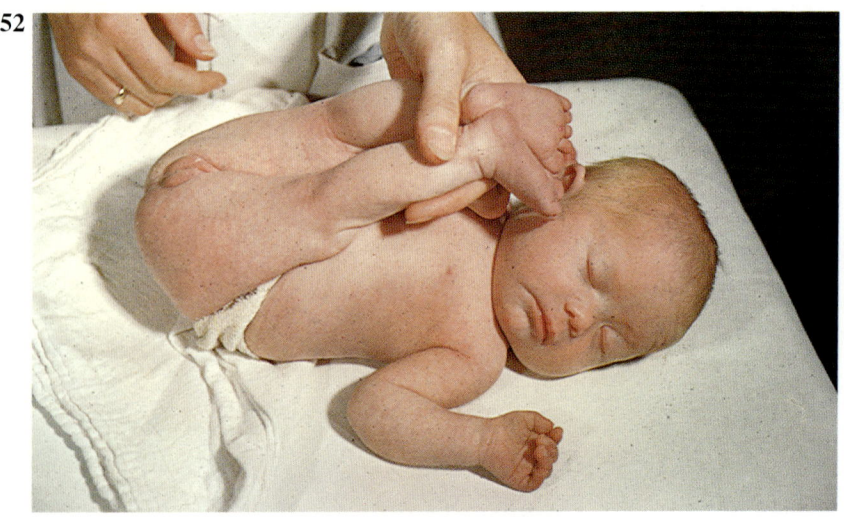

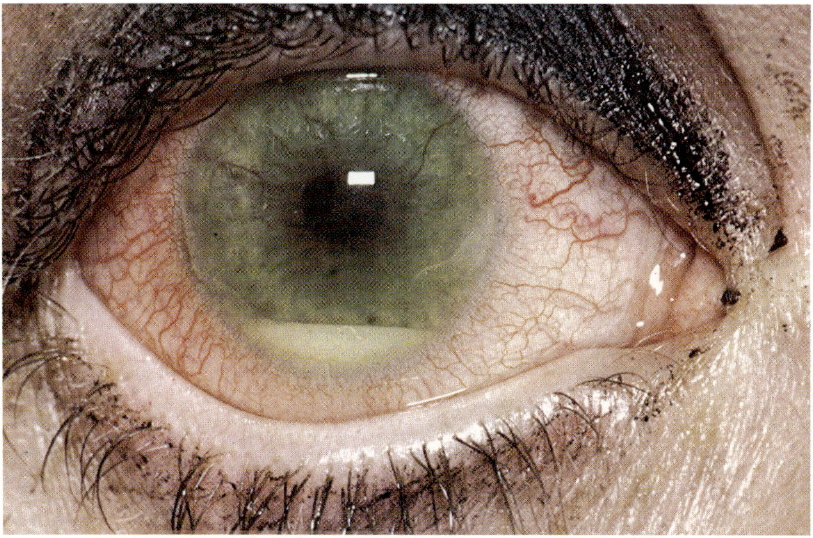

53 The patient gives a history that she attended for treatment some weeks before with sore red eyes and she was prescribed eye drops; her eye felt better and now suddenly feels worse.

a) What are the physical signs and what is the diagnosis?
b) How should it be treated?

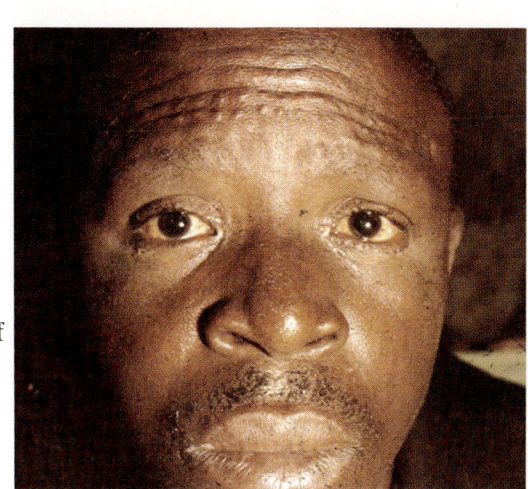

54 What is the cause of these bilateral, chronic, painless swellings of the sides of the face below the ears?

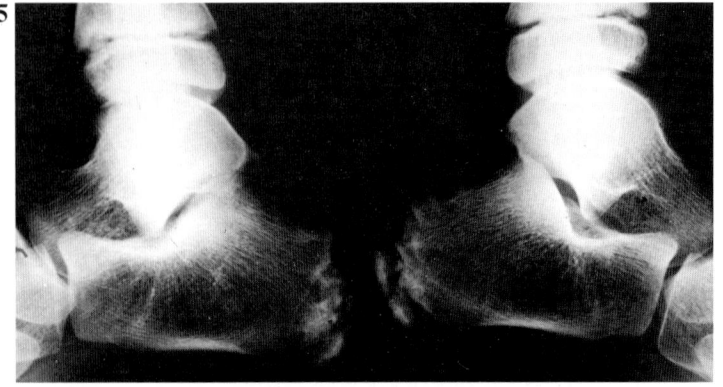

55 What is the significance of the appearances of the heels in these lateral radiographs of the ankles of a 12-year-old?

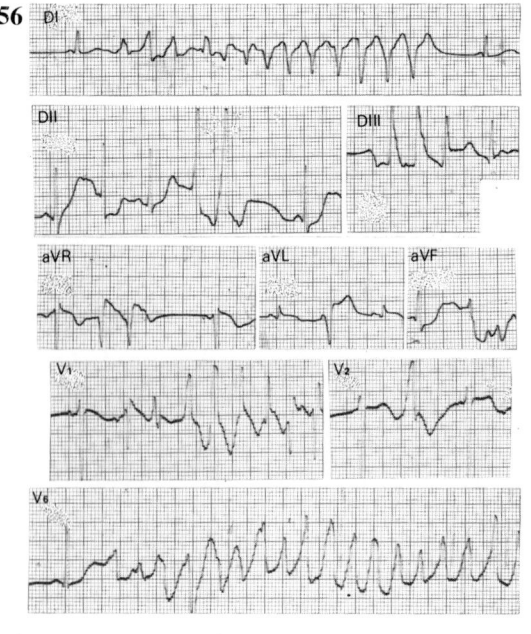

56 This is an ECG trace obtained:
  a) In a resuscitation after a fall.
  b) During cardiac surgery with hypothermia.
  c) When placing a pace-maker in a digitalised patient.

57 This young, intelligent man has a marked discrepancy in the length of his arms, which are deformed. From what does he suffer?

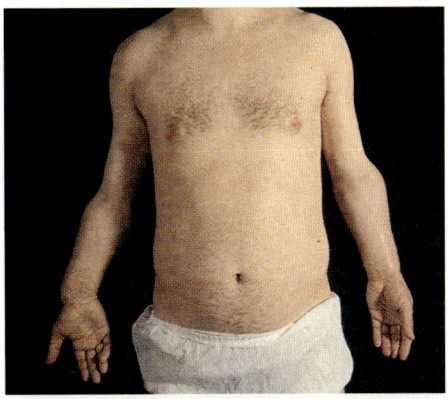
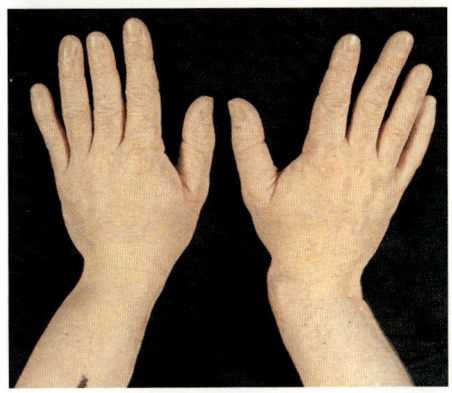

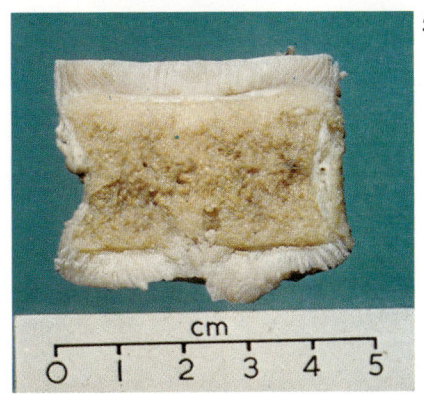

58 This type of trabecular change is associated with:

a) Osteomyelitis.
b) Fluorosis.
c) Renal osteodystrophy.
d) Secondary deposits of carcinoma of the prostate.
e) Osteogenesis imperfecta.

59

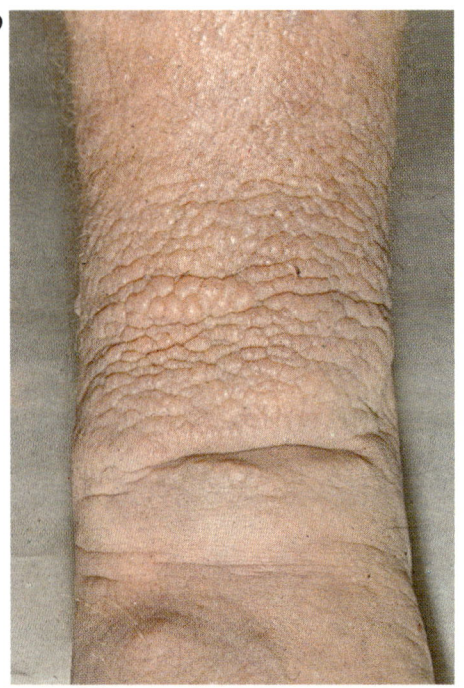

59 a) What is the likely diagnosis?
b) Name two clinical conditions with which this disorder may be associated.
c) What causes the thickening of the skin?
d) What is the characteristic immunological feature of this condition?

60

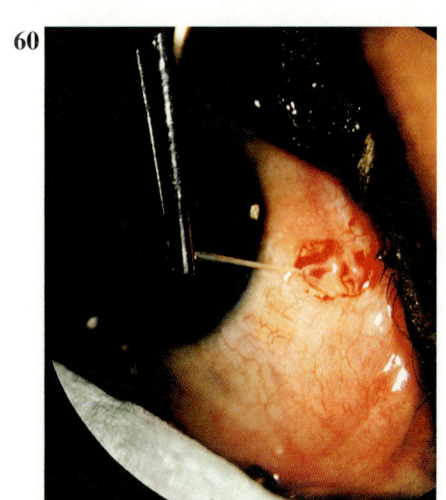

60 This patient from West Africa complained of feeling a worm crossing his eye. What is the likely diagnosis?

61 a) What is this condition?
b) What would you examine next?
c) What is the first consideration in treatment?

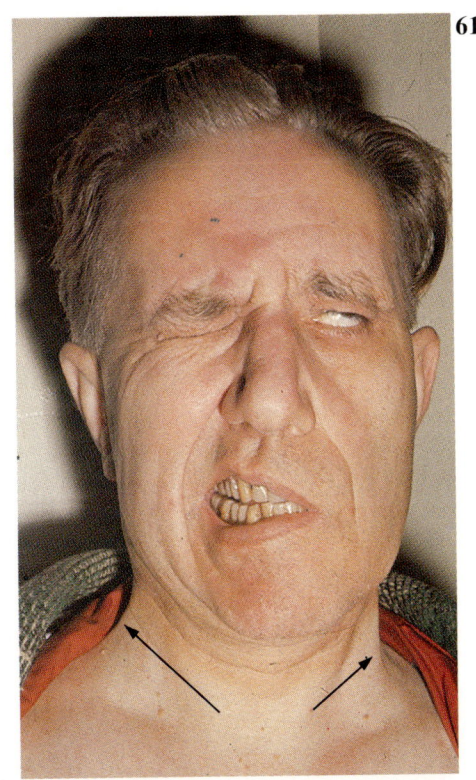

62 This lesion:

a) Is only found on the scalp.
b) Becomes malignant in over 50 per cent of cases.
c) Is inherited as an X-linked recessive.
d) Recedes rapidly with steroid therapy.
e) Has a characteristically nodular surface.

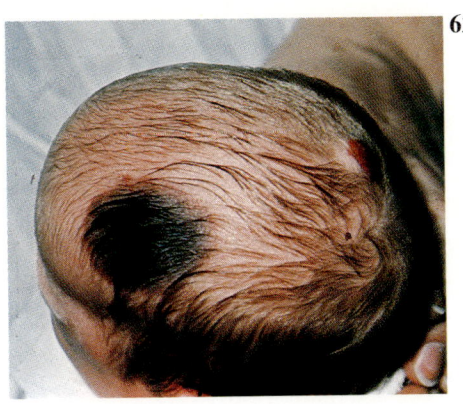

63

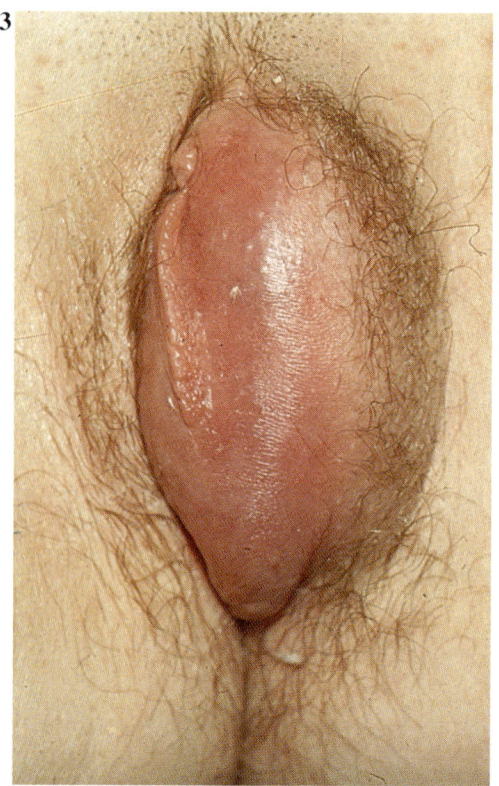

63 What is the diagnosis and treatment of choice?

64

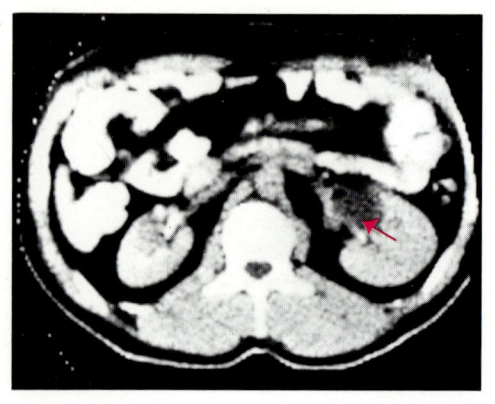

64 CAT scan of abdomen showing a solitary abnormality. What is it?

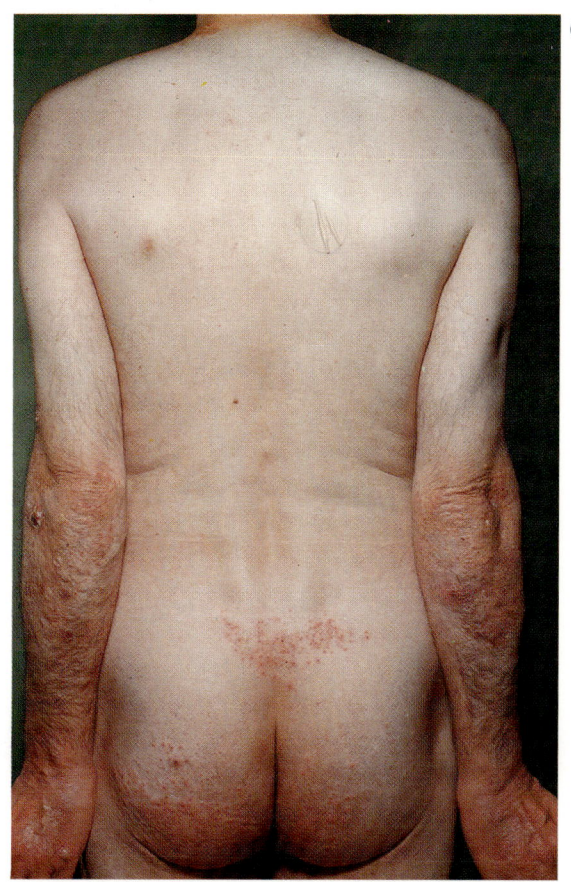

65 This 40-year-old man has a pruritic vesicular eruption.

a) What is the likely diagnosis?
b) What special investigations are indicated?
c) Is there any complication of this condition?
d) What is the treatment?

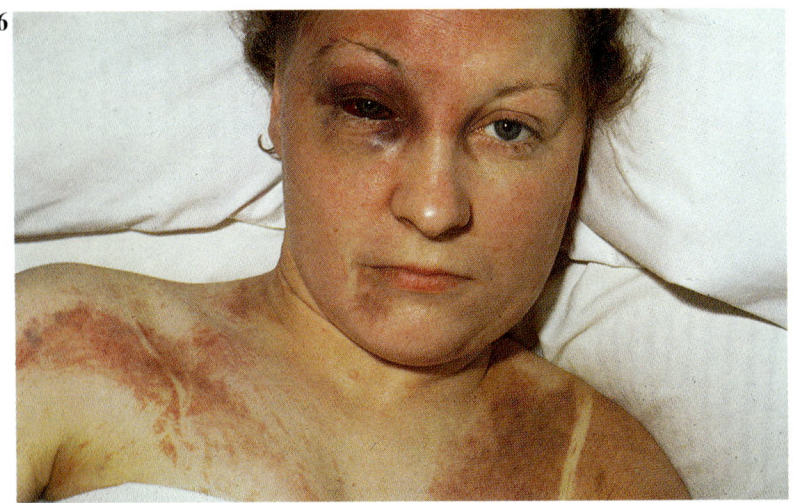

66 This woman, crushed in a crowd, is suffering from:

a) Fat embolism.
b) Henoch-Schönlein purpura.
c) Traumatic asphyxia.

67 What common viral infection of childhood takes a highly fatal form in malnourished patients with this florid rash?

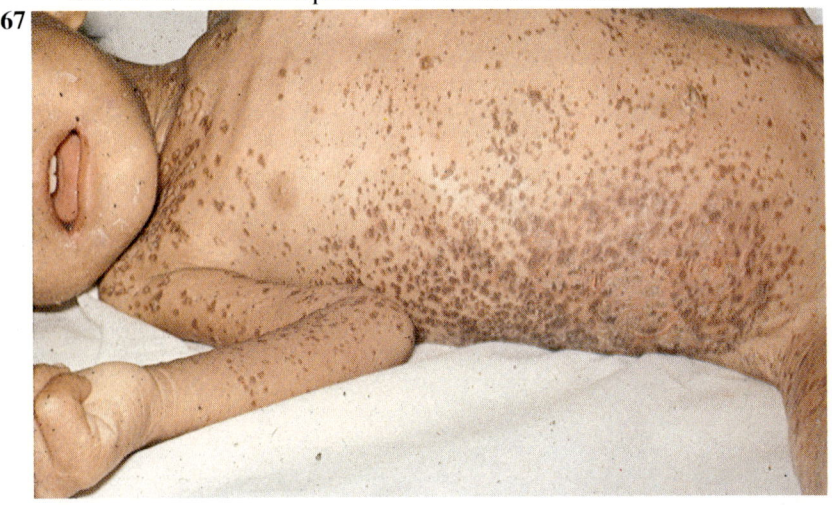

68 What is the significance of the deformities in the hand?

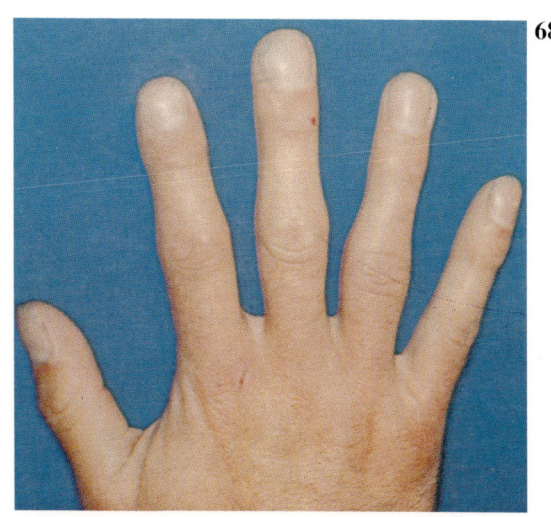

69 a) What is this condition?
b) What is its significance?

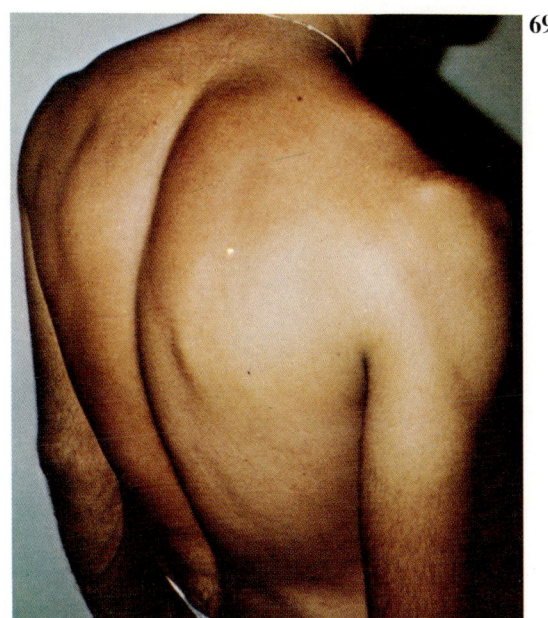

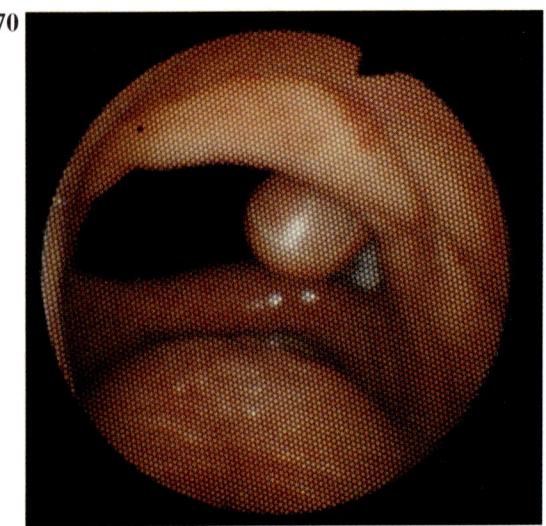

70 This picture shows the mouth, but viewed from the oral cavity, looking towards the patient's own finger, which is touching the lips. What abnormality is present which has enabled this photograph to be taken?

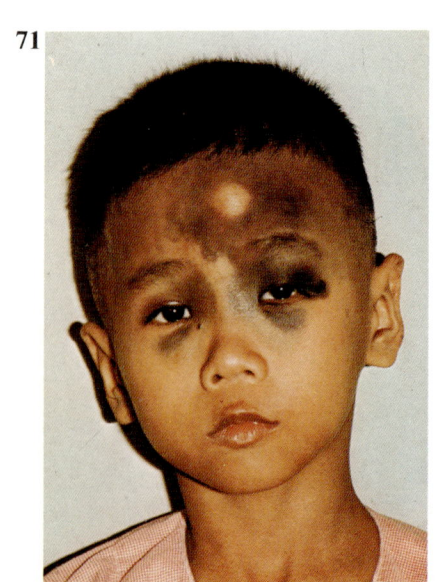

71 This patient is a Singaporean child who presented with fever and ecchymoses. What is the diagnosis?

72 The base of the heart viewed from above. Name the numbered parts.

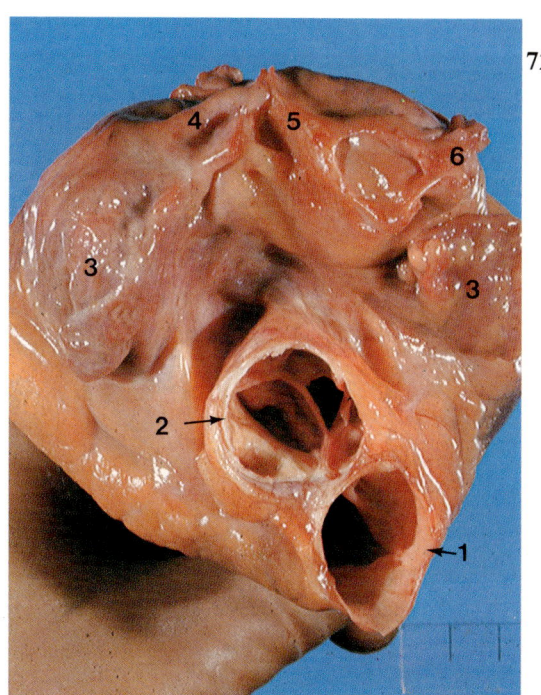

73 This complication is not uncommon during the acute stage of meningococcal meningitis.

a) What is it?
b) What is the prognosis?

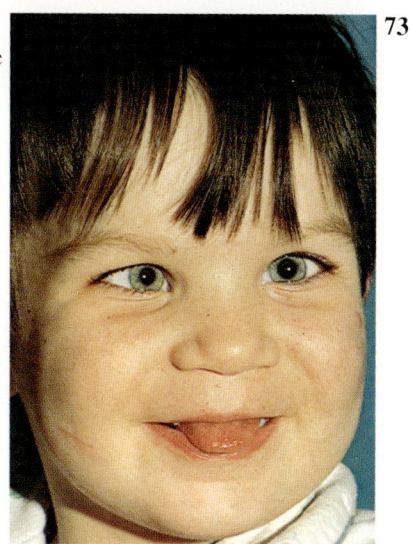

74 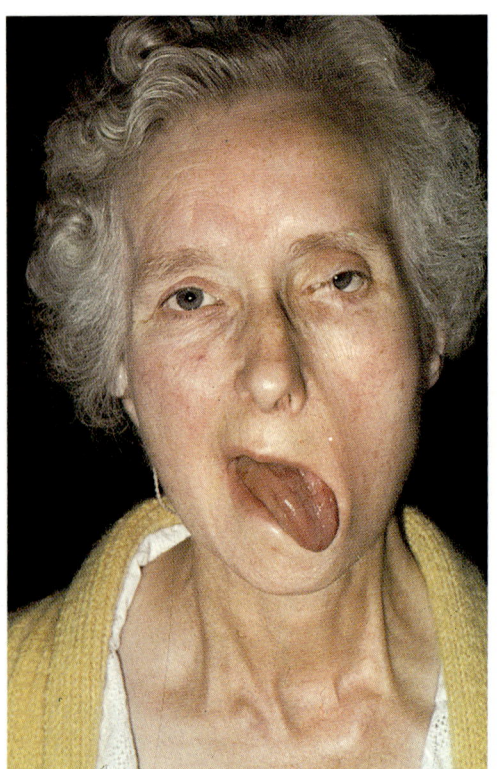 The abnormalities illustrated developed gradually.

a) What are they?
b) What do they suggest?
c) How would you try to confirm your diagnosis?

75 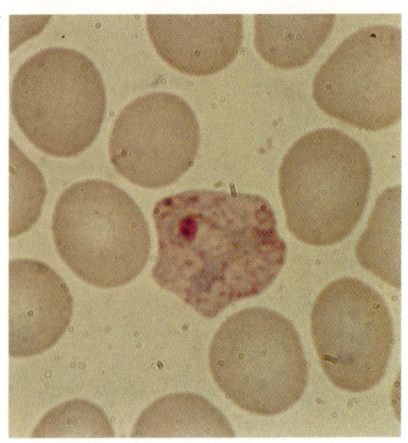 What is this parasite found in human blood?

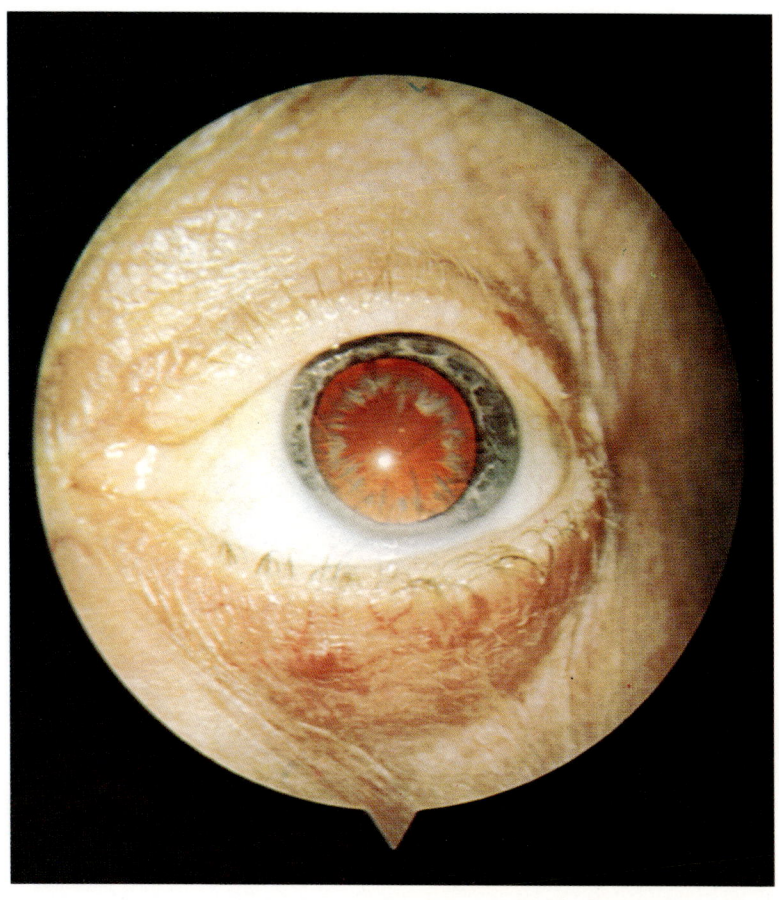

76 The patient complains of a gradual loss of vision in this eye.

a) What are the physical signs?
b) What is the diagnosis?

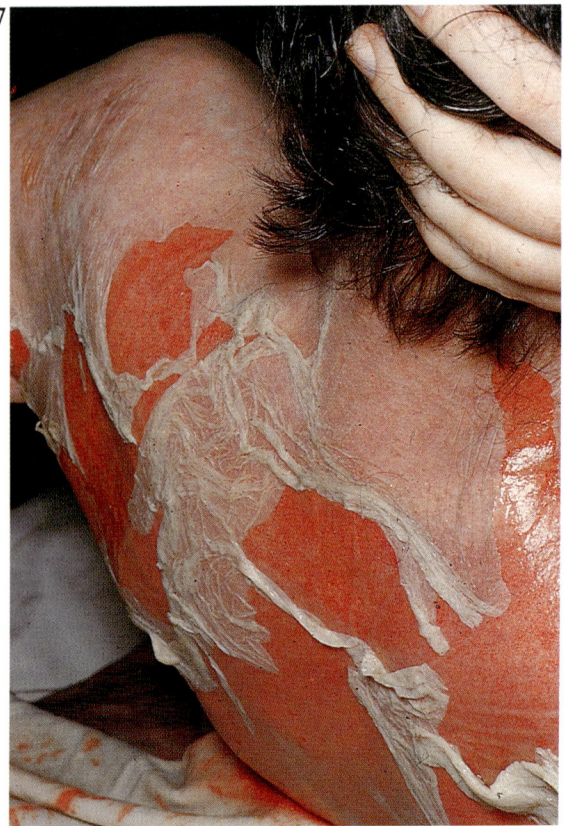

77 a) What is the diagnosis?
b) What is the most likely cause in adults?
c) If this occurs in an infant what is the likely cause?

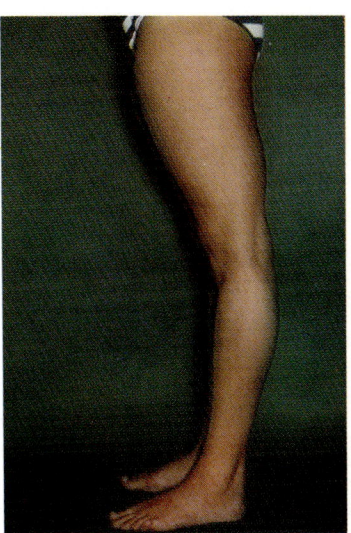

78
a) What is this condition?
b) What is the significance in a sporting aspect?

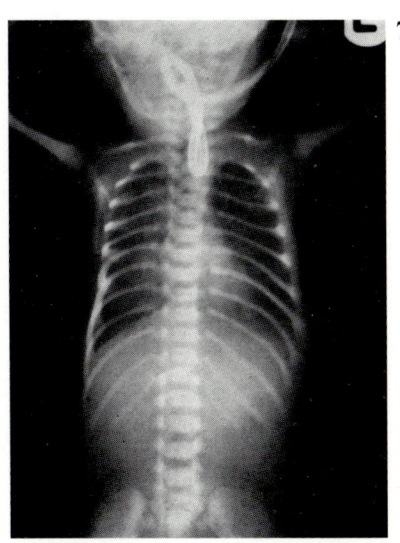

79
a) What does the X-ray of this newborn infant show?
b) What is the diagnosis?

80 This finding of a mosaic of cement lines is typical of:

a) Osteoporosis.
b) Osteomalacia.
c) Paget's disease.
d) Mucopolysaccharidosis.
e) Healing hyperparathyroidism.

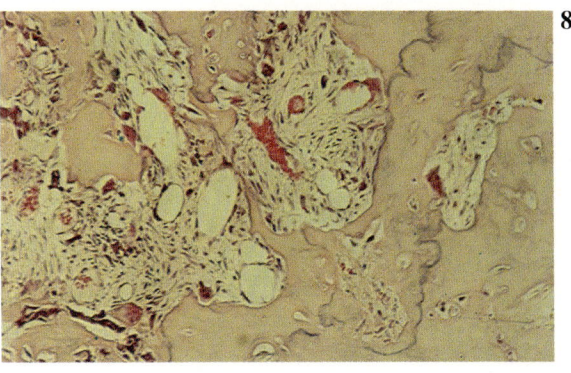

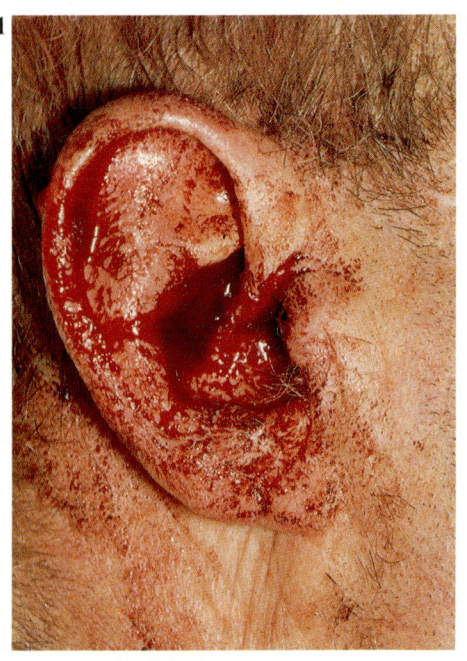

81 Bleeding from the ear, occuring after a severe head injury, is treated initially by:

a) Syringing out the external auditory canal with warm saline and careful otoscopy.
b) Antibiotics and follow-up by an ENT surgeon.
c) Packing with a ribbon gauze.

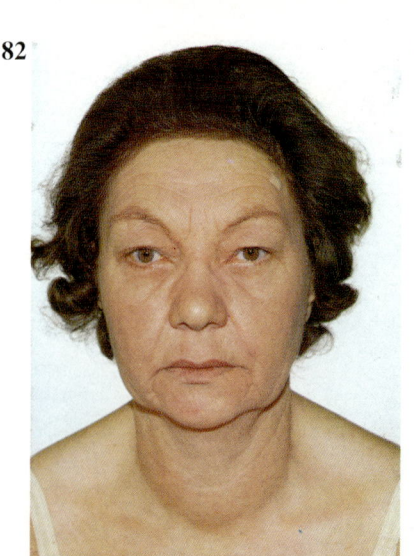

82 This middle-aged British woman complains of fatigue, weight gain and cold intolerance.

a) What is the probable underlying disorder?
b) What tests would be appropriate in order to confirm the diagnosis?
c) What immunological tests would indicate the cause of the underlying thyroid disease?
d) Name two likely causes of macrocytic anaemia in this patient.

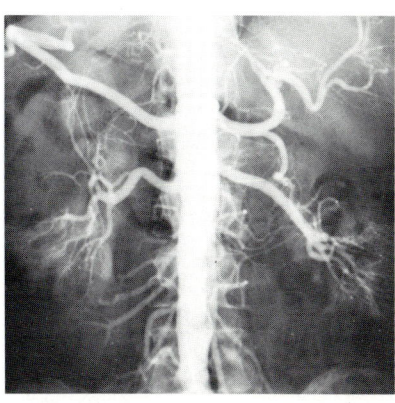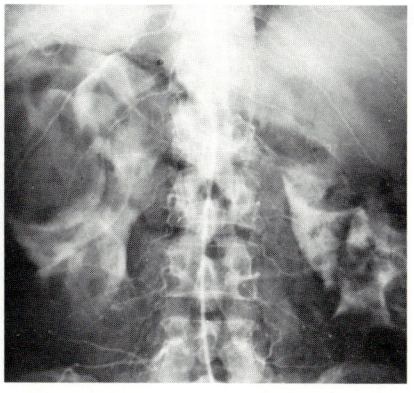

83 Patient presented with profuse haematuria and loin pain with normal renal functions.

a) What abnormality is present?
b) Comment on its progression.

84 Consider the cause and prognosis of this alarming posture.

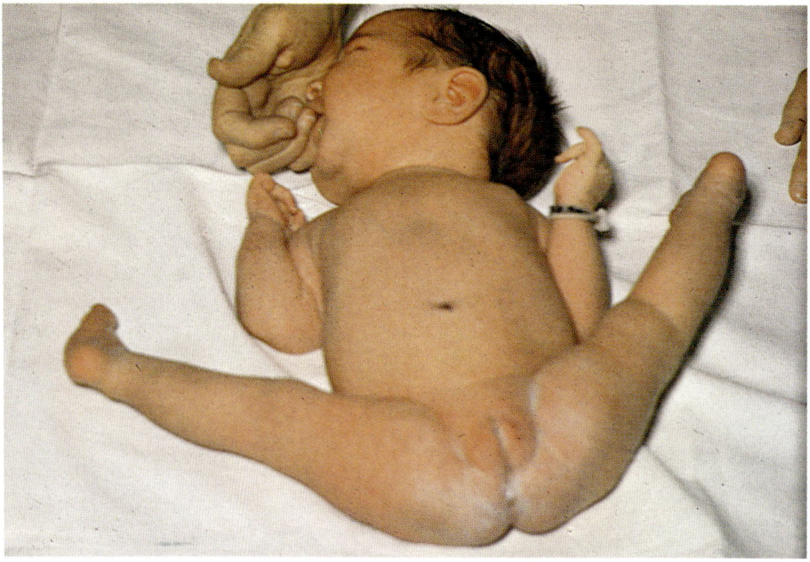

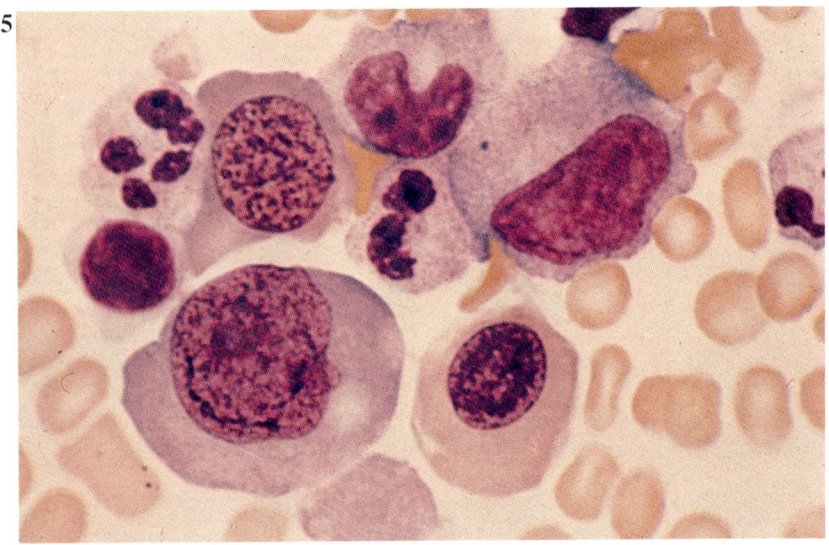

85 Identify the 8 nucleated cells shown from this bone-marrow aspirate, taken from a patient with severe macrocytic anaemia. What diagnosis would you consider likely?

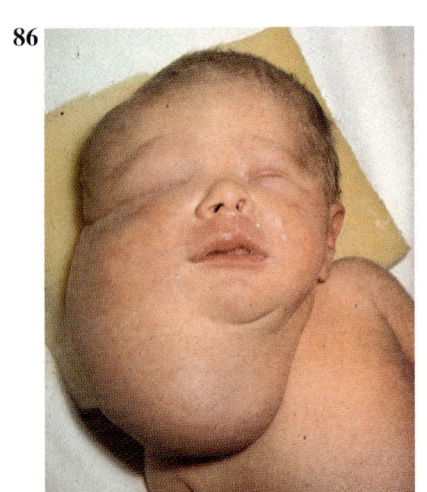

86 Mass affecting the right side of the face and neck of a newborn infant.

    a) What is the diagnosis?
    b) What is the treatment?
    c) What are the dangers of delayed treatment?

87

87 a) What abnormalities does this slide show?
b) What are the symptoms of this condition?
c) What signs does it produce?

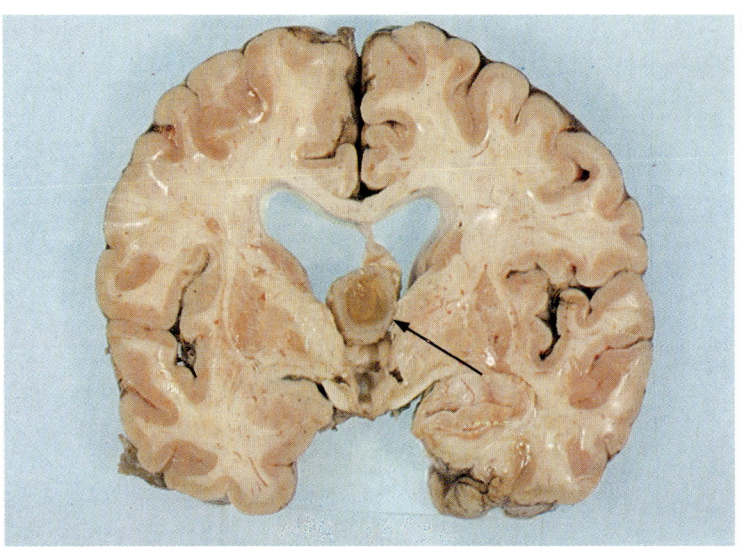

88 a) What is the probable diagnosis?
b) What other abnormality of the skin is usually seen in this condition?
c) If the patient was hypertensive, what associated condition might be expected?

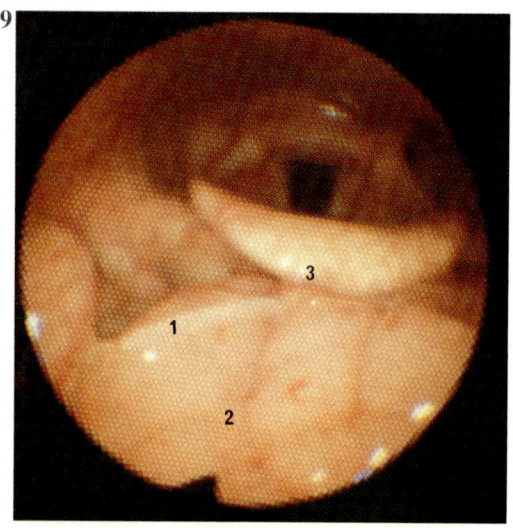

89 Why did this patient develop acute sore throat with otalgia immediately after a meal?

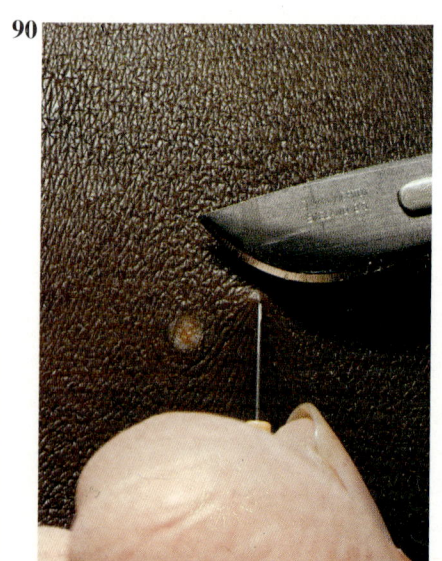

90 A patient from West Africa presented with severe pruritus and a high eosinophil count.

a) What is the diagnosis?
b) How do you confirm it?

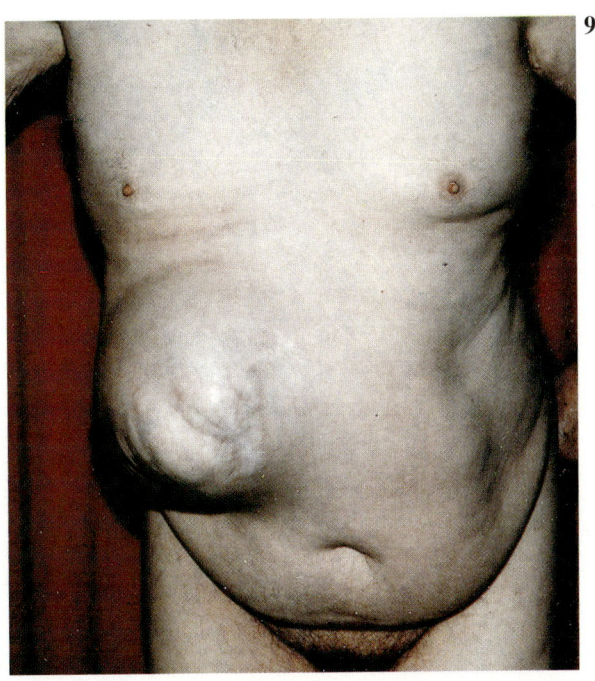

91 Several months following cholecystectomy this patient developed a progressively increasing but reducible swelling in the region of the operative incision.

a) What complication has occurred?
b) Which factors predispose to its development?

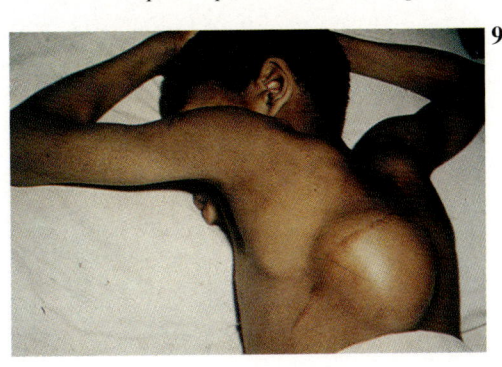

92 This child has a large fluctuant swelling in the left loin.

a) What is it?
b) What would be your first investigation?

93 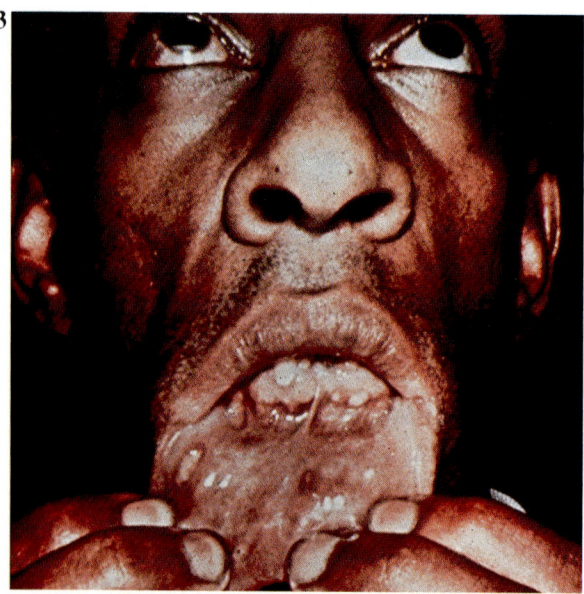 This patient demonstrates a painful red injected right eye with classical hypopyon (meniscus of white cells layering out in the anterior chamber). Upon everting the lower lip, he demonstrates aphthous ulceration of the buccal mucosa. The uveitis in the right eye and the aphthous lesions and the mucous membranes suggest what diagnosis?

94 a) What is the condition displayed at arthrotomy of the knee joint?
b) What is its significance?

95 a) What abnormalities does this film show?
b) What is the diagnosis?
c) What is the treatment?

95

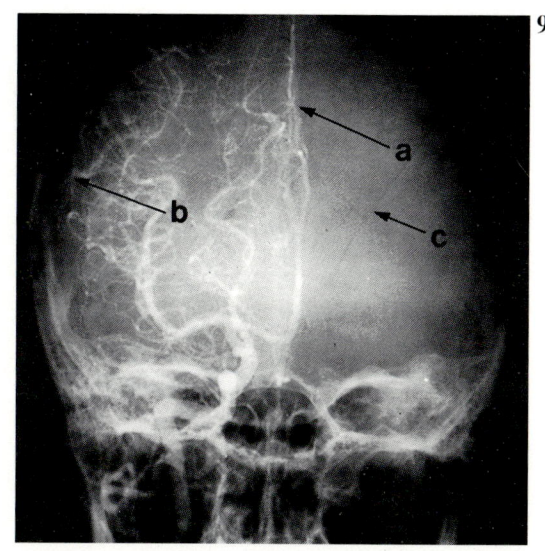

96 Name the two congenital abnormalities in this infant kidney.

96

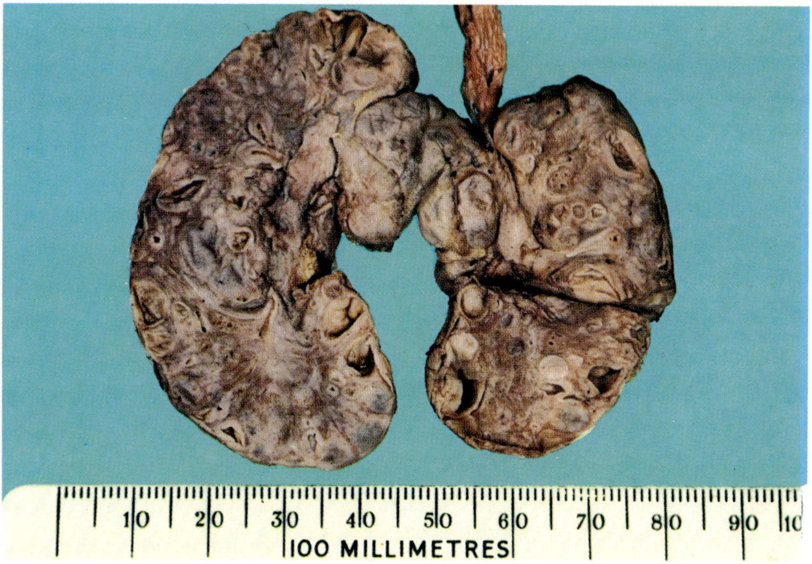

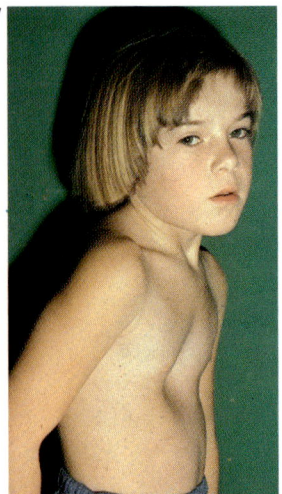

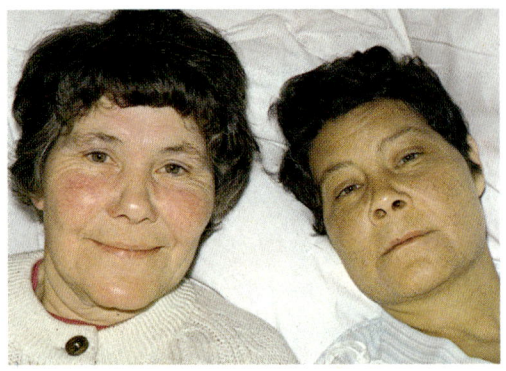

98 The patient (right) and her identical twin sister.

a) What is the probable diagnosis?
b) Is there any increased risk of her twin sister being affected?
c) What immunological test would help to determine the pathogenesis of this disease?
d) What radiological examination may be of diagnostic value?

97 a) What is the diagnosis?
b) What is the treatment of this condition in the 5-year-old girl?

99 a) What is this condition?
b) What is the mode of inheritance?

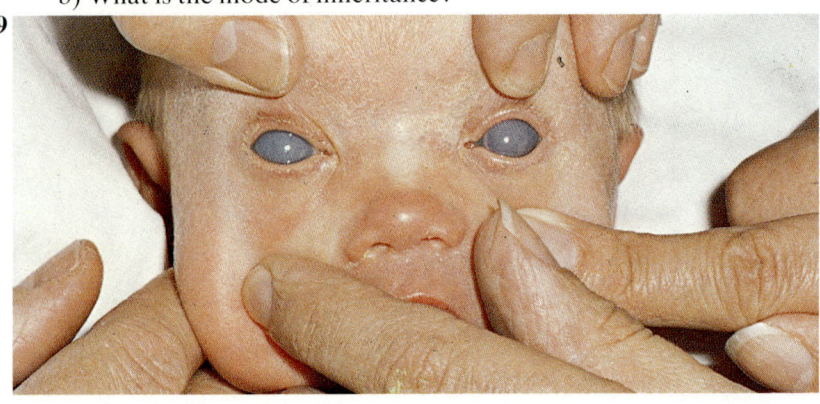

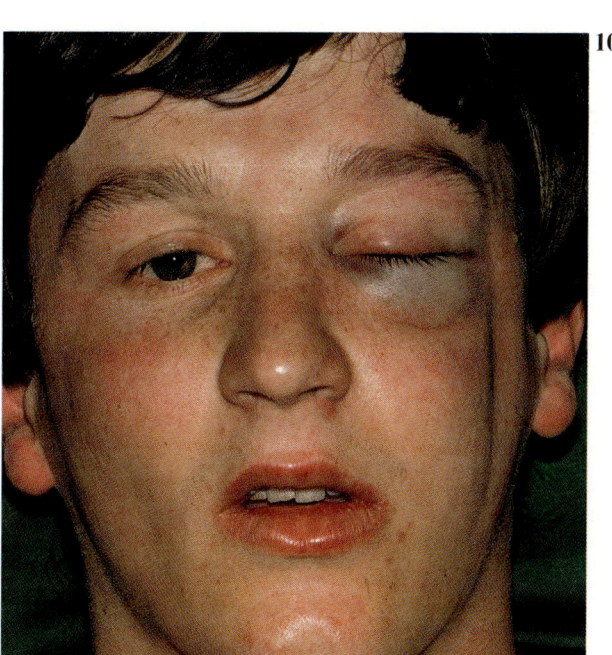

100 This man complained of diplopia and numbness of the left upper lip after an assault. The most likely diagnosis in this case is:

a) A depressed fracture of the left malar bone.
b) Fracture of the ascending ramus of the mandible.
c) Dislocation of the left temperomandibular joint.

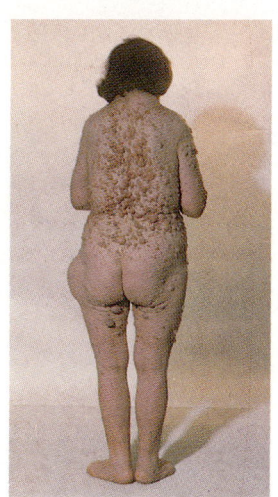

101 a) What is the diagnosis?
b) How is it inherited?
c) What orthopaedic complications might occur?
d) How often is a parent affected?

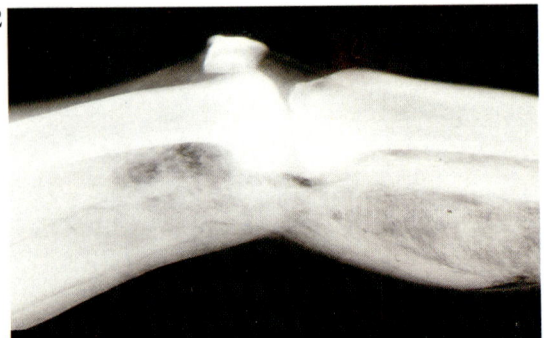

102 After a compound fracture of the lower tibia and fibula, crepitus was noted in the soft tissues below the knee joint.

a) What abnormality is shown in this plain radiograph?
b) Name the condition illustrated?
c) Which organisms are responsible for this condition?

103 The patient may be symptom-free and this physical sign may be noted on a routine ophthalmoscopic examination.

a) What is the relevant physical sign and probable diagnosis?
b) How should the patient be managed?

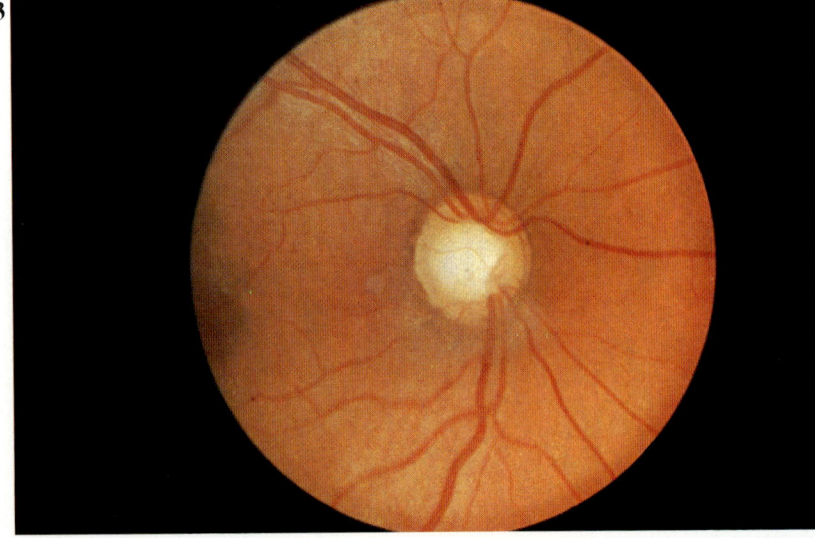

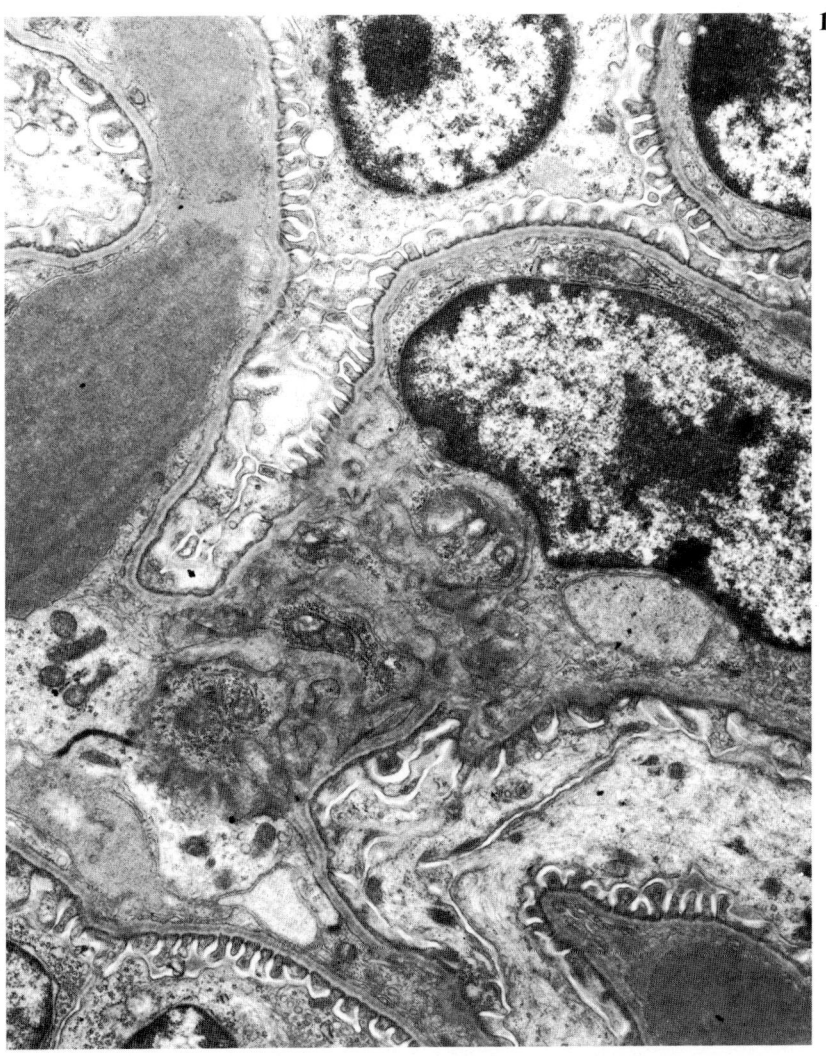

104 Name four types of cells represented in this micrograph of a normal glomerulus.

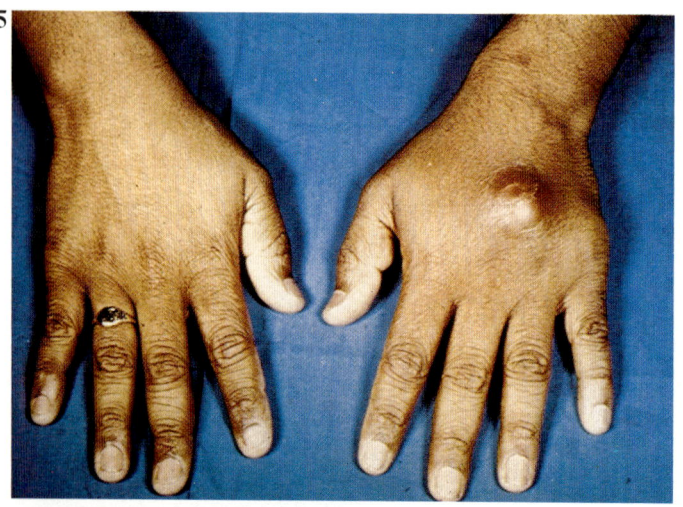

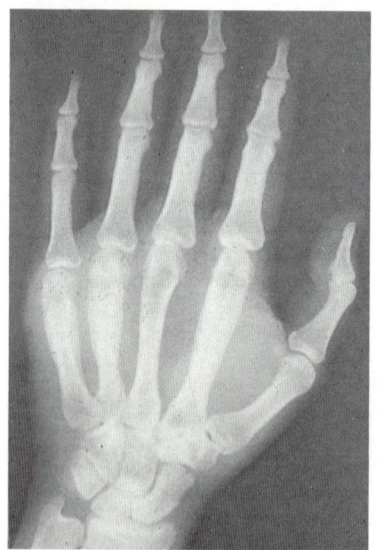

105 Painless swelling in the middle of the dorsum of the left hand. Radiographs show enlargement of the fourth metacarpal bone. What is the most likely diagnosis?

106 What are the two most likely diagnoses and which is the most likely diagnosis from the appearance?

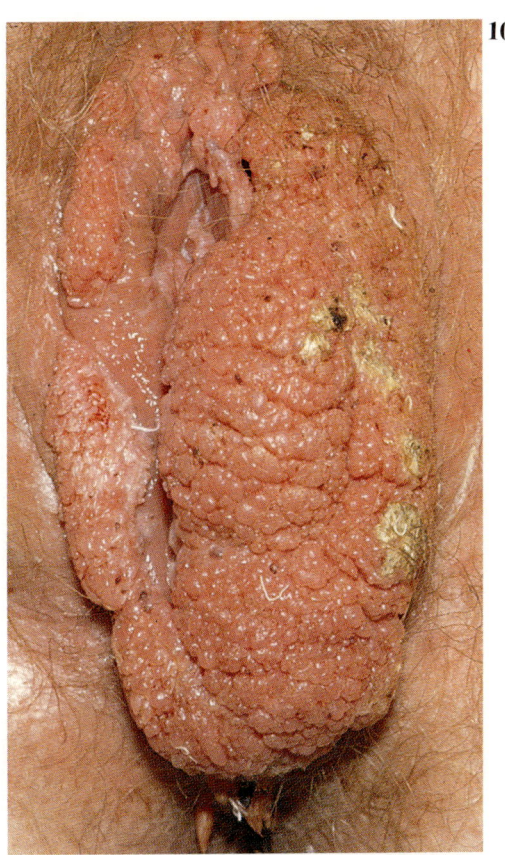

107 This person had been drinking surface water from a shallow pond. A year later this worm began to emerge from an ulcer in her lower leg. What is the diagnosis?

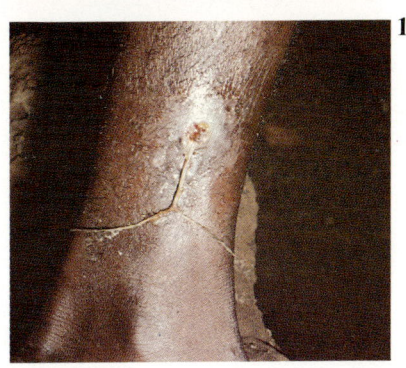

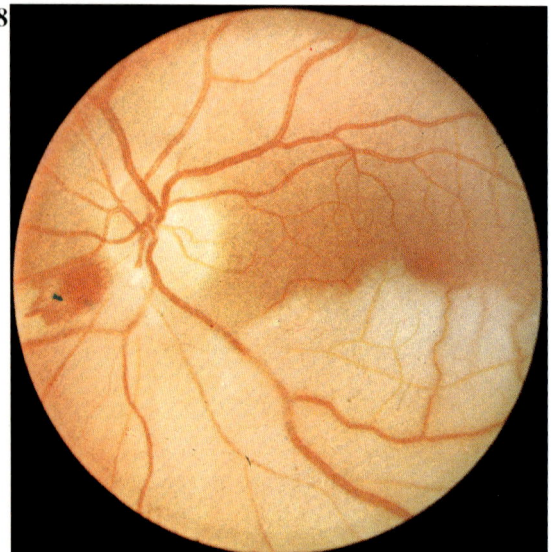

108 The patient complains of sudden loss of vision in one eye.

a) What are the physical signs?
b) What are the probable causes?

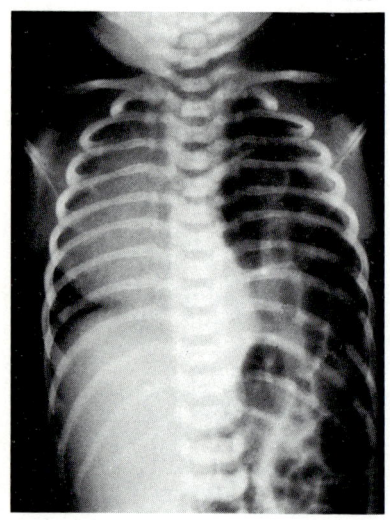

109 a) What does this chest radiograph show?
b) What action is required?

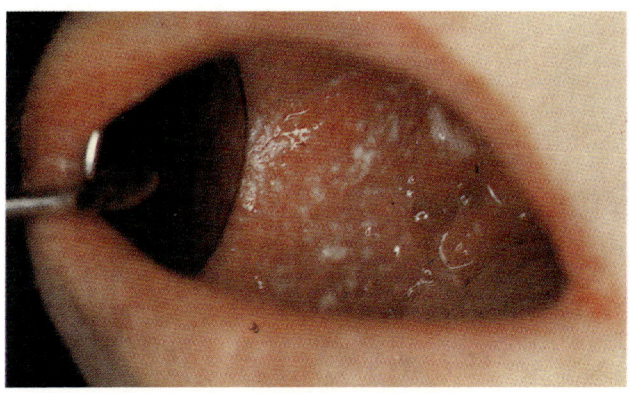

110 This is a common infective condition.

   a) What clinical diagnosis might be considered on the appearance alone?
   b) What relatively simple laboratory test might help to establish the diagnosis?
   c) What further steps should be taken following diagnosis of this condition?

111 Name the peculiar shape of the skull and its pathology.

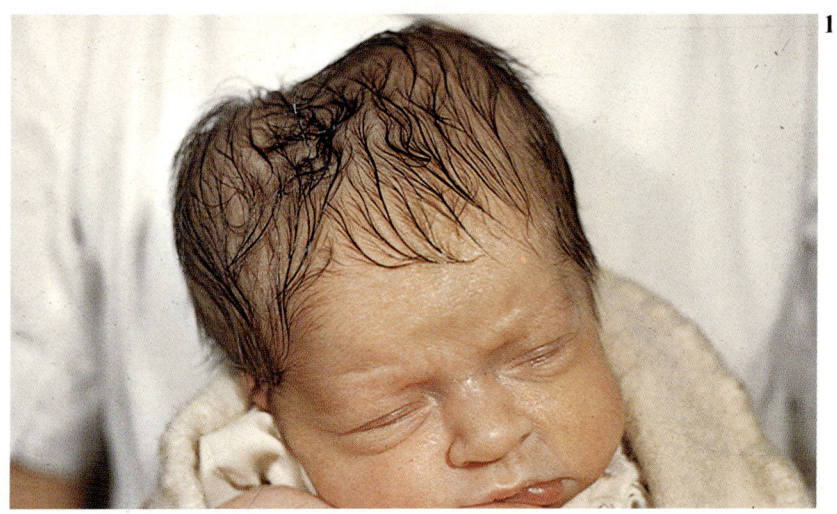

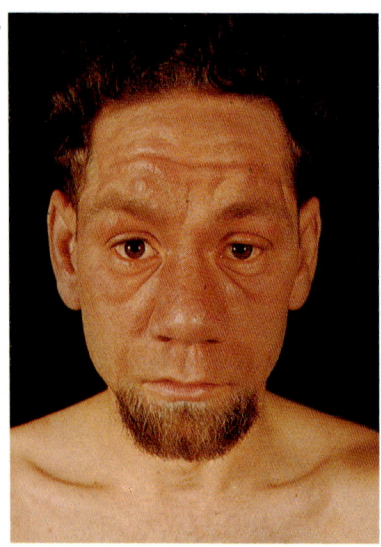
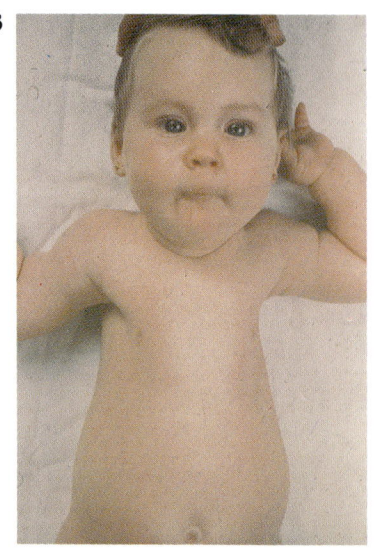

112 This man's face is characteristic of what disease?

113
a) What is the likely diagnosis in this floppy infant whose sib died from the same disorder?
b) What sign would you look for in the tongue?
c) What is the recurrence risk?

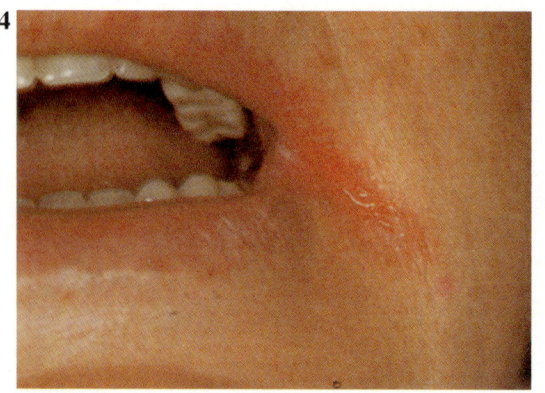

114
a) What is this condition?
b) What is its most common cause?
c) What other factors should be considered in the management of patients with this condition?

115

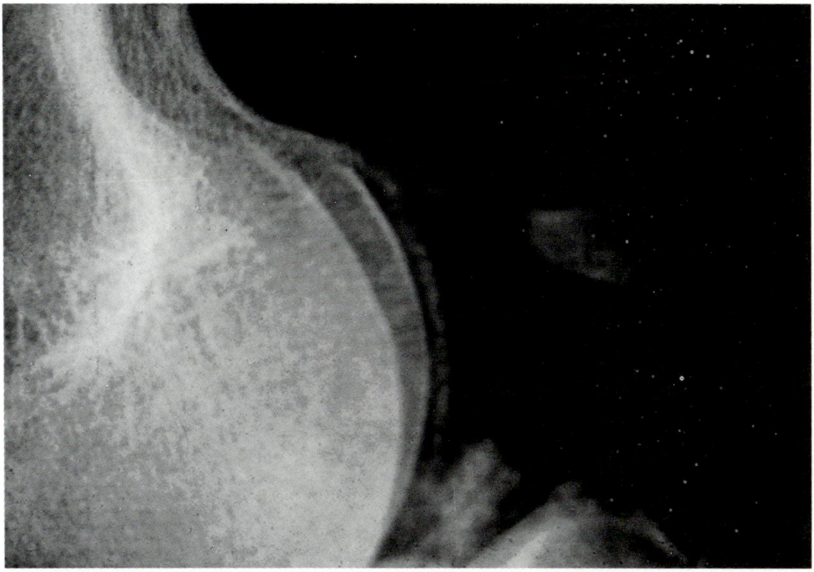

115 a) What does this X-ray of the femoral condyle show?
b) What is the diagnosis?

116 A transverse section of the apical portion of a heart shows thinning of the posterior wall.

a) Name the condition causing the thinning?
b) Which coronary artery is most likely to be involved?

116

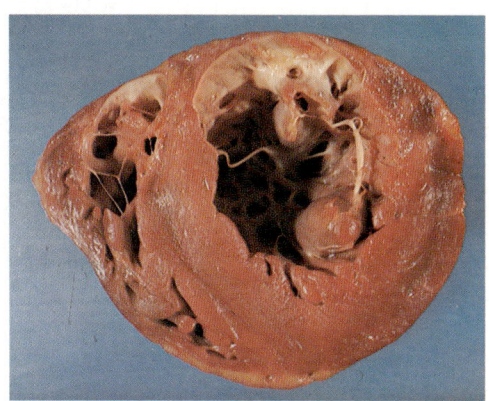

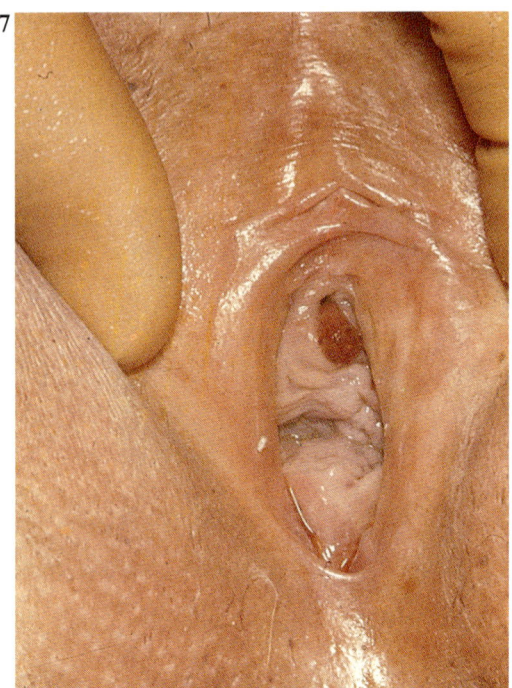

117 What are the possible causes of the red area in the region of the urethra?

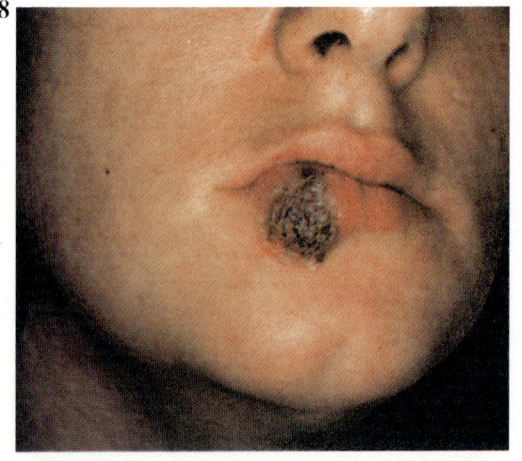

118 This is a painful lesion of the lip which has lasted for over two weeks.

a) What infective origins should be considered in the intial diagnosis?
b) Why is this particularly important to the practitioner to recognise the diagnostic possibilities?
c) Why is this an unusual lesion?

119

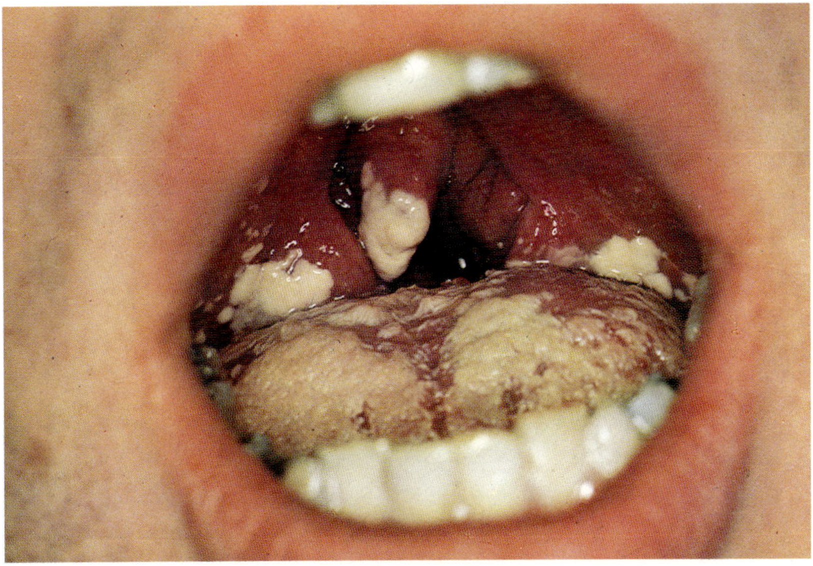

119 a) What is the name of this infection?
b) Name the organism and give its classification.
c) How is the infection spread?

120

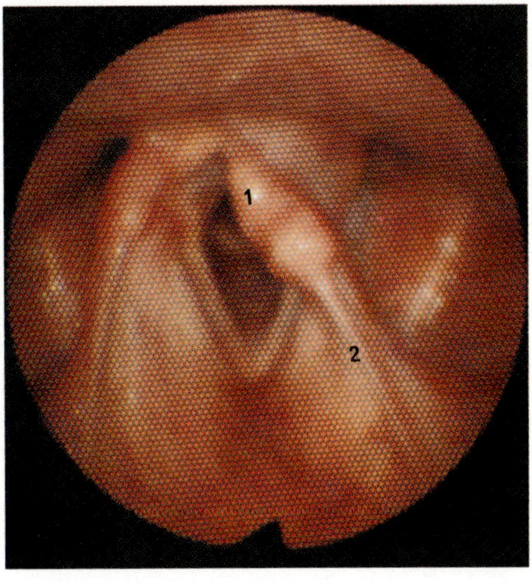

120 This 70-year-old patient was a heavy smoker who complained of loss of voice. What abnormality is present in the larynx?

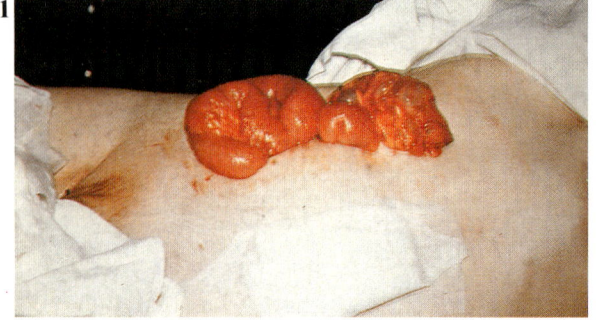

121 Ten days following laparotomy this patient has suffered a serious complication.

a) What is the condition called?
b) What factors predispose to its occurrence?

122 This patient has pain in the left arm with episodic blanching and coldness of the fingers of the left hand.

a) What is the test called?
b) What is the examiner trying to find out?

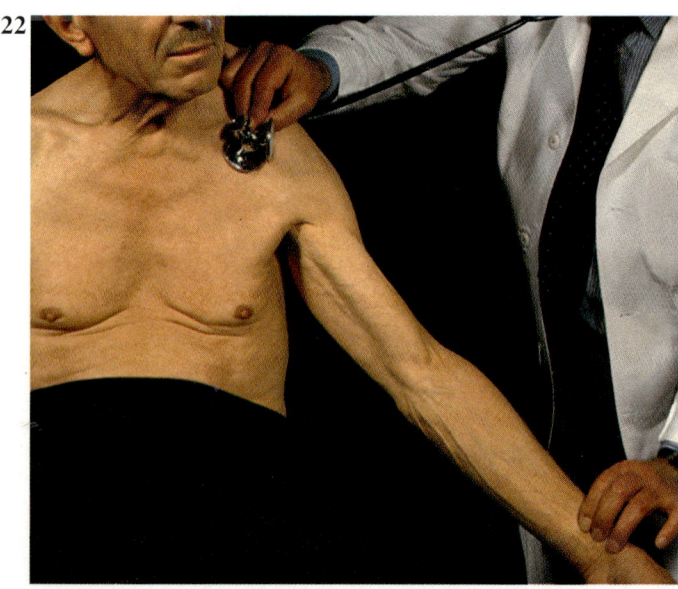

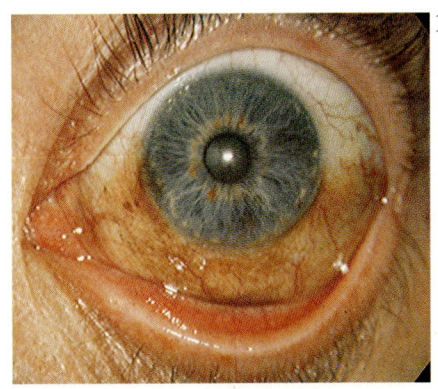

123 The patient complains of a long-standing discoloration of the lower part of the conjunctiva.

a) What is the physical sign?
b) What is the probable diagnosis?
c) How should it be managed?

124 a) What is the diagnosis?
b) Which other neurological conditions produce wasting of the small muscles of the hand?
c) How do you distinguish between these conditions?

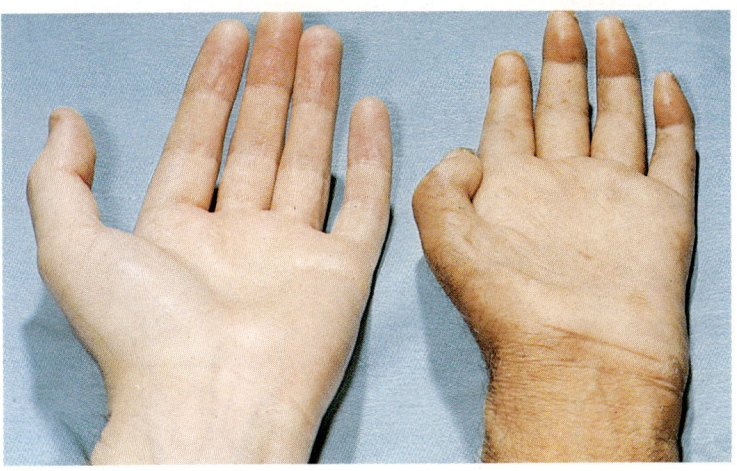

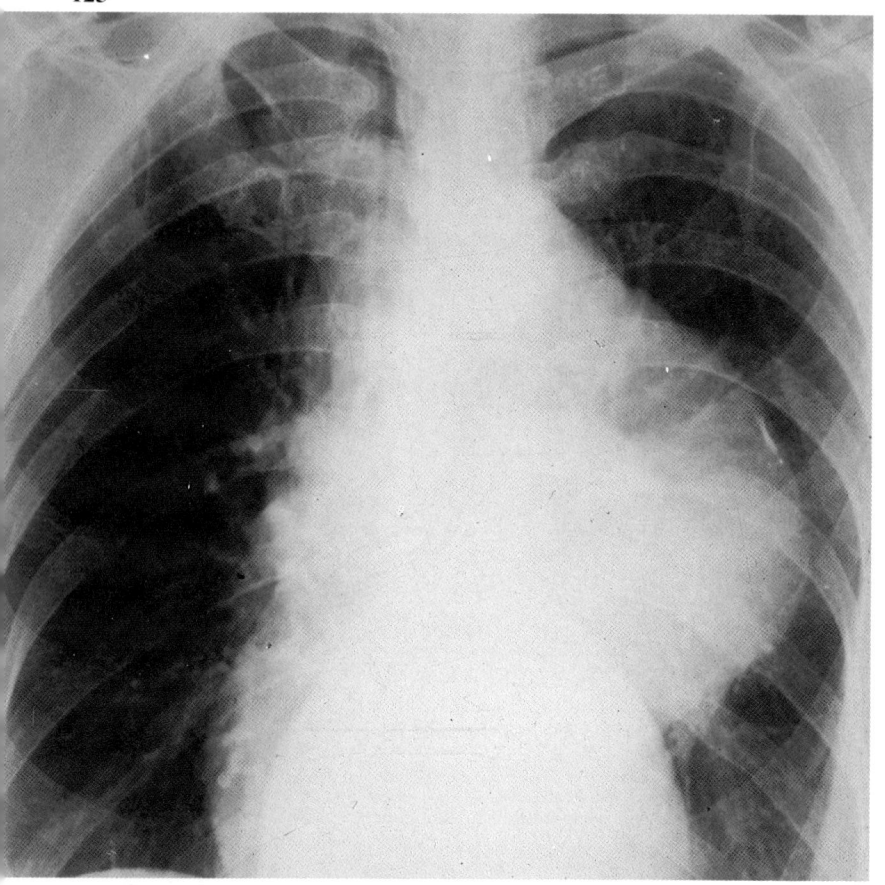

125 What does this X-ray chest show?

126 This is the classical presentation of a tongue lesion.

a) What would be your clinical diagnosis?
b) What treatment would you suggest?
c) What is the prognosis of this lesion?

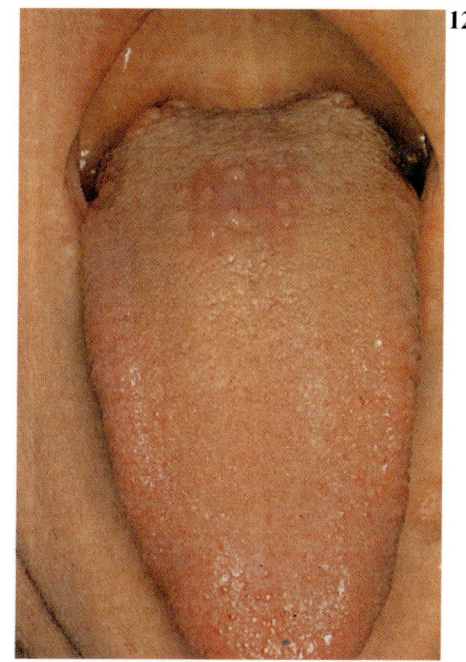

127 This shows contact between the liver and the lung following:

a) Congenital diaphragm agenesia?
b) A rupture of diaphragm, post-traumatic?
c) Migration of lung into the abdomen in sequestration?

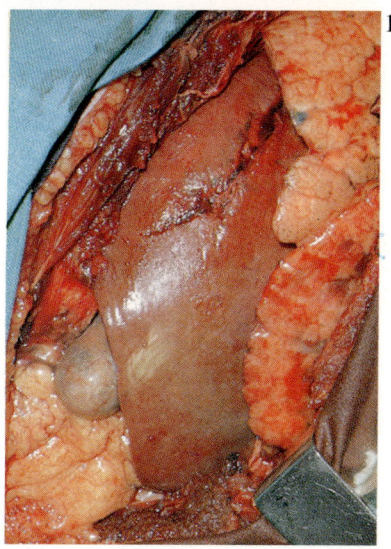

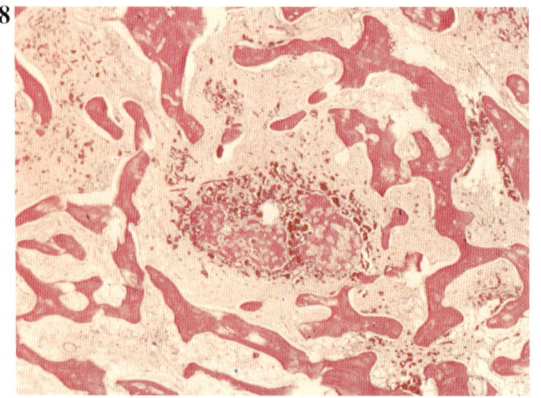

128 Differential diagnosis includes:
a) Osteomyelitis.
b) Osteoid osteoma.
c) Secondary deposit.
d) Myeloma.
e) Hyperparathyroidism.

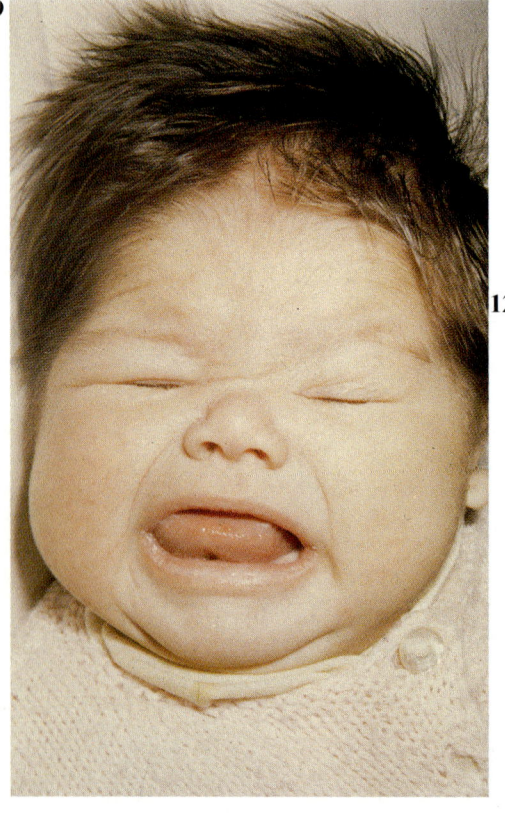

129 Which of the following is associated with hypothyroidism in infants?
a) Diagnosis is possible at birth.
b) Diarrhoea is commonly present.
c) Such infants have a typical high-pitched cry.
d) There is a high incidence of umbilical hernias.
e) There is poor weight gain, in spite of adequate feeding.

130 On coughing, this mass appeared through the introitus of the vulva.

a) What is the likely diagnosis?
b) Do you think it a recent event or has it been present for a considerable time?
c) What is the treatment of choice?

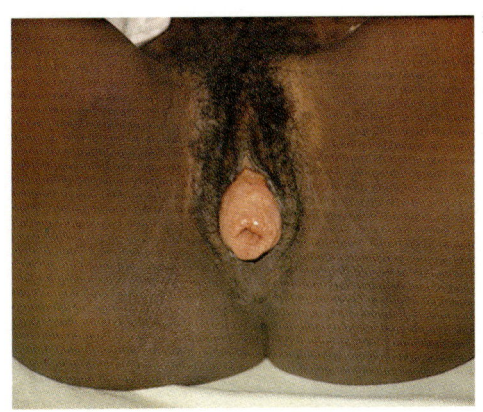

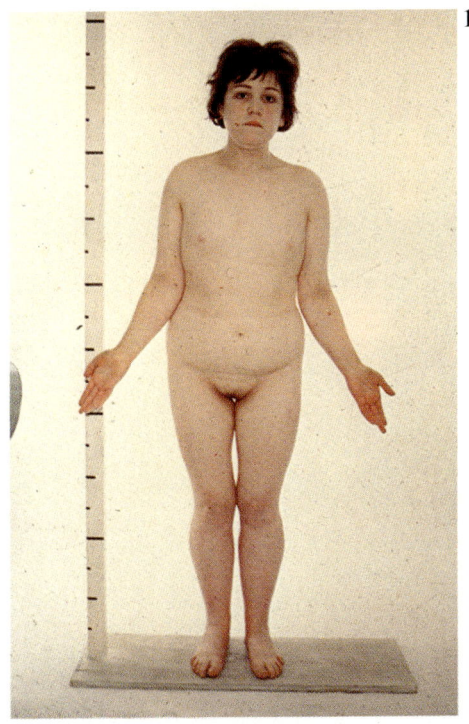

131 a) What is the probable diagnosis?
b) What are the endocrine features of this disorder?
c) What abnormality of the upper limbs is shown?
d) What is the essential diagnostic investigation?

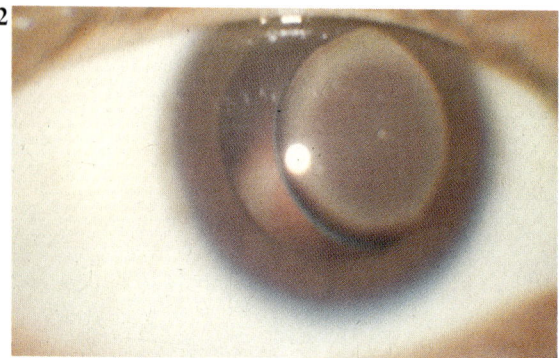

132
a) What is the abnormality?
b) Of which syndrome is it a manifestation?
c) Name another condition in which a similar ocular abnormality occurs and state how the two may be distinguished?
d) What cardiovascular abnormalities may be found in patients with the syndrome named in b)?

133 This lesion has appeared in a patient with lower bowel disease.

a) What is your initial clinical diagnosis?
b) What may be the relationship to skin lesions in these circumstances?
c) What other oral lesions may appear in lower bowel disease?

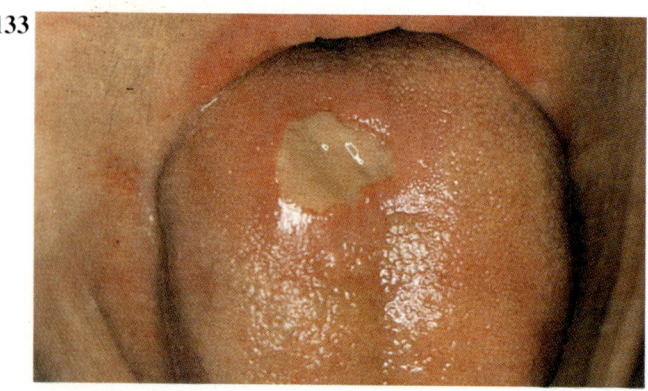

134

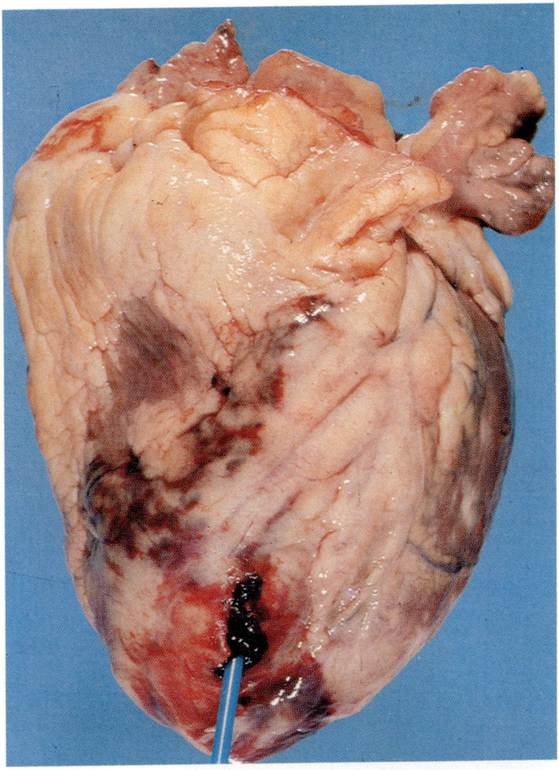

134 A rupture in the lower third of the anterior wall of the left ventricle. When is this type of rupture most likely to occur?

135

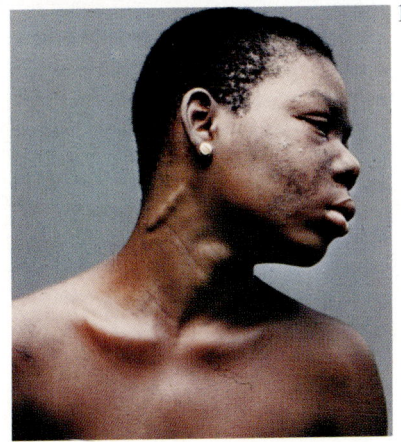

135 Gross thickening of the great auricular nerve was seen in this West African patient. What is the diagnosis?

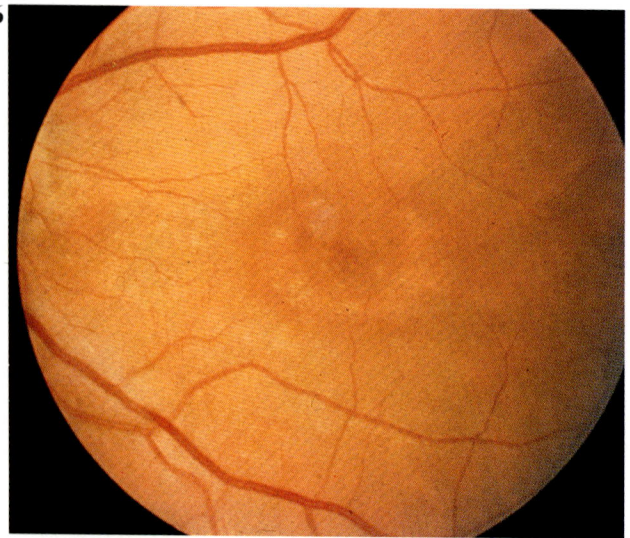

136 This patient with systemic lupus erythematous shows an iatrogenic disorder of the fundus.

a) Name the drug responsible for this iatrogenic effect.
b) Describe the fundus abnormality shown in the illustration.
c) What is the effect of this disorder on vision?

137 What complication of wound healing has occurred?

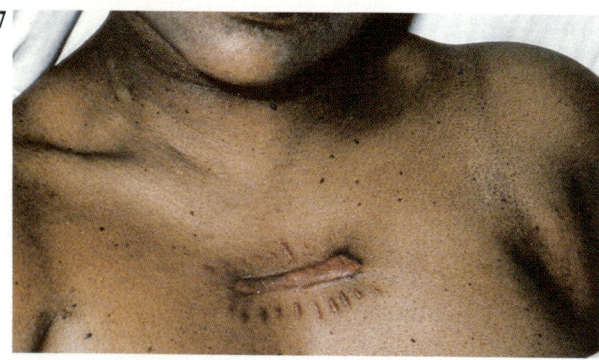

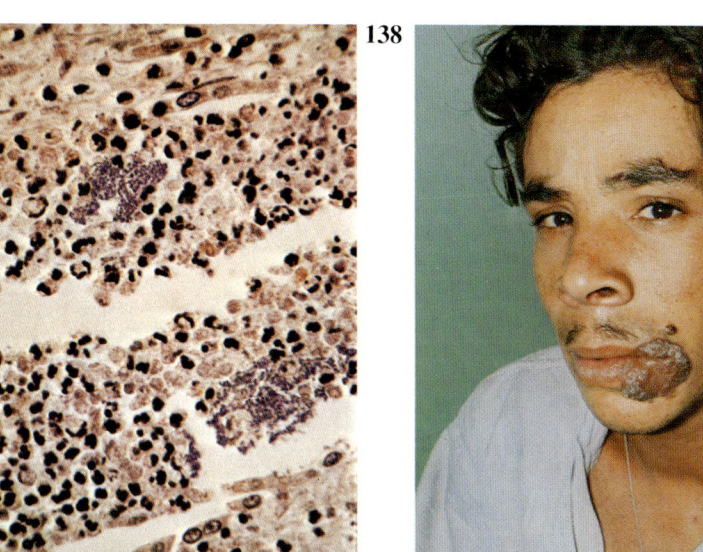

138 a) Pus and microorganisms in damaged kidney tubules are characteristic of which disease?
b) How may such infections reach the kidney?

139 A South American rural worker presented with this lesion. What is the likely diagnosis?

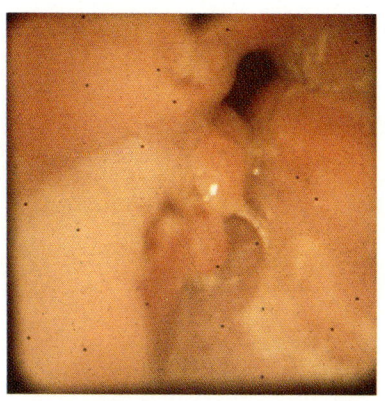

140 In lower oesophagus, this is possibly the consequence of:

a) Vomiting (Mallory–Weiss syndrome)?
b) Iatrogenic injury inflicted by bougienage?
c) Oesophagus varices sclerotherapy in the bleeding cirrhotic?

141

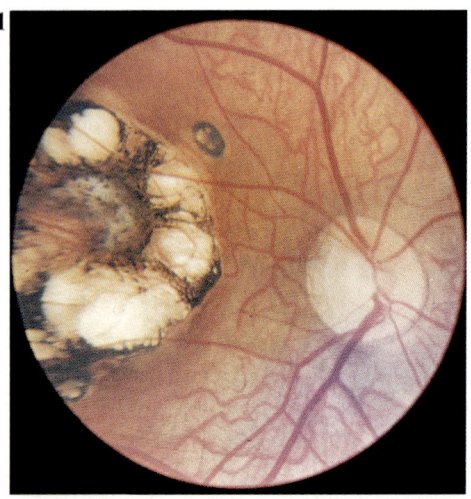

141 a) Name and describe the abnormality?
b) What is the most likely diagnosis?

142

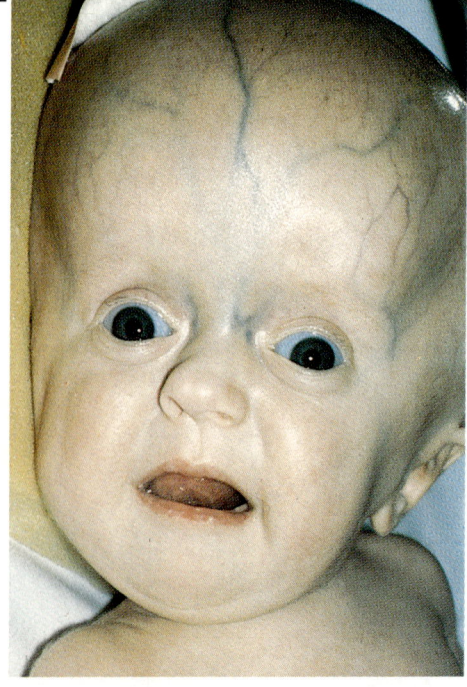

142 Which of the following conditions is hydrocephaly associated with?

a) Congenital rubella.
b) Myelomeningocele.
c) Potter's syndrome.
d) Achondroplasia.
e) Lacunar skull.

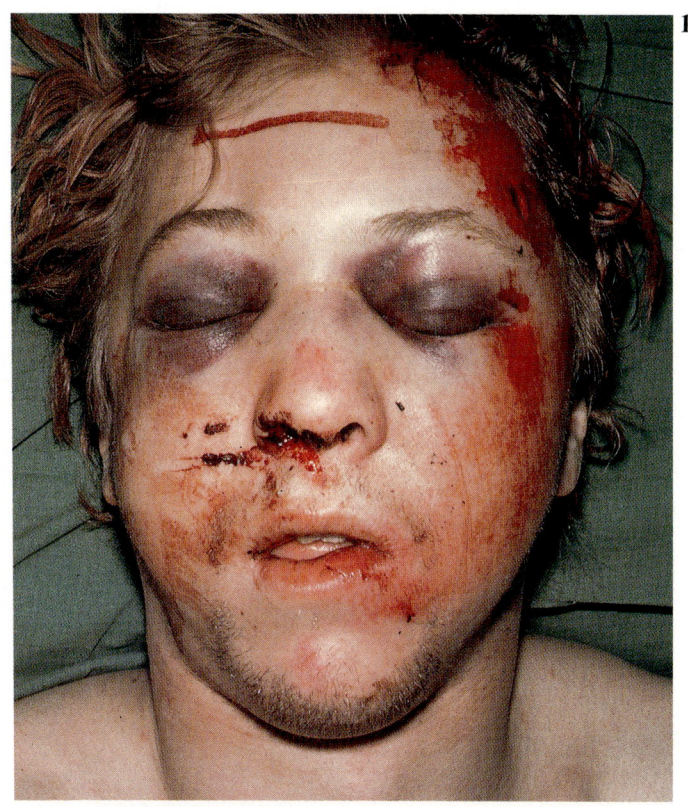

143 Following head injury, bilateral black eyes suggest:

a) Bilateral detached retinae.
b) Compound anterior cranial fossa fracture.
c) Subdural haemorrhage.

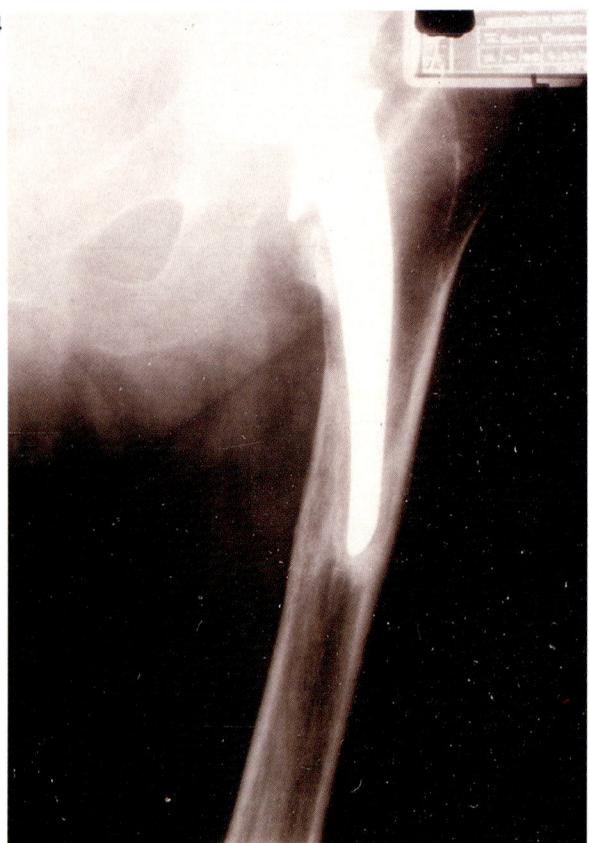

144 a) What complication of replacement arthroplasty is shown in this radiograph?
b) What is its usual cause?

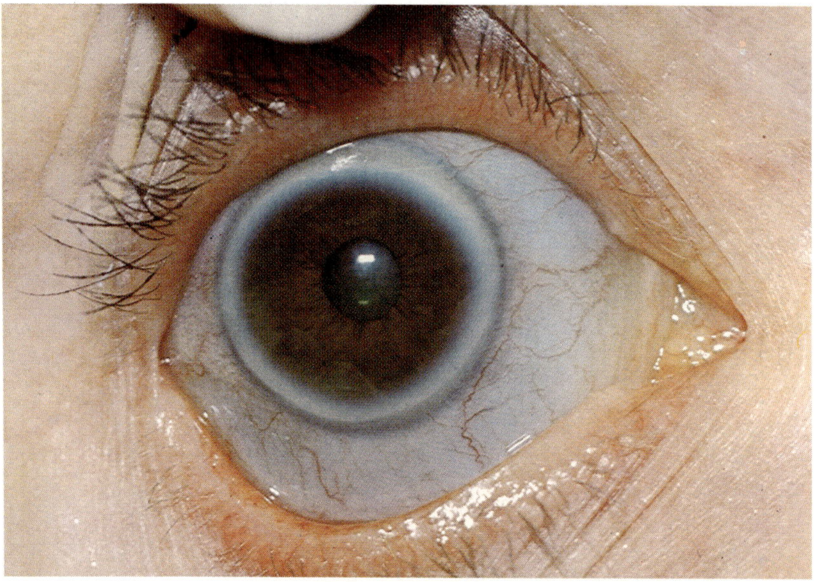

145

145 What diagnosis can you make from the appearance of this eye?

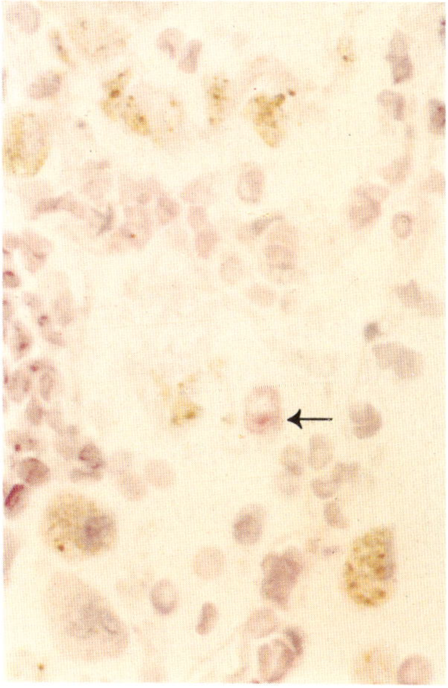

146

146 An adult patient with chickenpox developed serious respiratory distress during the fourth day of his illness.

a) What is the complication?
b) What is the lung pathology?

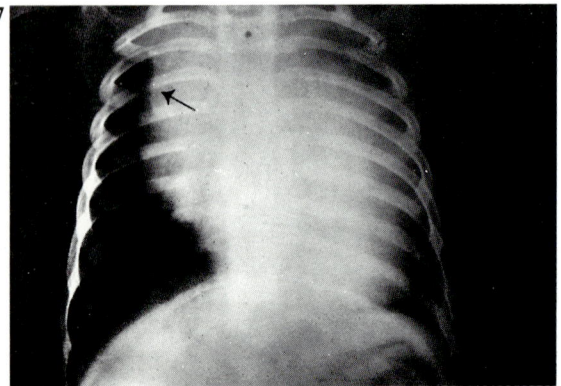

147 a) What is the most likely diagnosis of this superior mediastinal mass?
b) List the methods of presentation.

148 a) What disability does this patient have?
b) What is the cause?

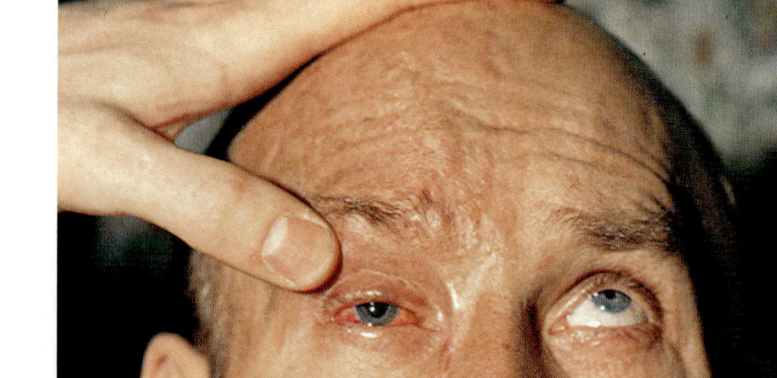

149 This young lady presented with a sun-sensitive eruption over her face and complained of breathlessness and arthralgia.

a) What is the diagnosis?
b) Why do you think she is breathless?
c) What single blood test would you perform?

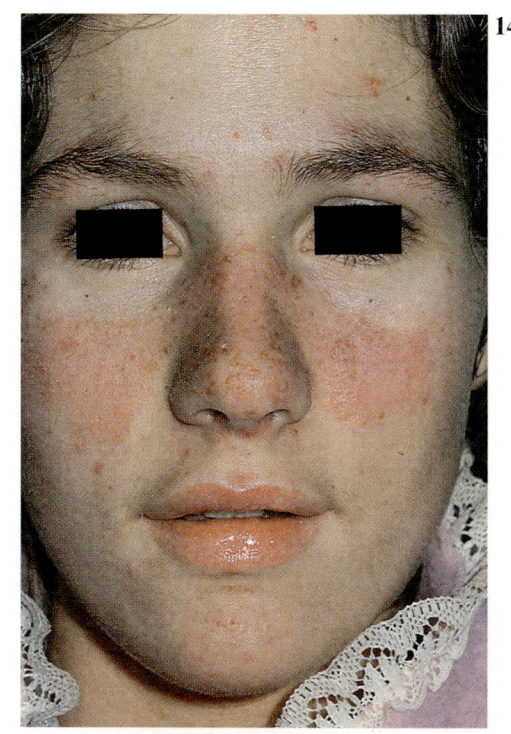

150 Aspect of a:

a) Trans-anal rectal prolapse when straining?
b) Trans-pyloric duodenal prolapse during normal antral function?
c) Gastro-oesophageal retrograde prolapse during vomiting?

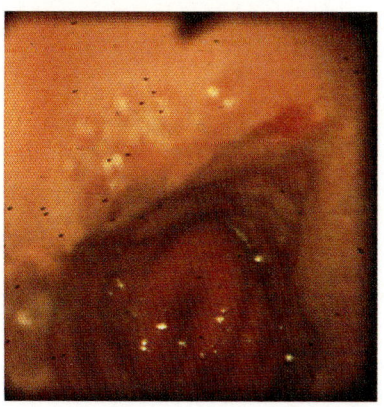

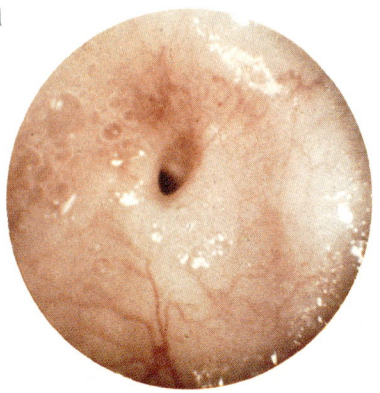 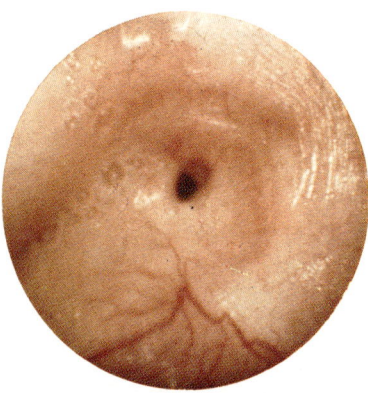

151 An oesophageal stenosis that could have been provoked by:

a) Levin's tube misplacement?
b) A blunt injury to the mid-chest?
c) A bleach burn sustained months previously?

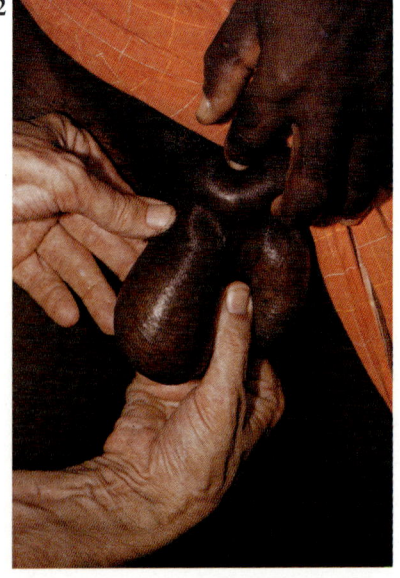

152 An African patient is found to have this hydrocoele.

a) Is there any parasite that can cause this lesion?
b) How can you confirm the diagnosis?

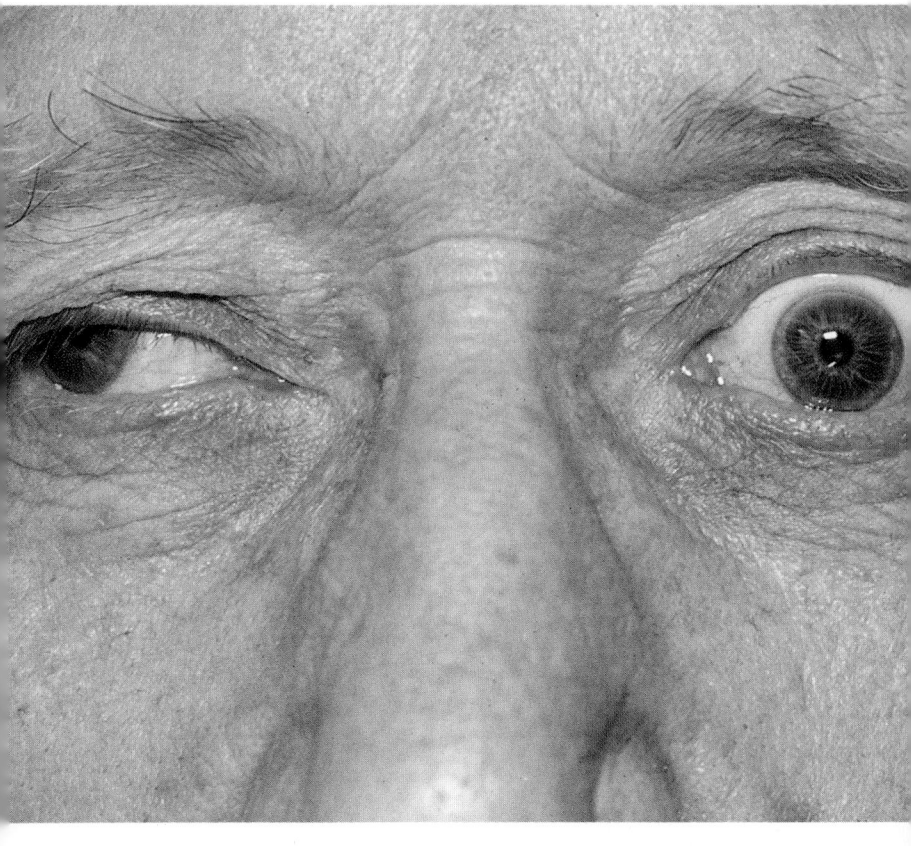

153 This ocular abnormality occurs in association with:

a) Myasthenia gravis?
b) Third cranial-nerve palsy?
c) Fourth cranial-nerve palsy?
d) Cerebrovascular disease?
e) Diabetes mellitus?

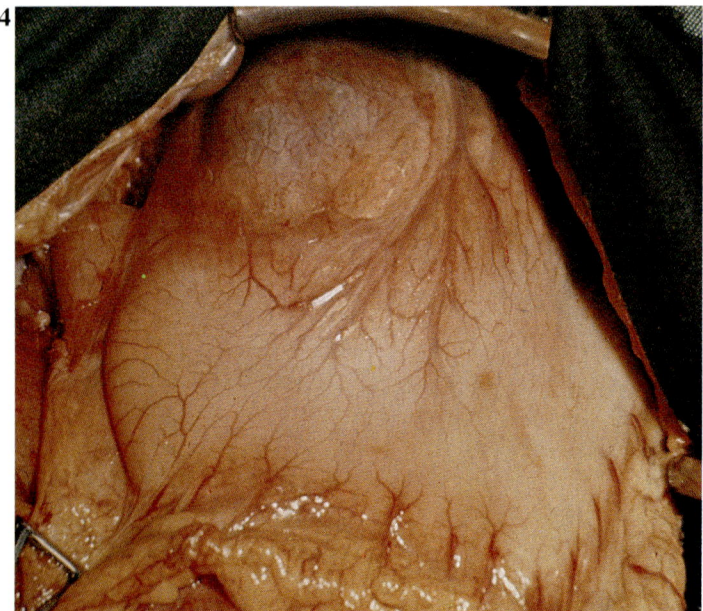

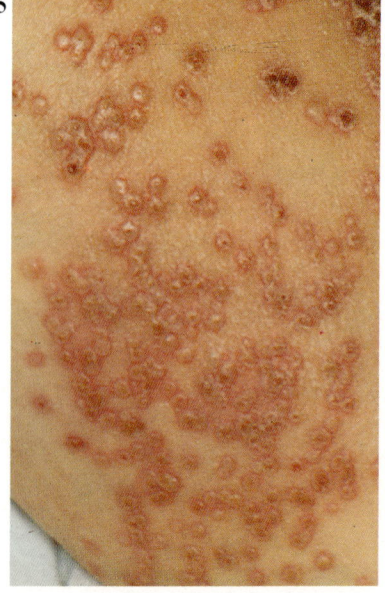

154 In a child, such a pseudocyst of the pancreas:

a) Can develop after trauma.
b) Can be marsupialized to the stomach.
c) Can usually appear secondarily.

155 Eczematous patients are particularly prone to this condition.

a) What is the name of the disease?
b) Name the organism responsible.

156

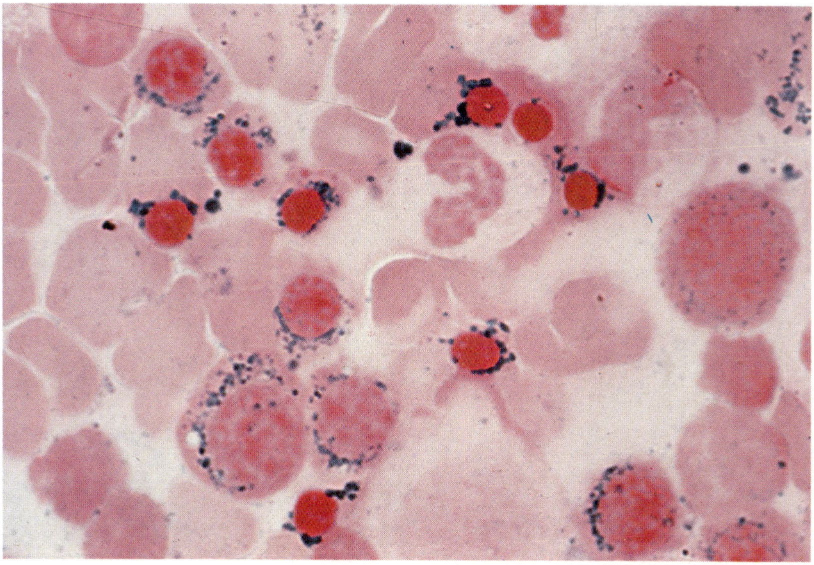

156 a) What does this Prussian blue-stained bone-marrow smear demonstrate?
b) What is the likely diagnosis?

157 a) To what group of conditions does this belong?
b) What is the recurrence risk?
c) How should the next pregnancy be handled?

157

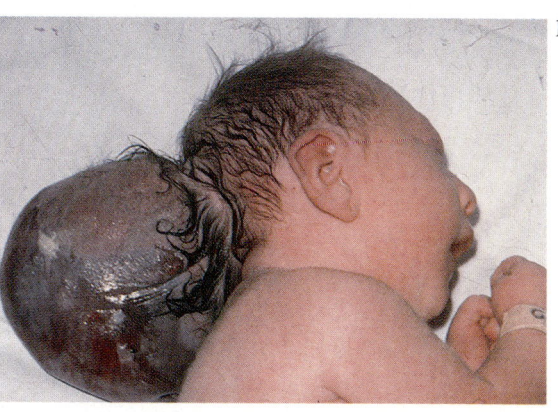

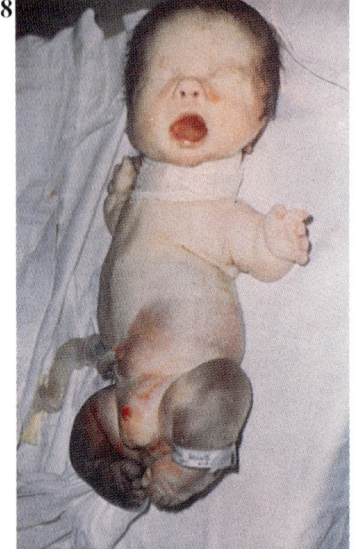
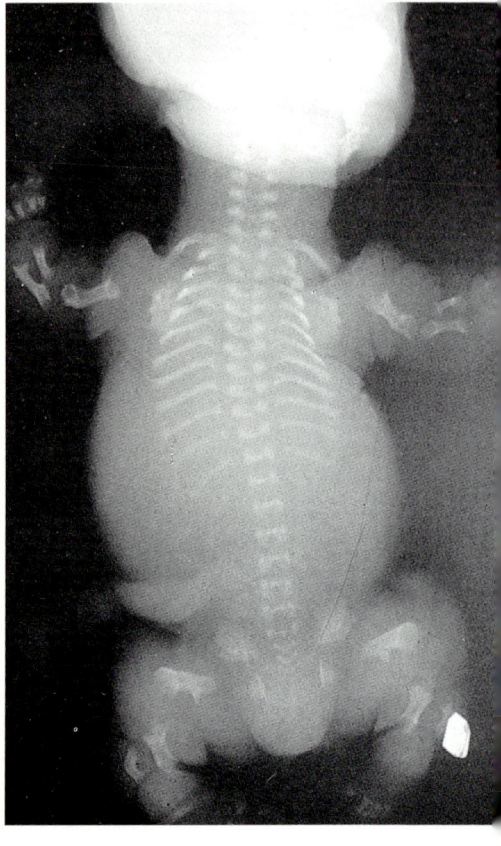

158
a) What is the diagnosis?
b) What is the recurrence risk?
c) Is it always lethal in the first 6 months of life?
d) What radiological features do you notice?

159 What abnormality is present in the larynx and hypopharynx of this pregnant lady, and in what other conditions may it occur?

159

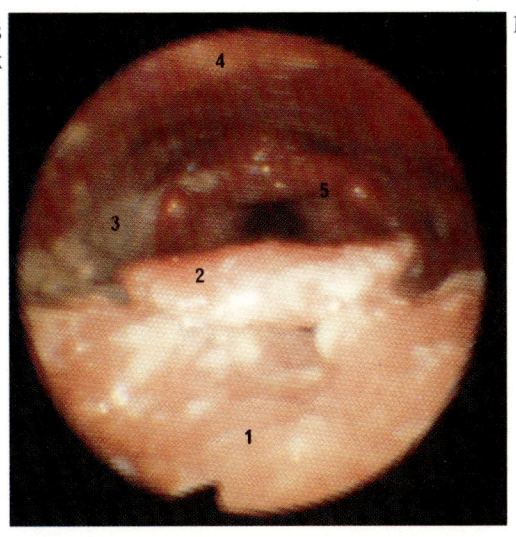

160 Name four renal structural changes which characterize benign hypertension of limited severity.

160

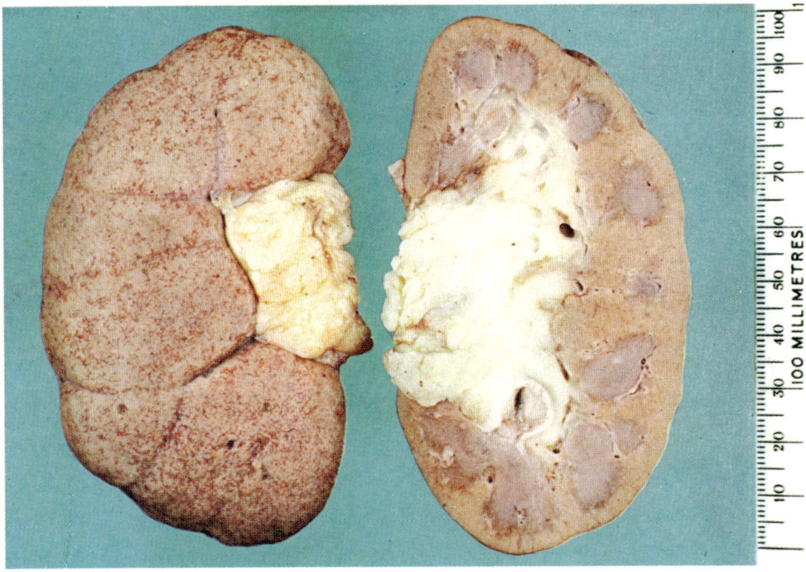

161

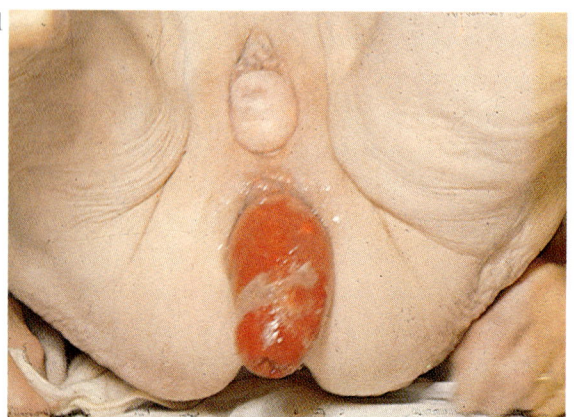

161 What lesions are present in this elderly patient? Are they benign, or malignant conditions?

162 This plain X-ray of the skull is from a patient who presented with chronic headaches, palpitations, excessive sweating and dyspnoea on exertion. What is the abnormality?

162

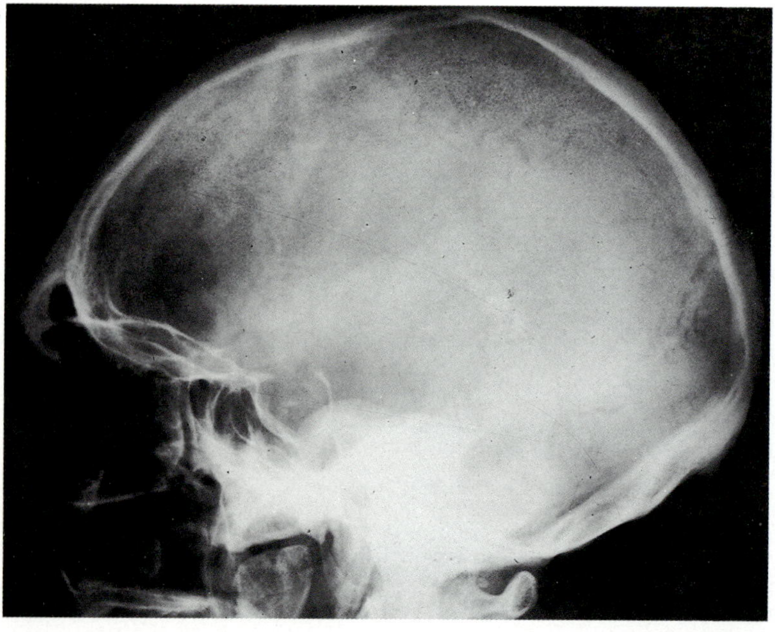

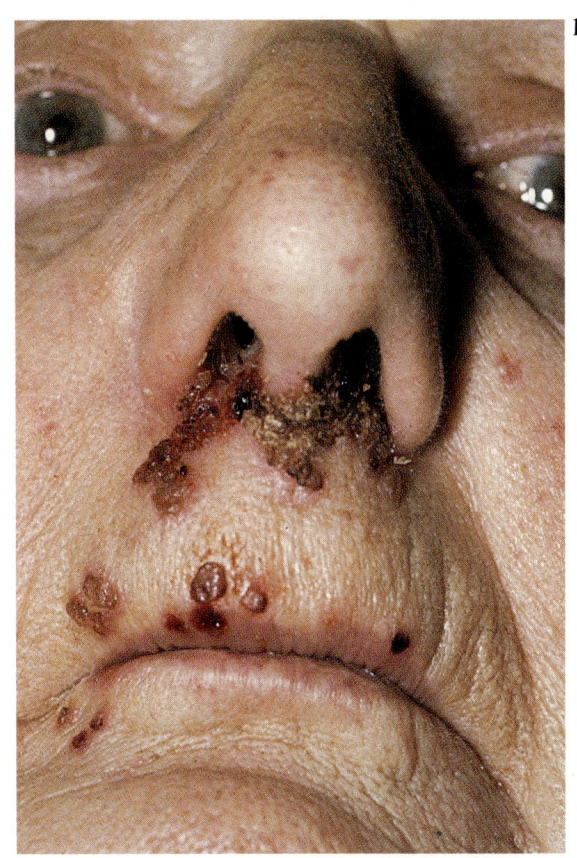

163 This skin rash in an elderly man is likely to be:

a) Acute psoriasis?
b) Drug allergy?
c) Eczema?
d) Herpes zoster?
e) Herpes simplex?

164

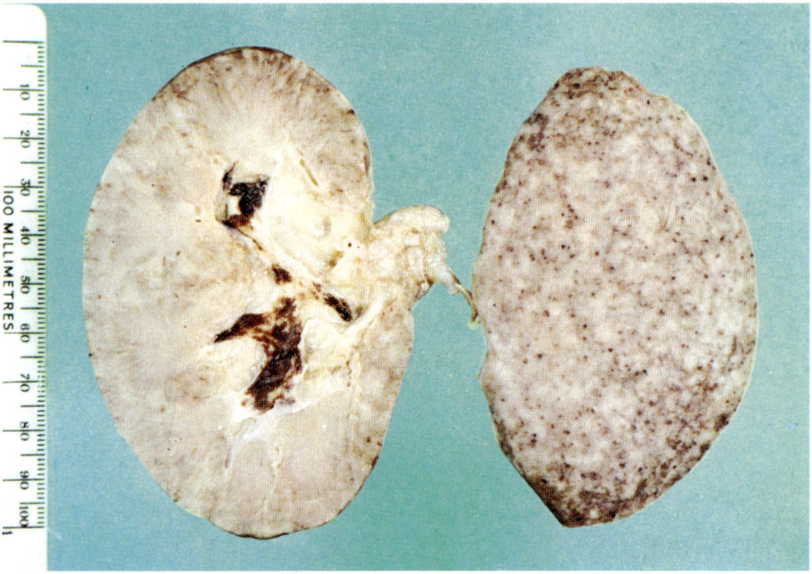

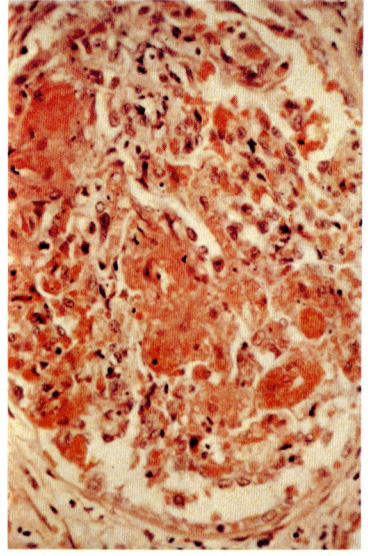

164 a) Which clinical condition do you associate with these renal changes?

b) What is their main clinical effect?

165
a) Name the condition.
b) What is the cause of the irregular pupil?
c) What is the aetiopathology of the condition illustrated?
d) List (i) systemic, (ii) intra-ocular abnormalities associated with this condition.
e) What complication follows?

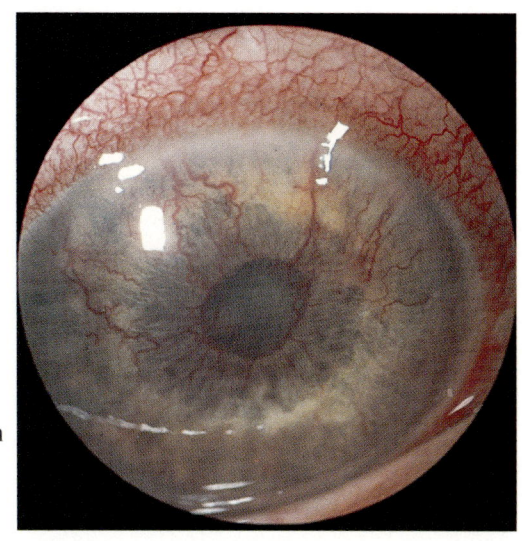

166 What is this parasite found in human blood in a febrile patient from East Africa?

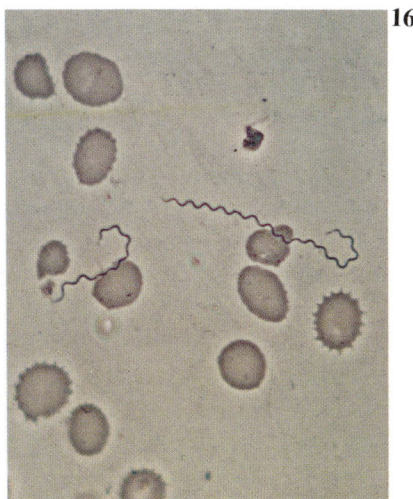

167
a) What is the diagnosis?
b) How is it inherited?
c) What is the risk if both parents are normal?

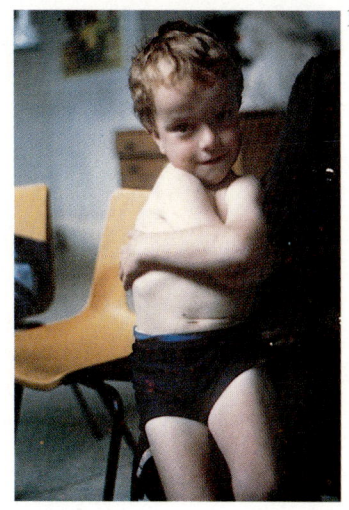

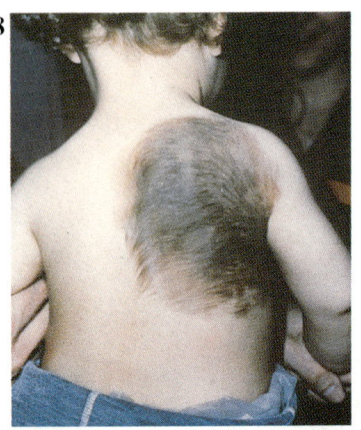

168
a) What do you call the lesion?
b) Is it genetically determined?
c) It is always benign?

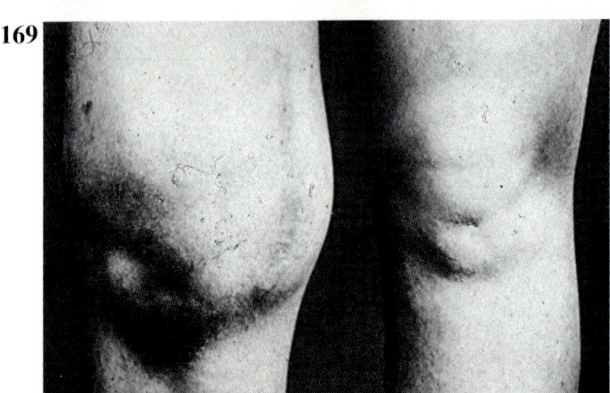

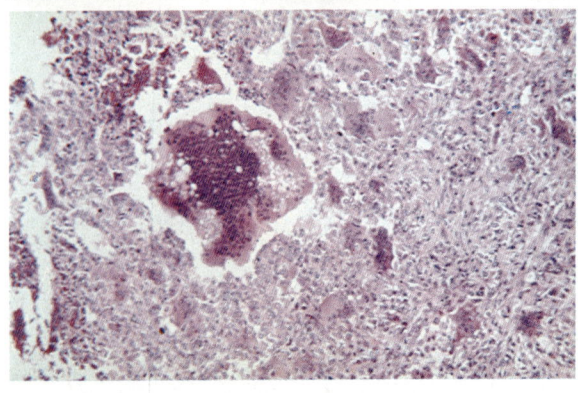

169 Painful swelling arising at the lower end of the right femur in a teenager. Radiographs show a typical lesion abutting against the articular surface. Histological examination shows that there are numerous small multi-nucleated cells of varying size lying in a stroma of round or oval cells. What is the diagnosis?

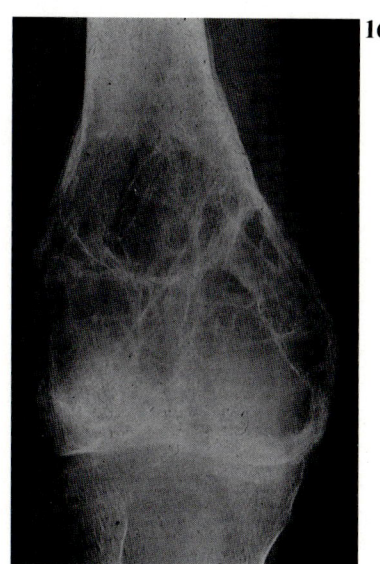

170 a) What is this condition?
b) What is the cause?
c) How would you confirm the diagnosis?

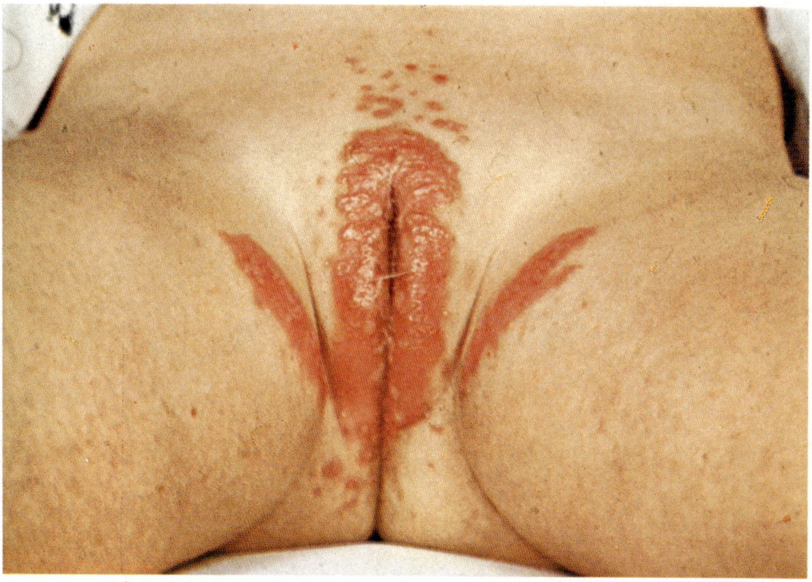

171 This West African child has oedema, ascites and gross proteinuria related to a parasitic infection. What is the diagnosis?

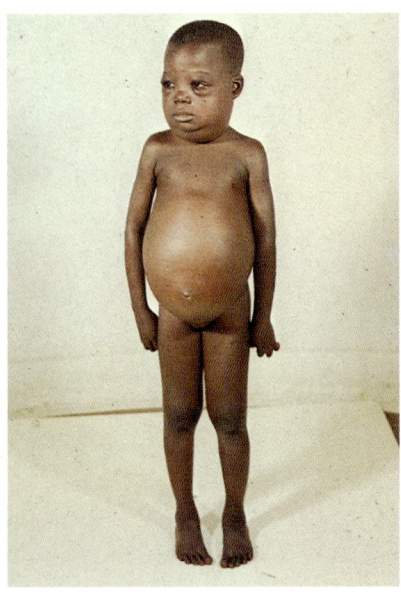

172 This patient complained of severe hypersensitivity over the shaded area of the left thumb

a) What is this condition called?
b) What is it due to?
c) How is it produced?

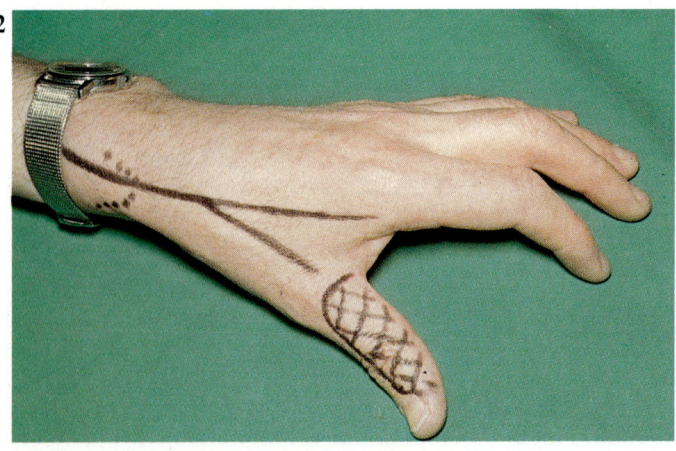

173 This elderly patient has patches of hypopigmentation, which usually occur in association with:

a) Myxoedema?
b) Pernicious anaemia?
c) Diabetes mellitus?
d) Beriberi?
e) Digoxin intoxication?

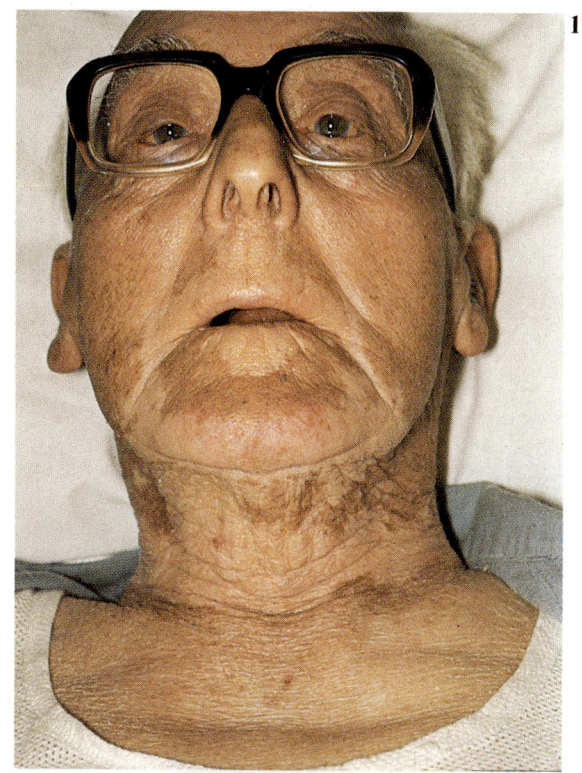

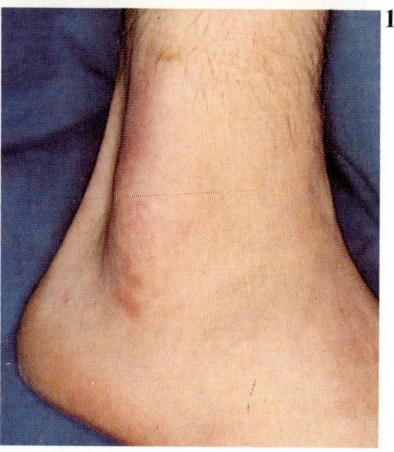

174 This patient complained of a gradual onset of pain and swelling over the outer side of the ankle in the region of the bony prominence. There is no history of injury. What is the condition?

175

176

175 a) What is this parasite seen in the gland aspirate of an African patient?

b) What disease does it cause?

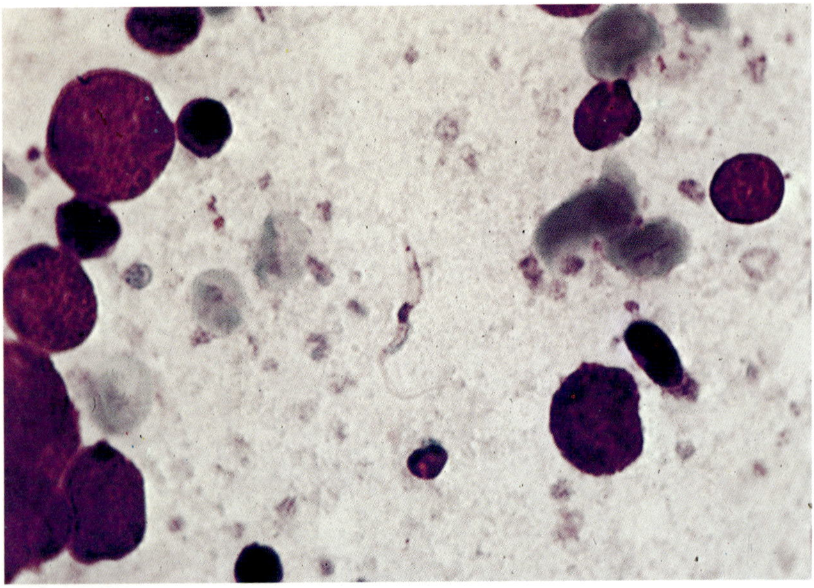

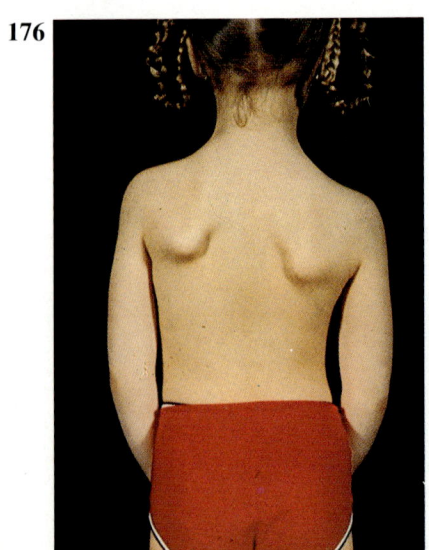

176 This otherwise healthy child has one scapula higher than the other.

a) What is the diagnosis?

b) What investigations would you perform?

177 This is an ophthalmoscopic appearance of the fundus of a middle-aged hypertensive man who suffered with recurrent transient cerebral ischaemic attacks. What does this show?

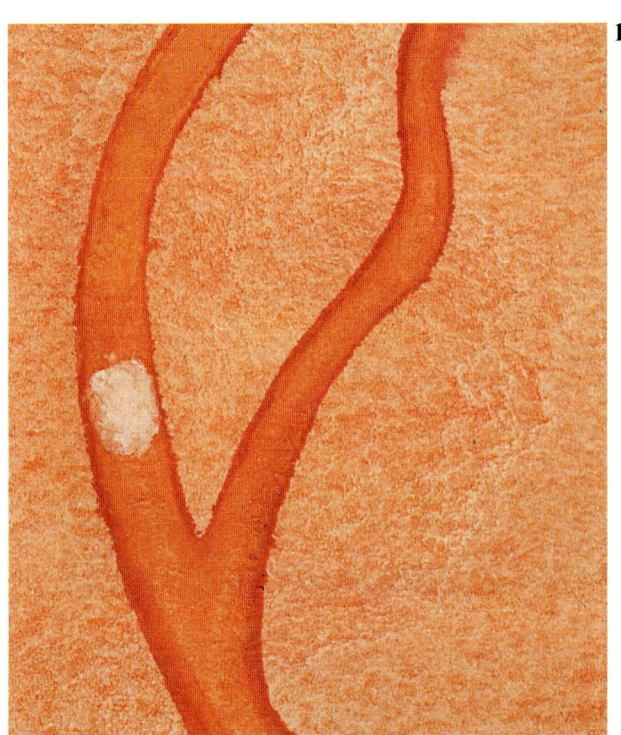

178 a) What is this condition?
b) What are the commonly associated anomalies?

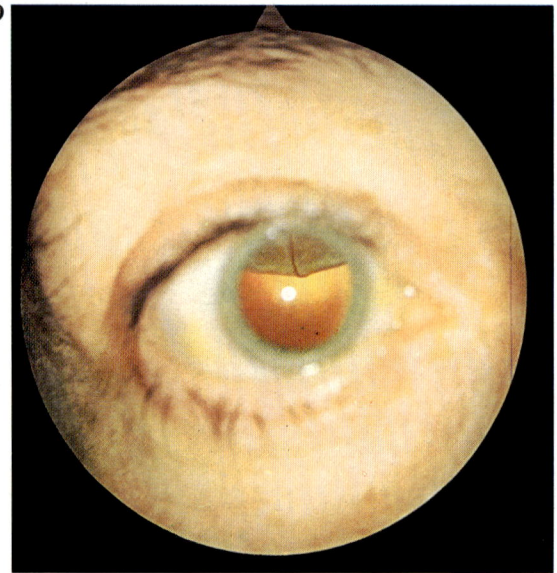

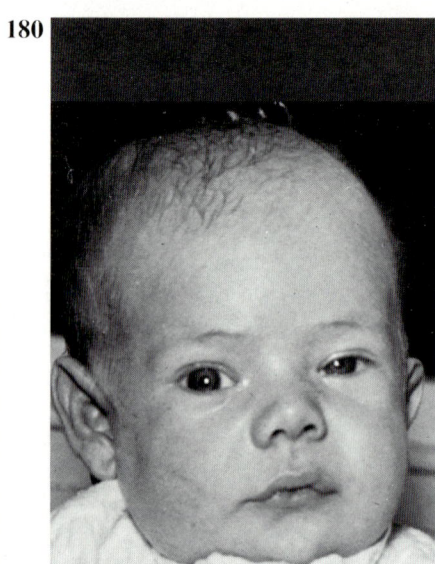

179 The patient complains of flashing lights, black spots and a curtain or shadow coming over his vision, in this case from below upwards. The visual acuity may be normal at this stage.

a) What are the physical signs?
b) What is the diagnosis?
c) How should it be managed?

180 What is the diagnosis of the baby's eye condition?

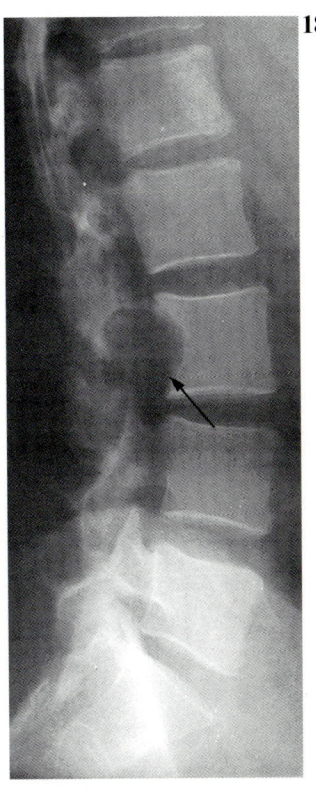

181 a) What does this X-ray show?
b) What is the diagnosis?
c) How would such a patient present?

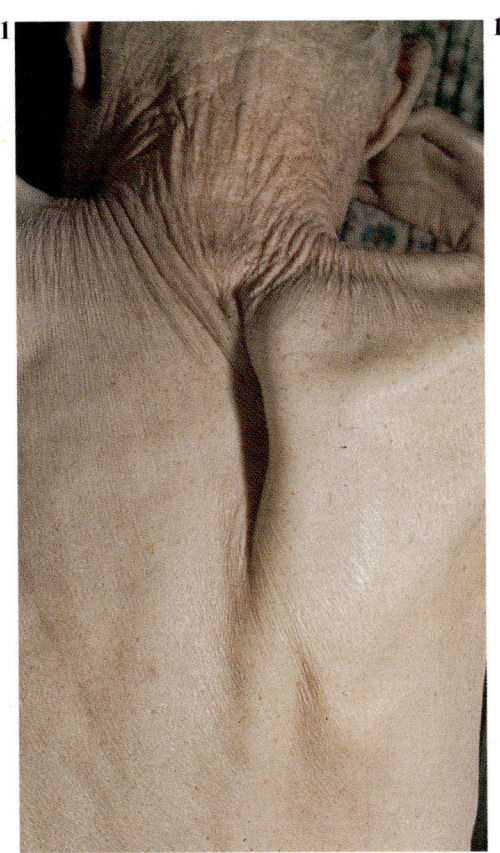

182 This elderly man has winging of right scapula. The causes are:

a) Carcinoma?
b) Paralysis of serratus magnus?
c) Paralysis of teres minor?
d) Lesion of long thoracic nerve?
e) Lesion at C2?

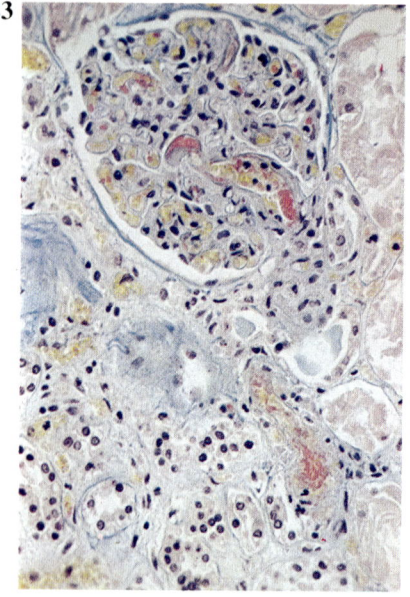

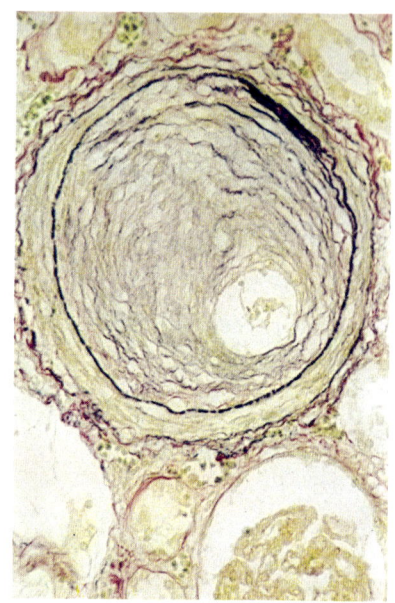

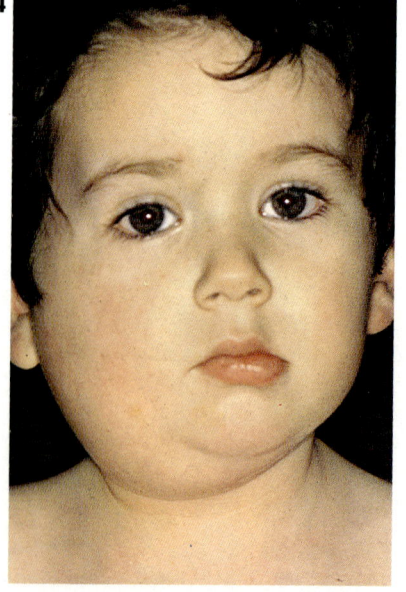

183 a) Which systemic disorder is associated with these glomerular and arterial changes?
b) What is the most common urinary abnormality in this disease?

184 a) Which organism causes this disease?
b) How is it spread?
c) What proportion of attacks are subclinical?

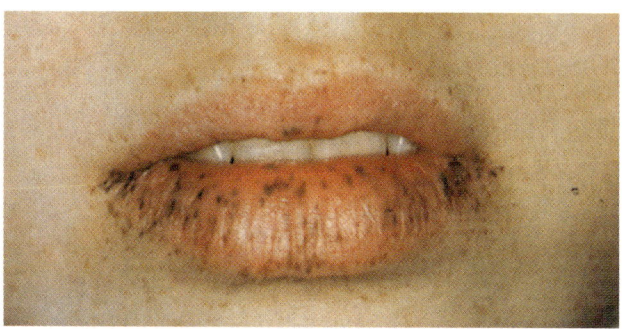

185 These melanotic macules are circumoral markers of a syndrome affecting the intestine.

a) What is the syndrome?
b) What gut lesions are present in this syndrome?
c) What genetic factors are involved?

186 This abnormality is commonly seen with:

a) Syphilitic aortic aneurysm?
b) Hypertension?
c) Trauma?
d) Advancing age?
e) Atheroma?

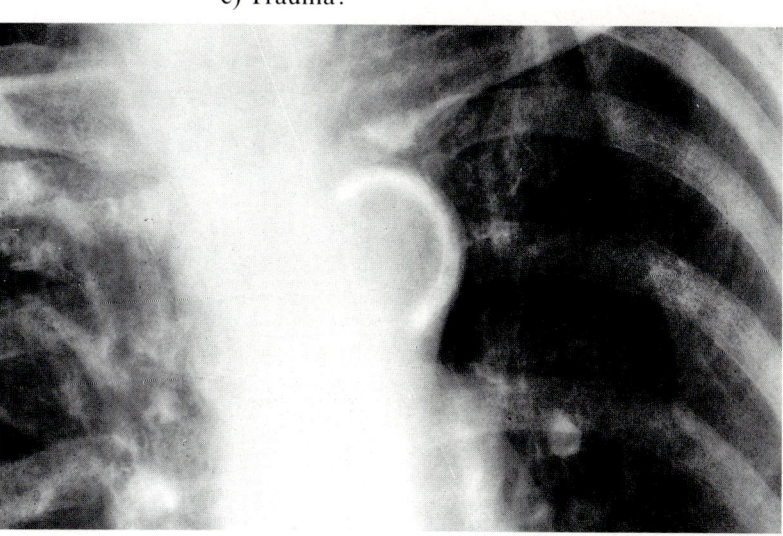

187 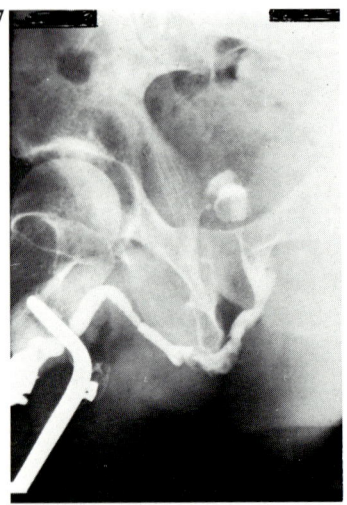 Ascending urethrogram of a patient with bleeding per urethram.

a) What is the abnormality?
b) What is its cause?

188 The patient says something has blown into his eye. The visual acuity may be normal but there may be a considerable amount of lacrimation and photophobia.

a) What is the physical sign?
b) How is it best treated?

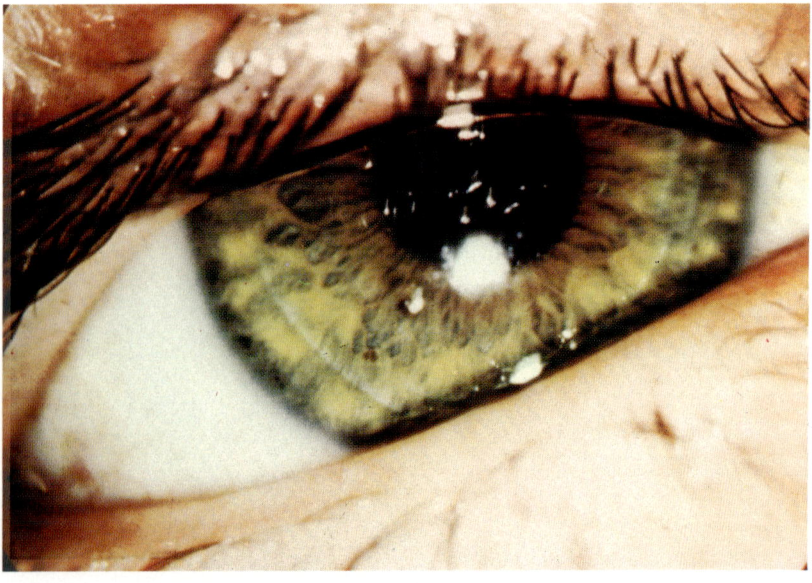

189

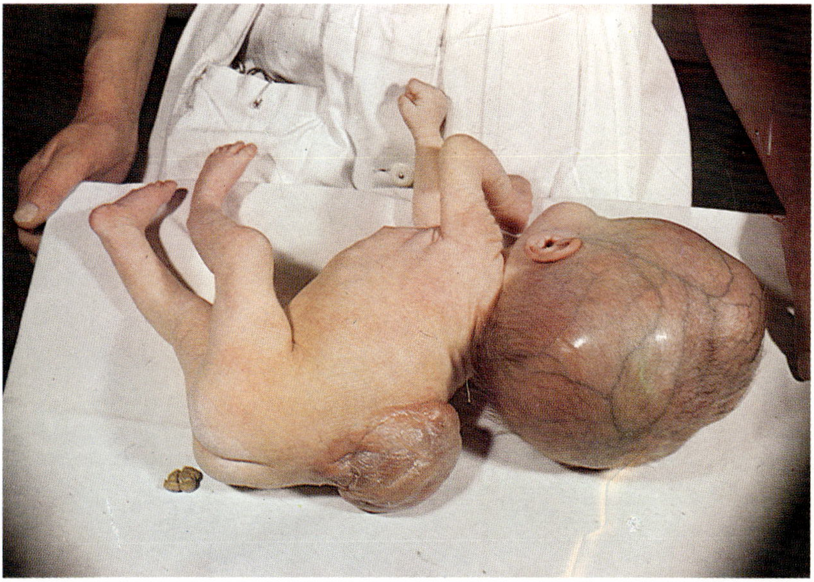

189 What afflicts this infant apart from the large hydrocephalus and paraplegia of the limbs?

190 What has caused inflammation of the distal part of this vermiform appendix?

190

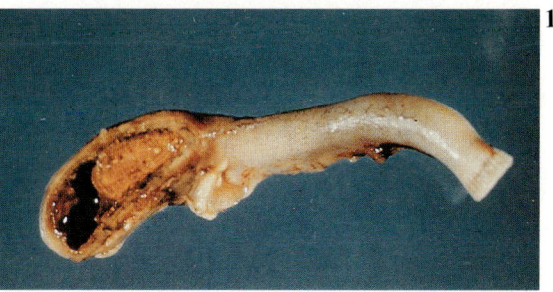

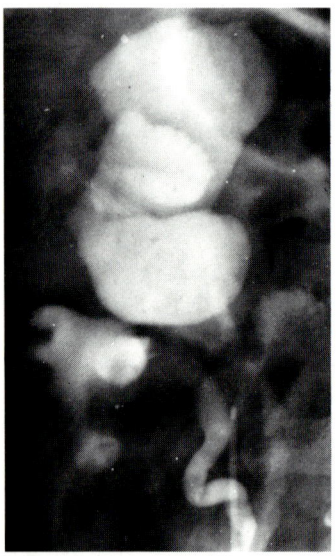

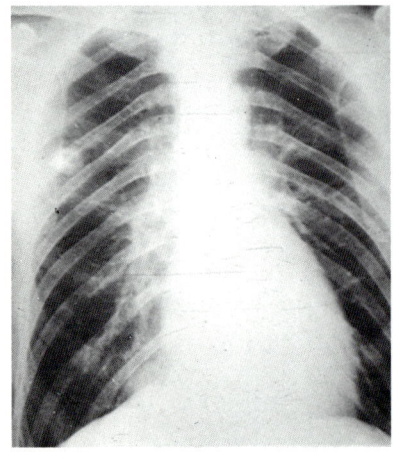

192 a) What does this chest X-ray of a patient with rheumatoid arthritis show?
b) What is the likely diagnosis?

191 a) What is the likely cause of the gross dilatation of the upper moiety of this duplex kidney?
b) Comment on the lower moiety.

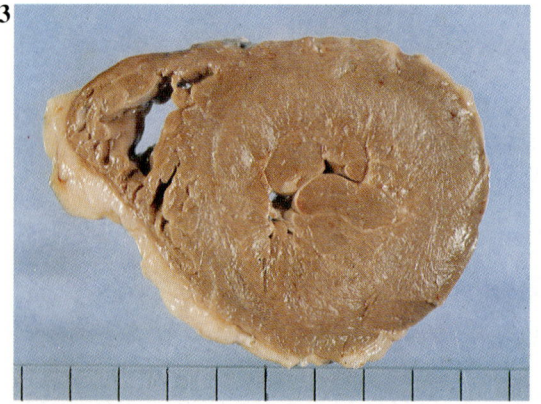

193 A transverse mid-ventricular slice of the heart. Name the type of hypertrophy and its cause.

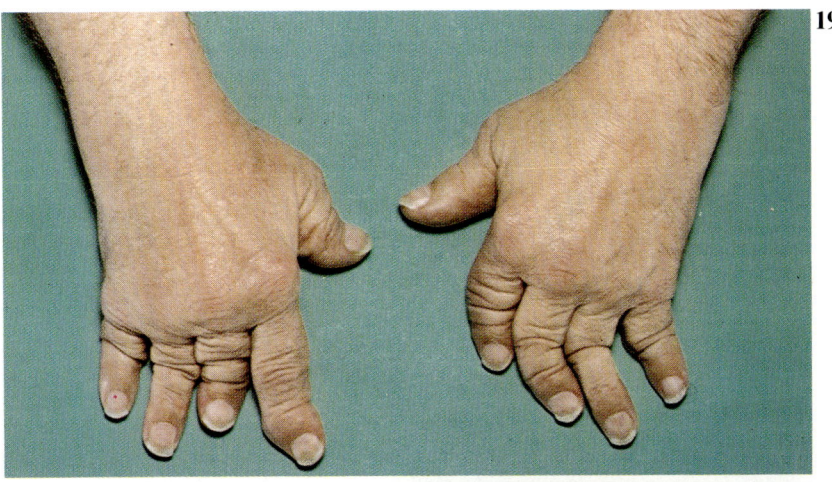

194 a) What is this deformity known as?
b) In what conditions may it occur?

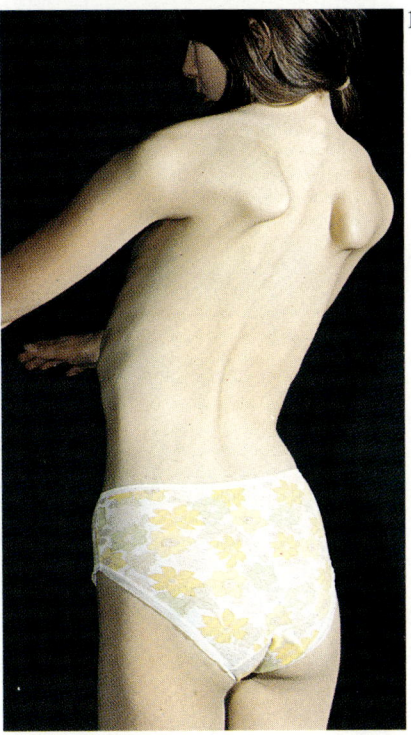

195 A 13-year-old girl, always a poor runner, whose gait had deteriorated over the previous 12 months. She also had difficulty in holding her hands up to do her hair, and complained that her 'stomach was sticking out'.

a) What is the diagnosis?
b) How is the condition usually inherited?
c) What is the prognosis?

196 This shotgun wound of the chest:

  a) Is an exit wound.
  b) Is a contact entry wound.
  c) Is an entry wound fired from 3 metres distance.

197 The patient complains of a severe injury to the eye caused by a fist, squash ball, etc.

  a) What is the physical sign?
  b) How should the patient be managed?

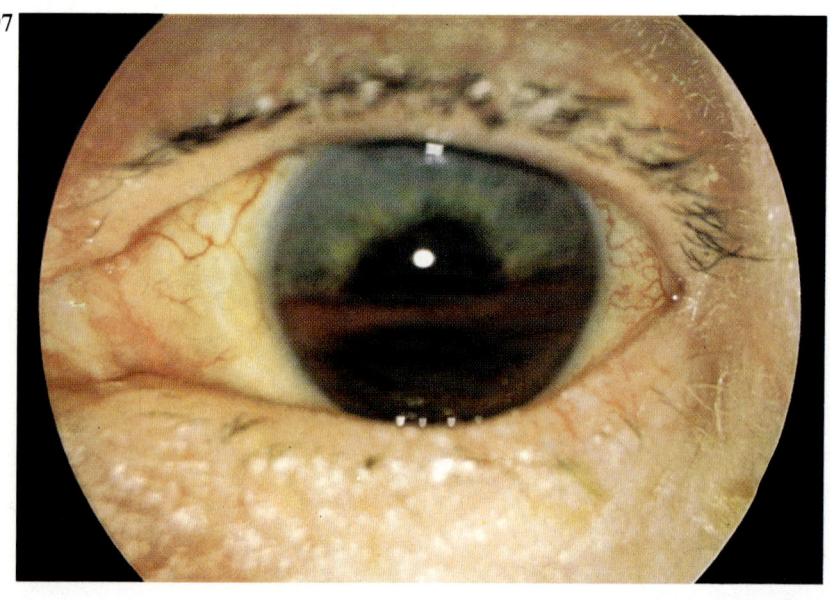

198 This patient has acute arthritis. The diagnosis is:

a) Dermato-myositis?
b) Psoriasis?
c) Bacterial endocarditis?
d) Tabes dorsalis?
e) Tophaceous gout?

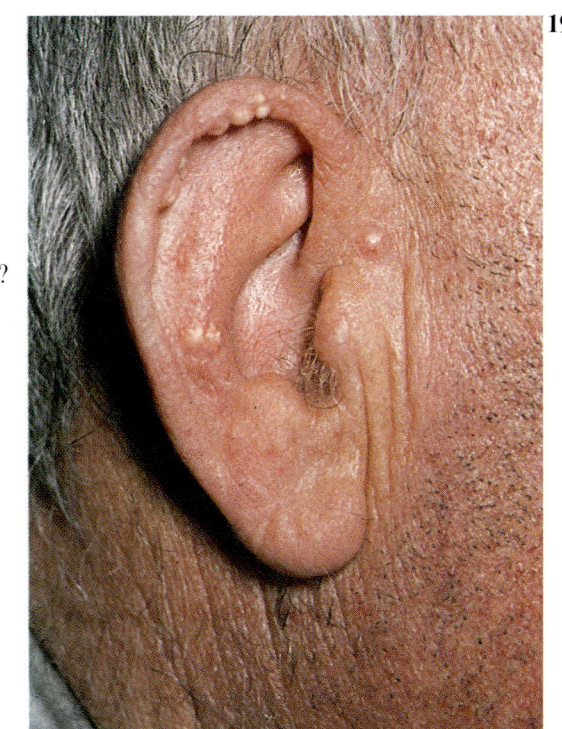

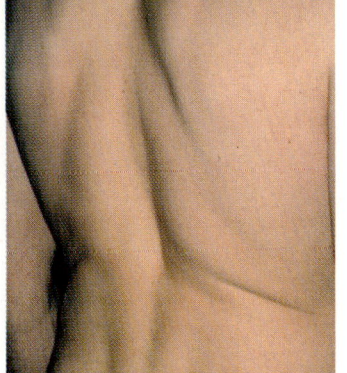

199 What is the significance of this appearance in the lumbar spine in a patient with low back pain?

200

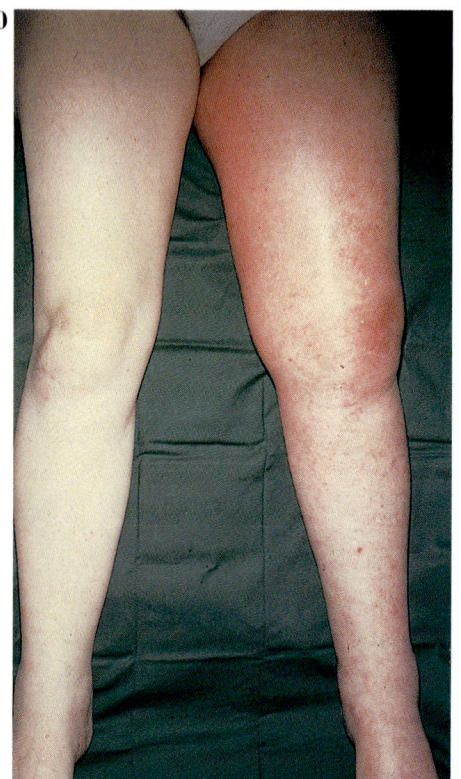

200 This woman reported her left leg became swollen after a minor injury 10 days ago. The most likely diagnosis includes:

a) Deep vein thrombosis.
b) Haematoma of thigh muscle.
c) Femoral artery embolism.

201 What is peculiar to this lumbo-sacral tumour?

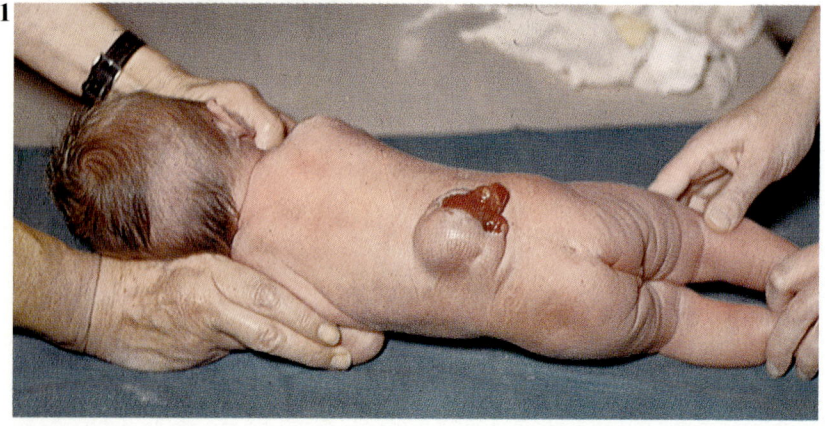

202 A peripheral blood smear.

a) What are the red-cell abnormalities shown here?

b) What is the likely underlying disease?

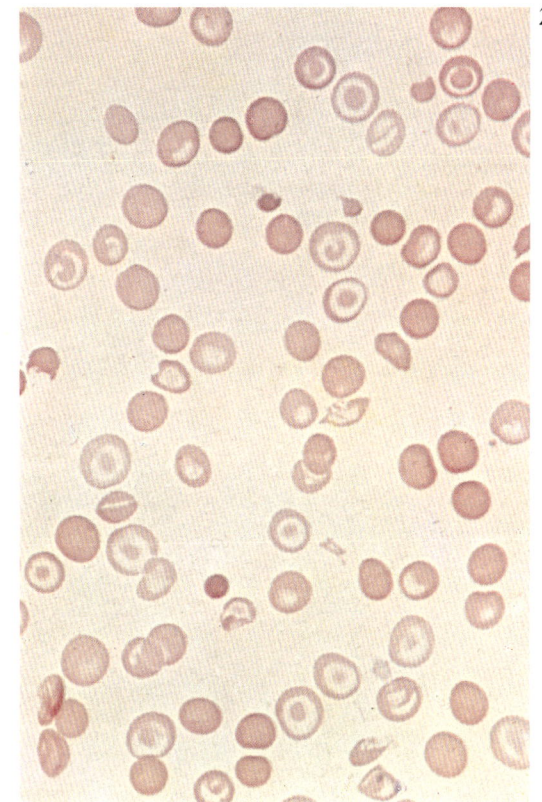

203 a) What lesion is shown in this picture?

b) With what endocrine condition is it most commonly associated?

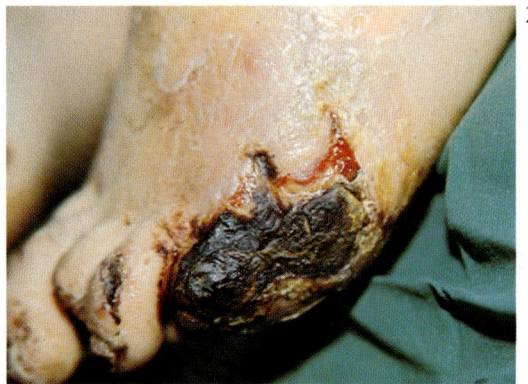

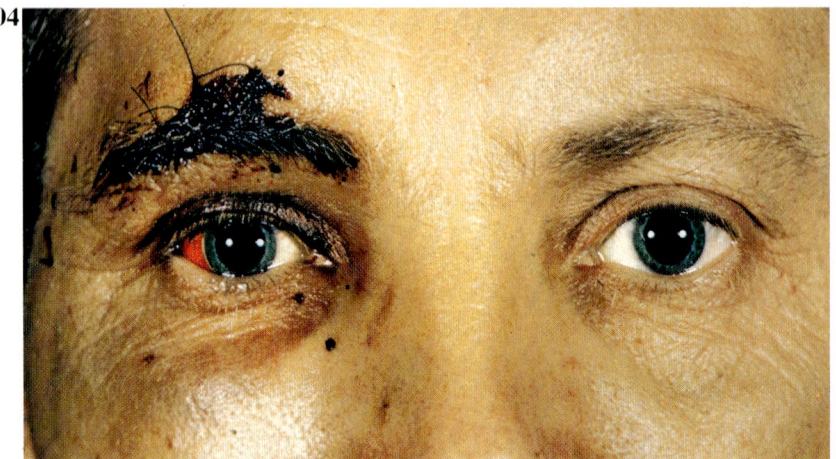

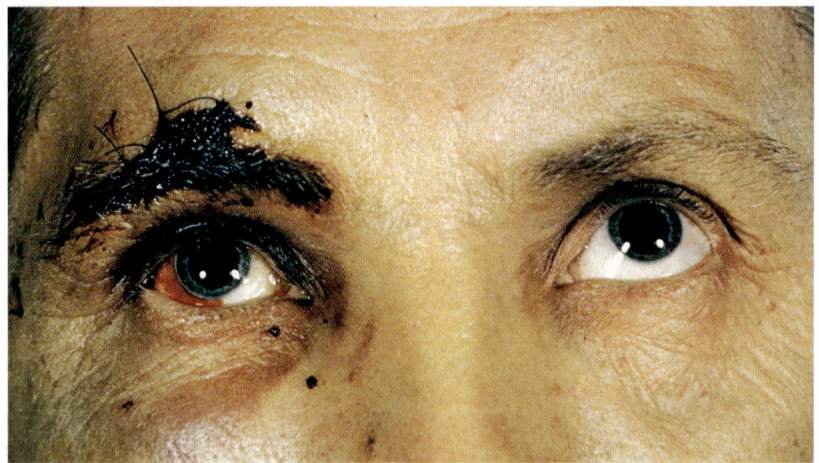

204 The patient sustained a 'black eye' and a laceration which has been sutured. After the swelling subsided he complained of double-vision on movement of his eyes.

a) What are the physical signs?
b) How is the treatment best managed?

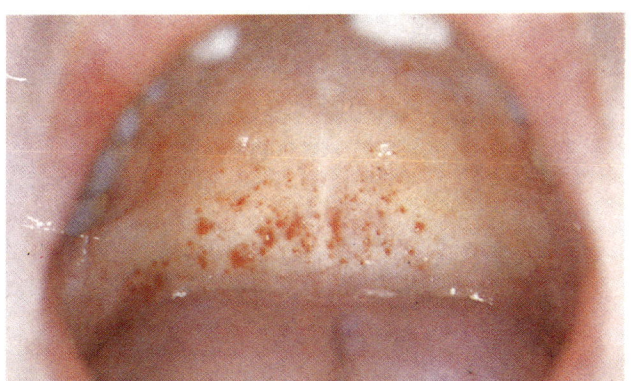

205 These petechial haemorrhages on the palate may mark a haematological abnormality.

a) What may this be?
b) What other oral lesions may occur in this condition?
c) What other common conditions may transiently give rise to a similar appearance?

206 These burns are most likely to have been caused by:

a) Lightning. b) Molten metal. c) Boiling water.

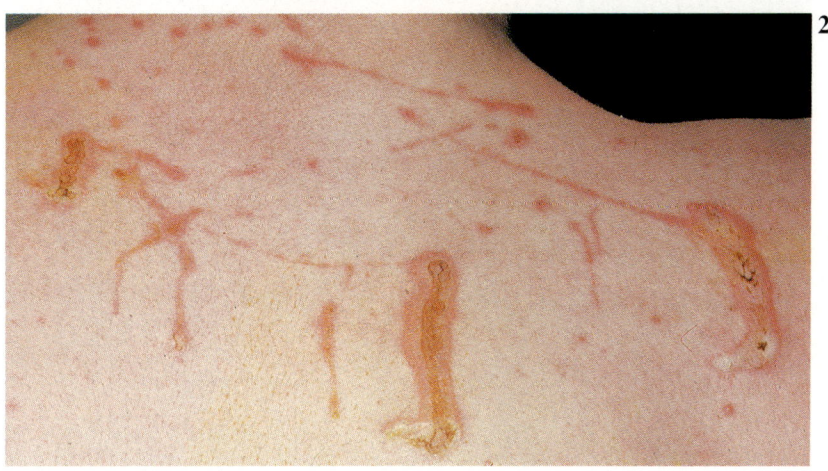

207

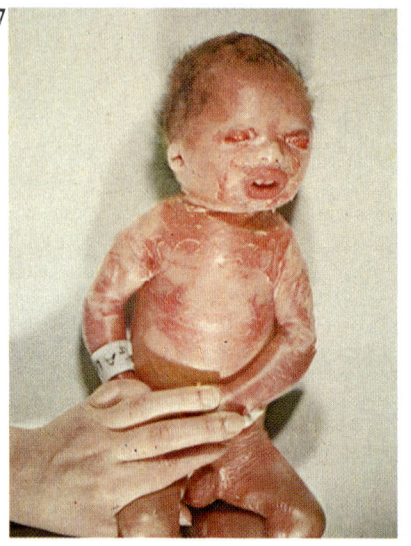

207 This baby is encased in a collodion-like membrane. The face, eyes and ears are compressed, distorted and oedematous. What is the diagnosis and prognosis?

208 These burn blisters are typical of:

a) Chemical burns.
b) Electrical burns.
c) Thermal burns.

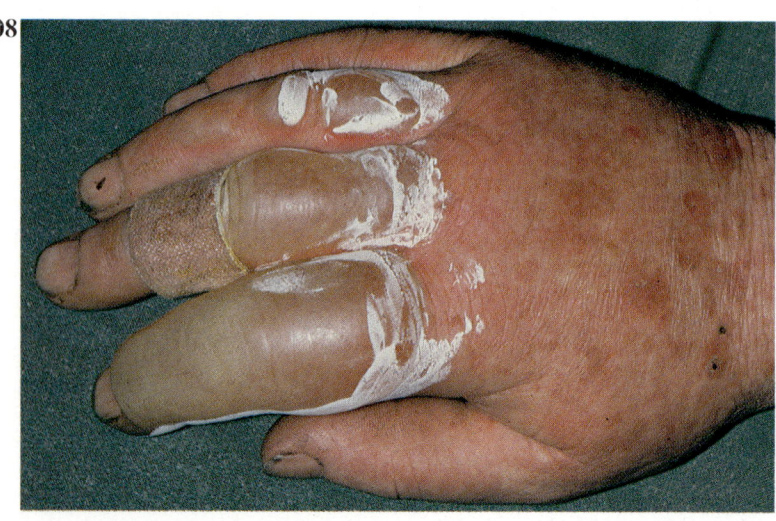

209 Name two of the features which characterize this form of diabetic glomerulopathy.

209

210 a) What does this X-ray show?
b) Name four conditions in which it may occur.

210

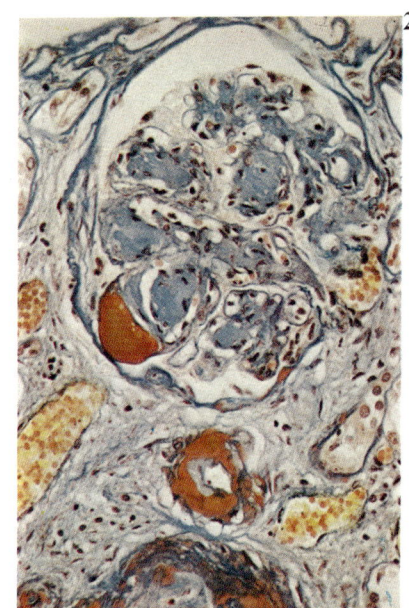

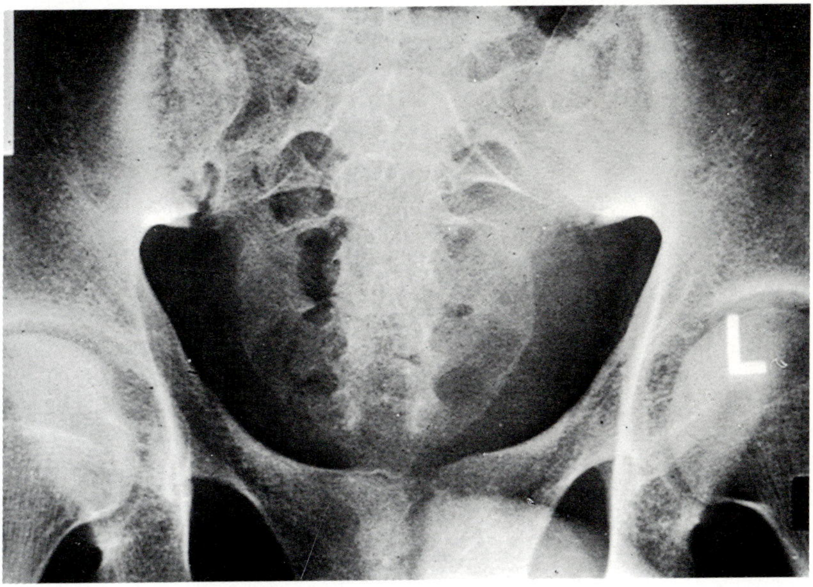

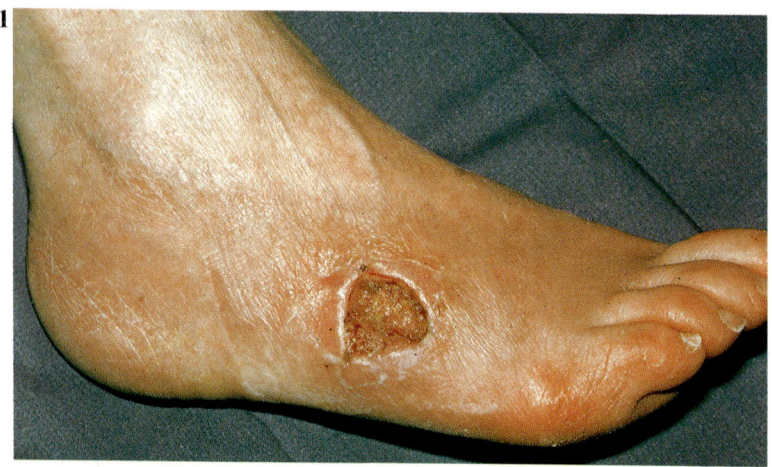

211 This wound in an elderly woman has given rise to increasing neck stiffness. The most likely diagnosis is:

a) Rheumatic fever.
b) Tetanus.
c) Gas gangrene.

212 a) What does this optic fundus demonstrate?
b) Give two causes?

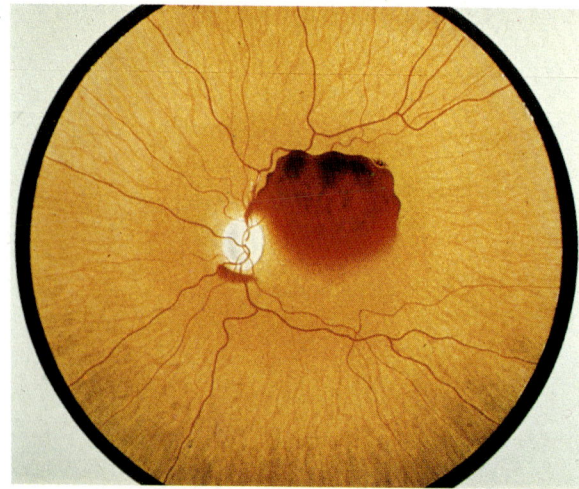

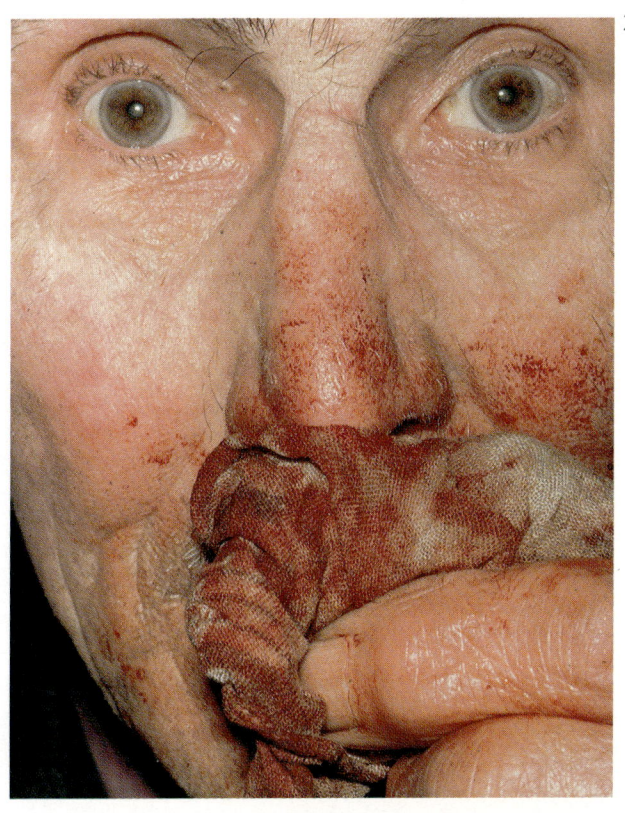

213 This elderly patient may suffer from:

a) Henoch-Schölein purpura.
b) Chronic lymphatic leukaemia.
c) Sinusitis.

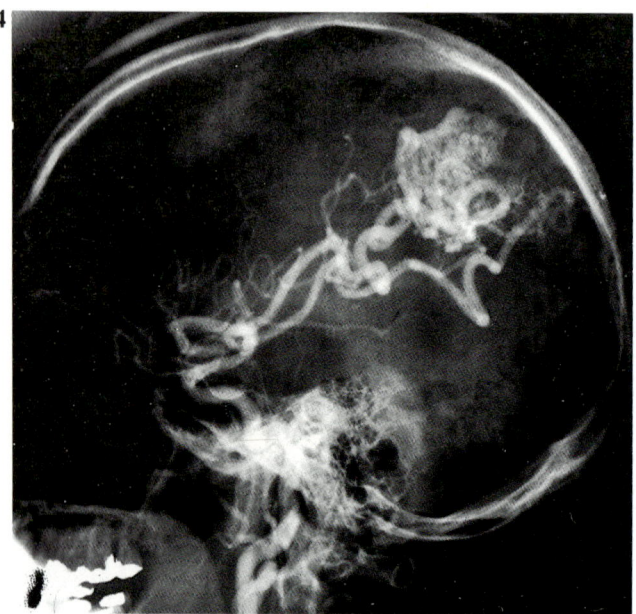

214
a) What is this lesion?
b) How do such lesions present?
c) How are they treated?

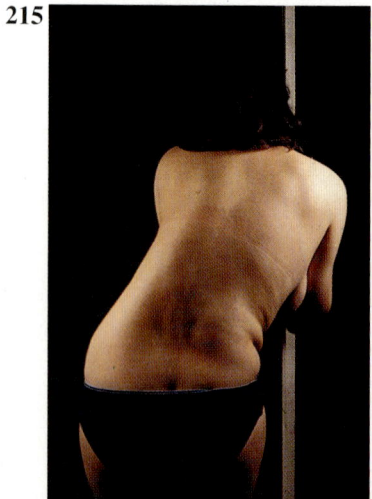

215 This patient has severe pain in the left leg; on attempting to bend forwards her body tilts over to the right.

a) What is this sign called?
b) To what is it due?

216
a) Describe the abnormal feature.
b) What is the likely diagnosis?
c) Describe the likely progression of this condition, its ocular complications and symptoms.
d) Name a procedure which may arrest this progression.

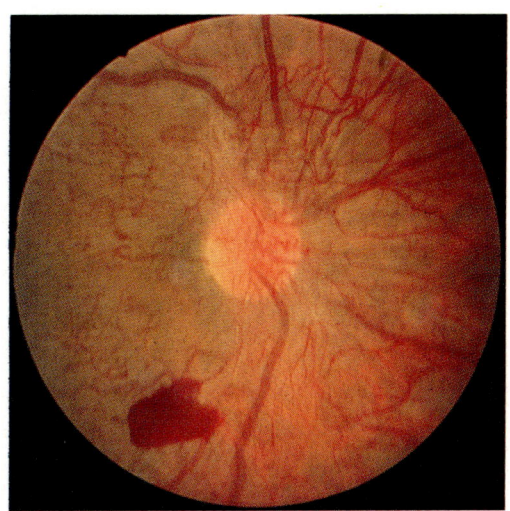

217
a) What are the main constituents of staghorn calculi?
b) Are they more likely to:
   (i) be unilateral or bilateral?
   (ii) formed in an acid or alkaline urine?
c) What are their clinical manifestations?

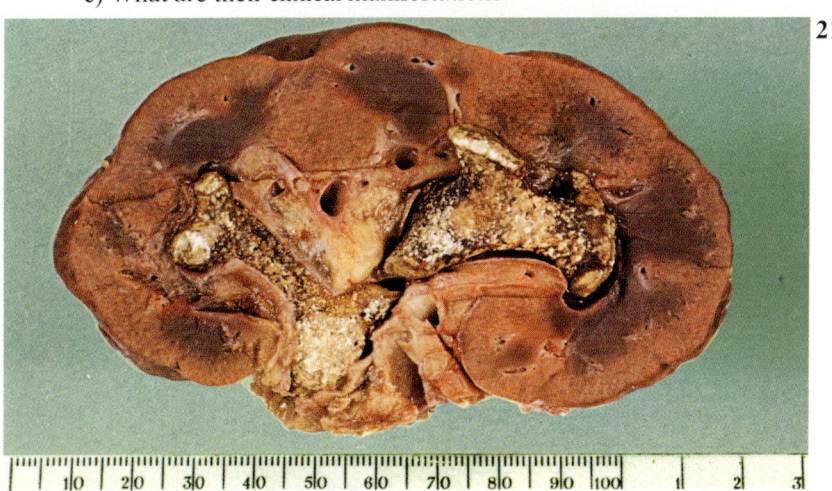

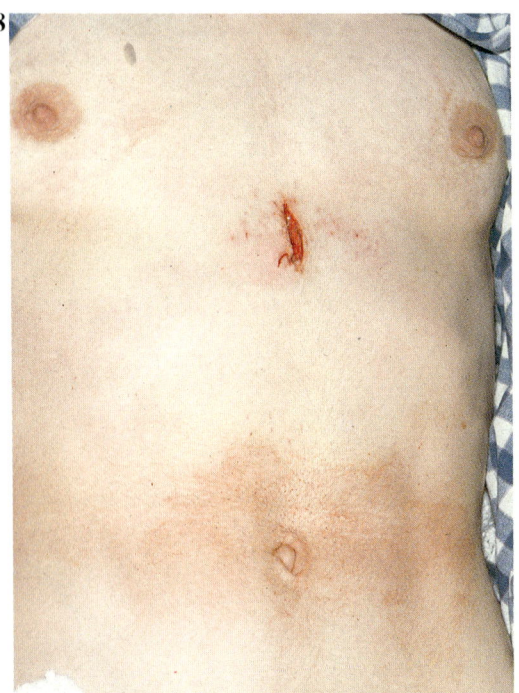

218 The best investigation for this self-inflicted stab wound is:

a) Injection of contrast medium and radiography to outline the track.
b) Laparotomy.
c) Probing.

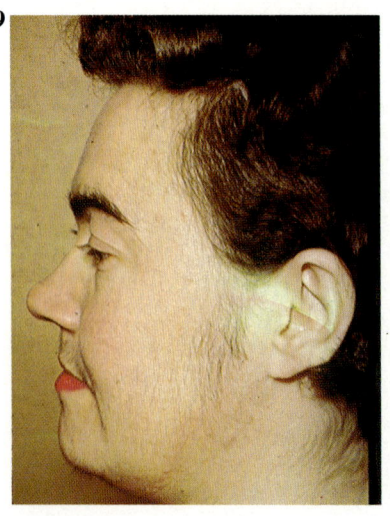

219 a) What physical sign is shown here?
b) Into what diagnostic category do most such patients fall?
c) What clinical features may lead you to suspect significant underlying organic disease?
d) What drugs may be responsible for this abnormality?

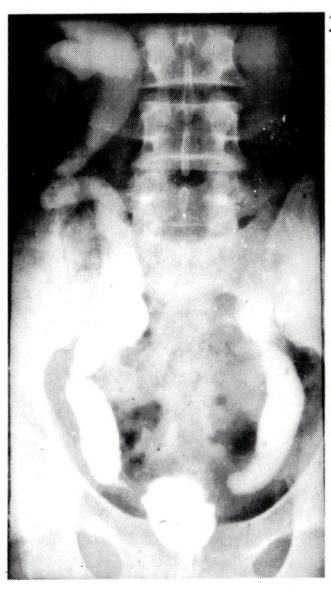

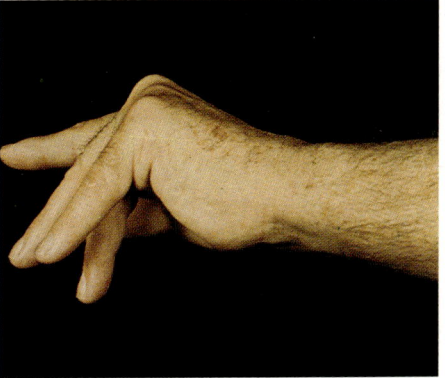

221 Take a *very careful* look at the position of the fingers in this hand. What is the diagnosis?

a) Ulnar nerve paralysis?
b) Median nerve paralysis?
c) Division of flexor tendon?
d) Other?

220 a) What tropical condition may give rise to appearances of the IVU?
b) What abnormalities are present?
c) What is the differential diagnosis?

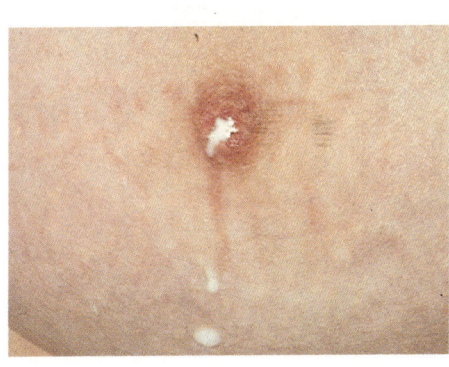

222 Galactorrhoea is lactation in the absence of an appropriate physiological stimulus.

a) Is it always associated with an elevated prolactin level?
b) Name three drugs which may cause galactorrhoea.
c) Which thyroid disorder may be associated with it?

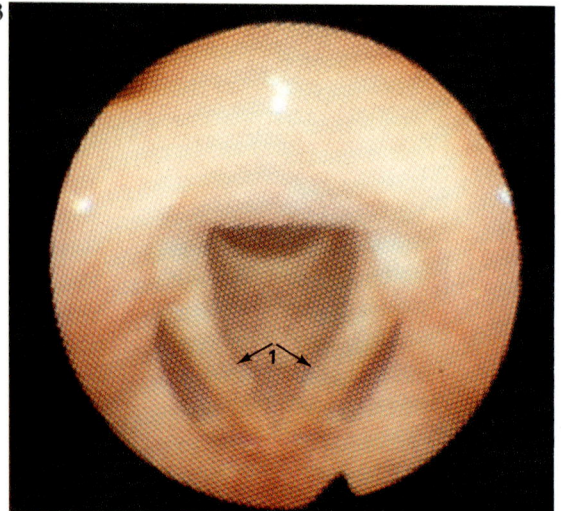

223 What are these lesions which are situated at the junction of the anterior ⅓ and the posterior ⅔ of the true vocal cords, and in whom do they more commonly occur?

224 This patient had previously suffered an extensive deep venous thrombosis in his right leg. What is the likely cause of the ulcer now present?

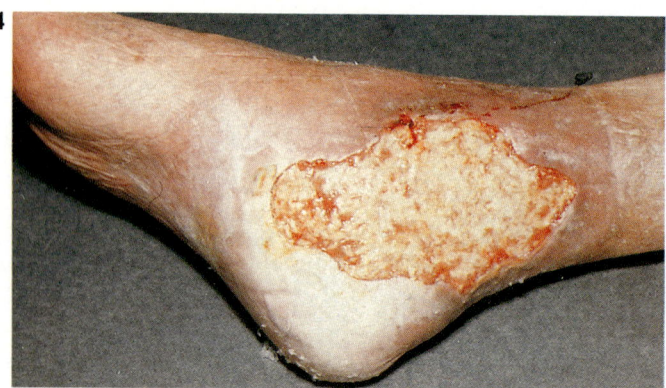

225

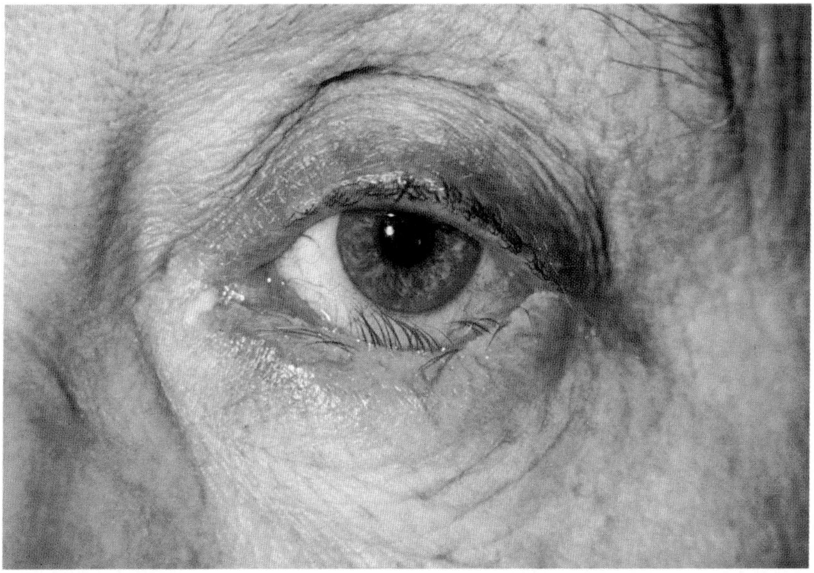

225 The patient complains of a sore, running, red eye which may have gone on for some months.

a) What is the physical sign?
b) What is the diagnosis?
c) How is it best managed?

226

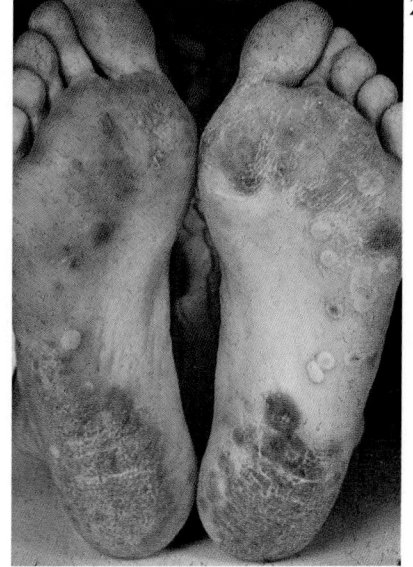

226 Pustular rash on the soles of the feet of a young man with swollen knees. What is the diagnosis?

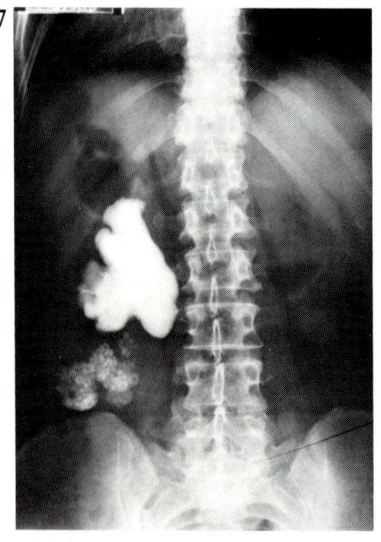
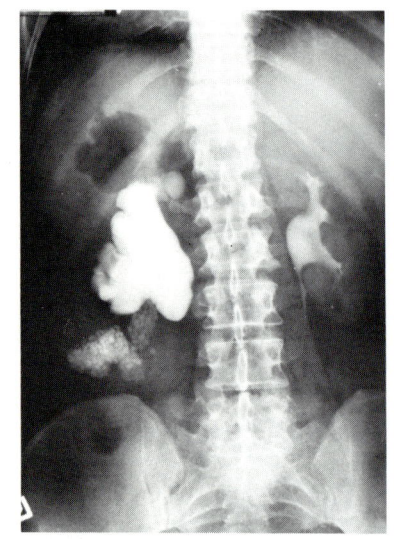

227 a) What abnormalities are present on these plain and IVU films?
b) What could be the underlying cause?

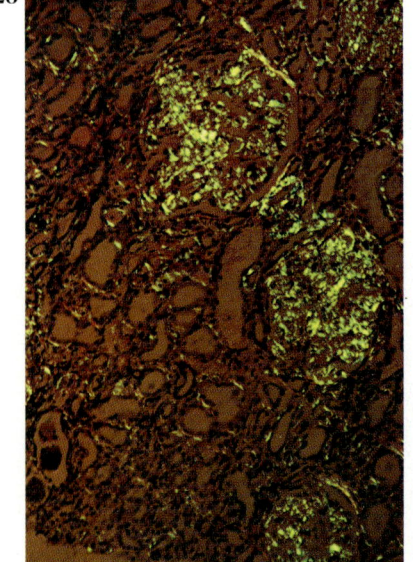

228 The section illustrated was taken from a renal biopsy from a nephrotic patient.

a) Which technique has been applied?
b) What does it demonstrate?

229 a) What abnormality does this slide show?
b) What is the cause?
c) What are the characteristic findings?

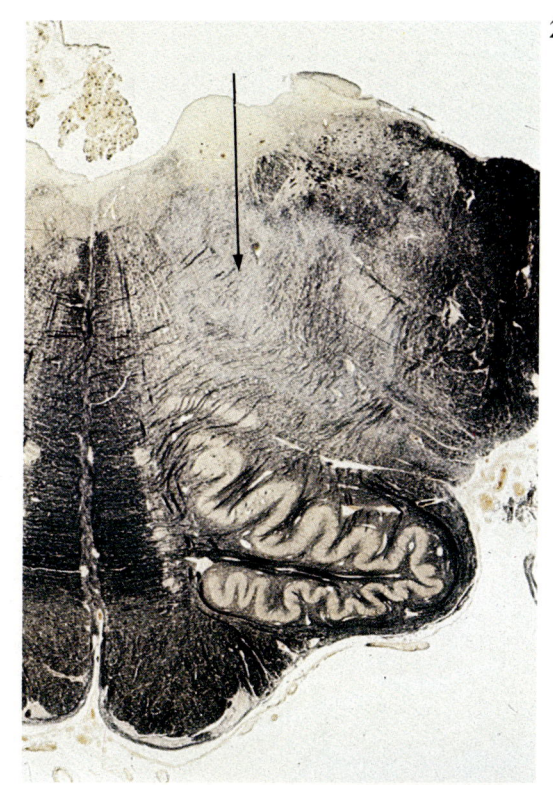

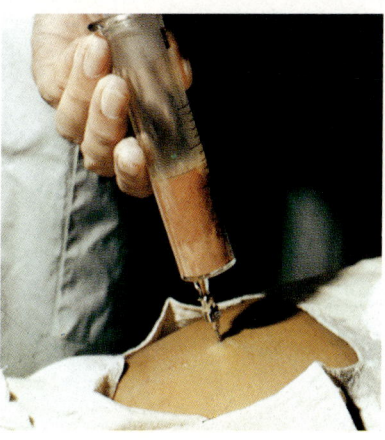

230 A Thai patient presented with fever, tenderness over the liver, and hepatomegaly. On aspiration this characteristic fluid was withdrawn. What is the diagnosis?

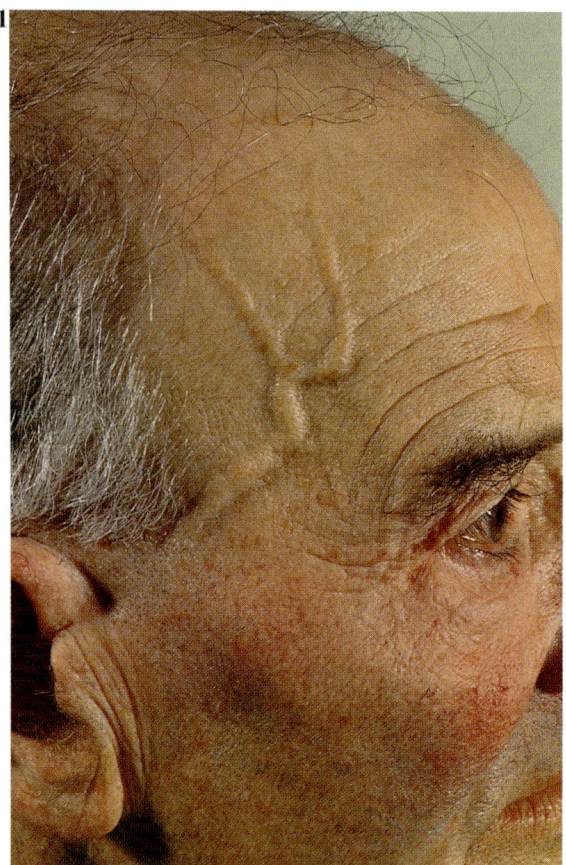

231 a) Why is this elderly man complaining of a severe headache?
b) What two investigations would you perform?
c) What is the complication?
d) Is there any treatment?

232 This elderly female patient has finger-tip ischaemia and necrosis. The causes are:

a) Systemic sclerosis?
b) Ecchymosis?
c) Cervical spondylosis?
d) Dysproteinaemias?
e) Polyarteritis?

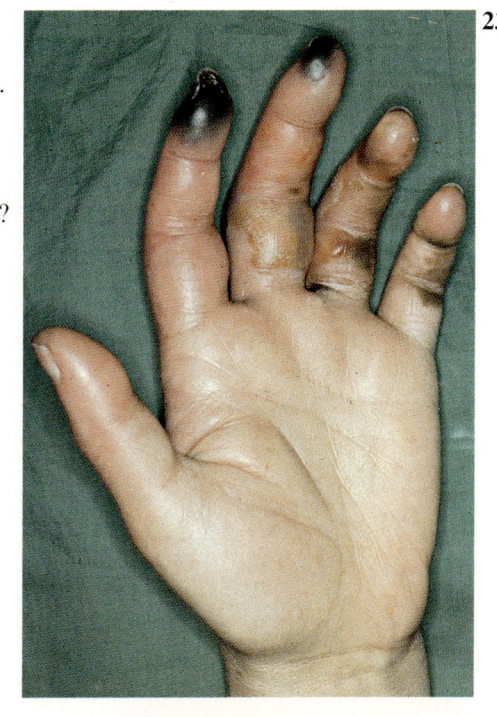

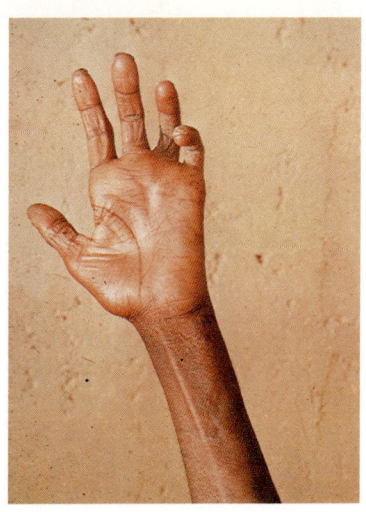

233 This Indian patient complained of weakness, loss of sensation in the hand and on examination there was wasting of the thenar and hypothenar eminences. What is the diagnosis?

234

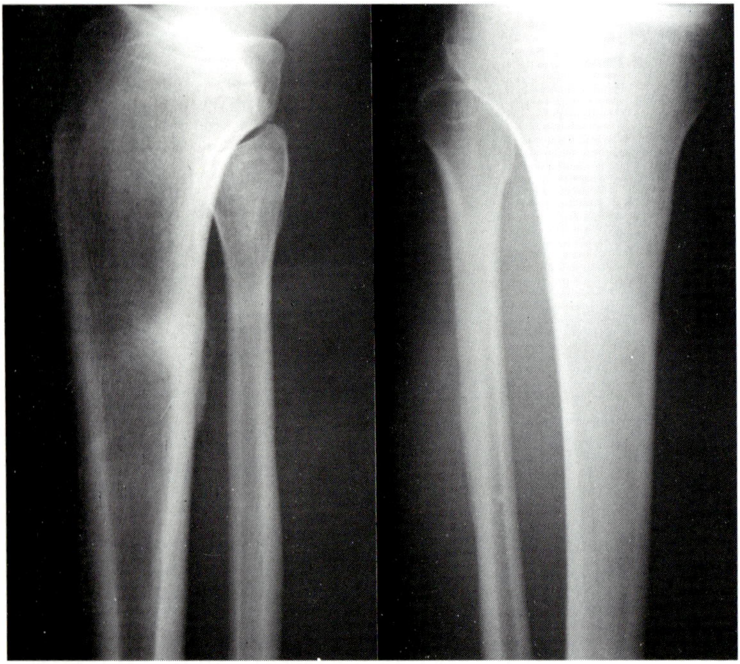

234 a) What changes do these X-rays represent?
b) What is their significance?

235

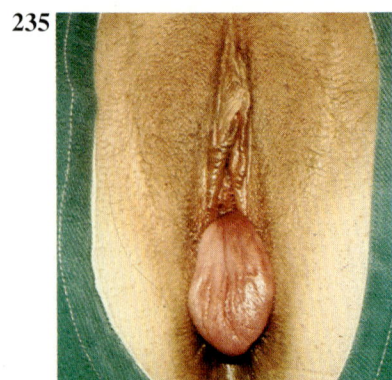

235 a) What is the likely diagnosis?
b) What is the likely presenting symptom?
c) What is the treatment?

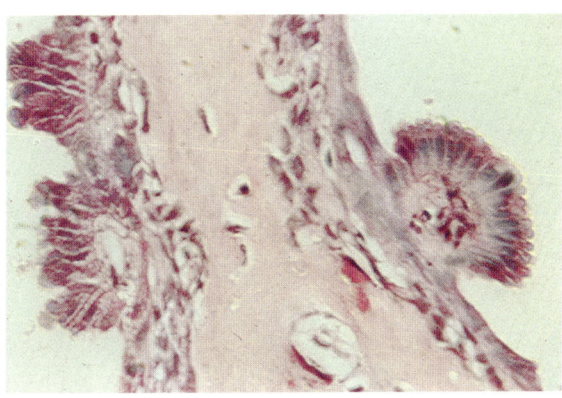

236 This section shows features characteristic of:

a) Hyperparathyroidism.
b) Osteoclastic bone resorption.
c) Metastatic seedlings.
d) Fibrosarcoma.
e) Actinomycosis.

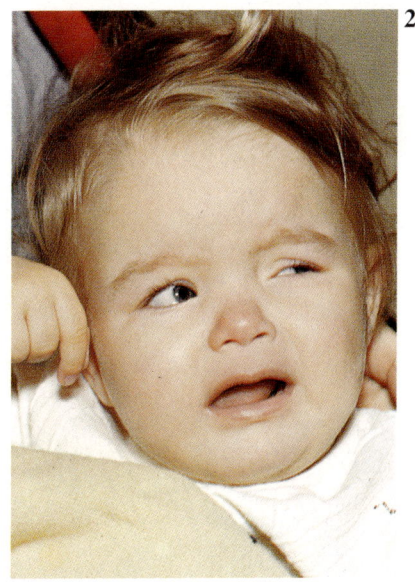

237 This infant has a left-sided cataract, narrowing of the palpebral fissure, a congenital heart defect and is generally retarded. What is the pathology?

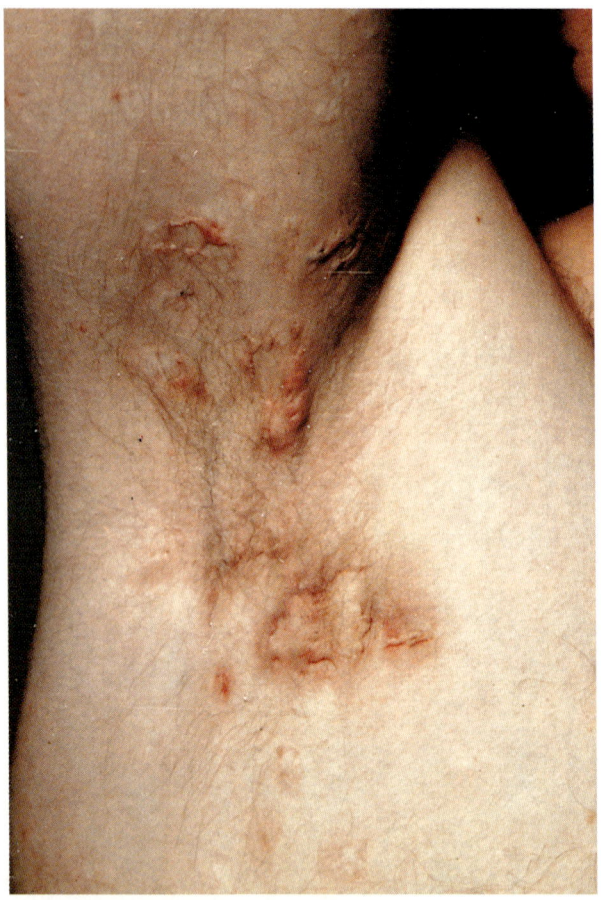

238 a) What condition affecting the axillary skin is seen in this picture?
b) In which sweat glands does the condition arise?
c) Which other areas of the body are often affected?

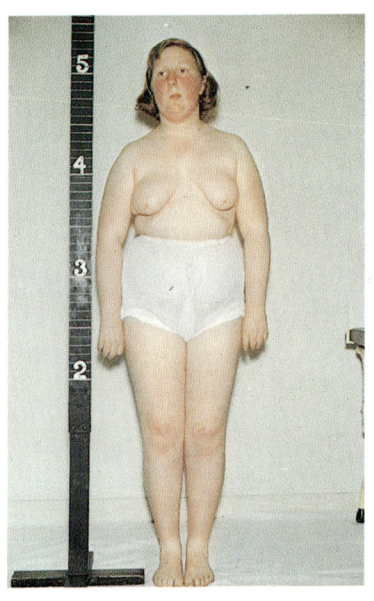

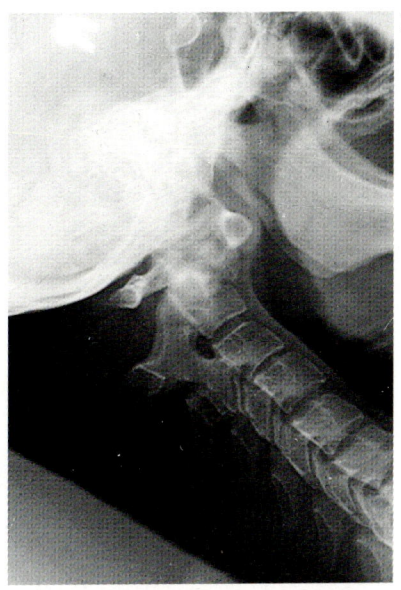

239 This 11-year-old girl shows precocious development of secondary sex characteristics, a high coloured face and striae. The hormonal assay was normal. What is the diagnosis?

240 a) What does this X-ray of the cervical spine show?
b) What is the most common cause of the condition?

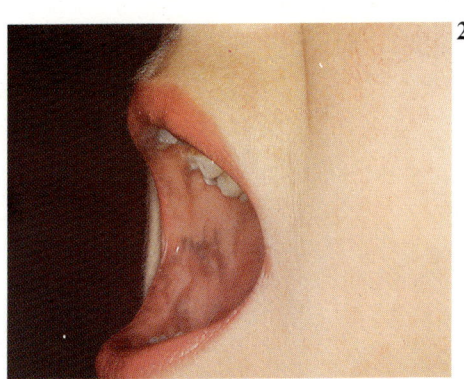

241 a) What is the diagnosis?
b) How may patients present?
c) What is the complication?

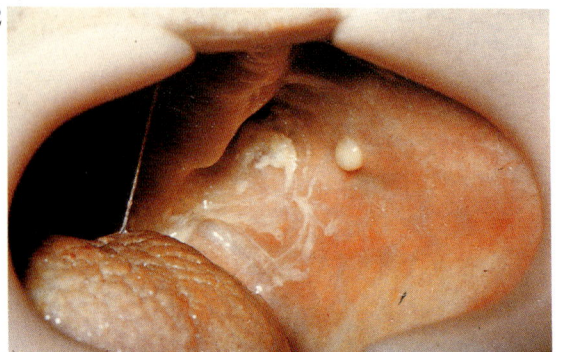

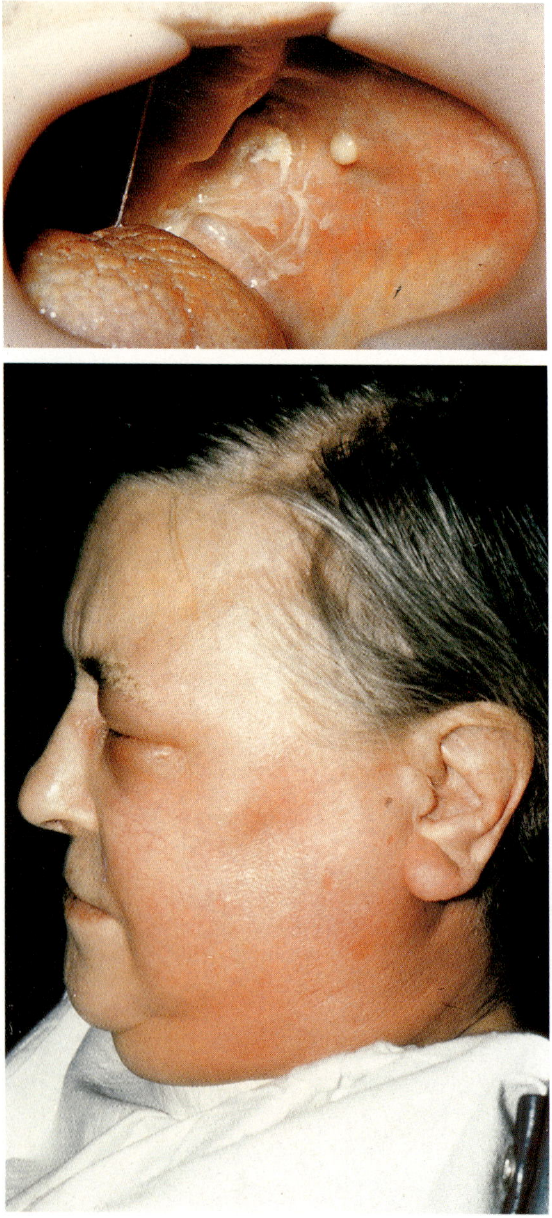

242 The intra-oral view is from the same patient seen in the main picture.

    a) What is this condition called?
    b) In which patients is it typically seen?
    c) What is the usual causative organism?

243 The myocardium of a primary cardiomyopathy.

    a) Name the type.
    b) Describe the histological features present.

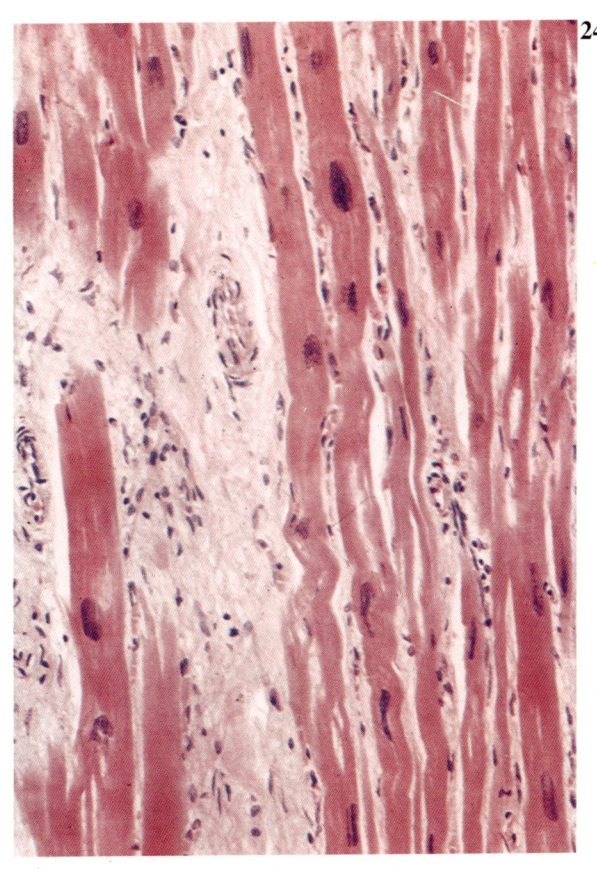

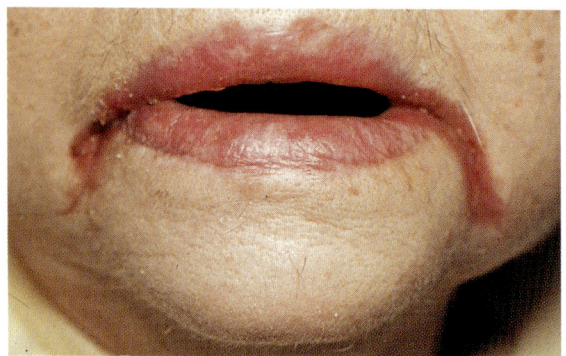

244 This sign occurs in association with:

a) Vitamin C deficiency?
b) Magnesium deficiency?
c) Vitamin D intoxication?
d) Multiple vitamin deficiency?
e) Vitamin A intoxication?

245 Photomicrograph of a thyroid-gland tumour excised from a 33-year-old man. (*H&E × 220.*)

a) What is the tumour?
b) From what cells does it arise?
c) What other tumours and abnormalities may occur in patients with this type of thyroid neoplasm?

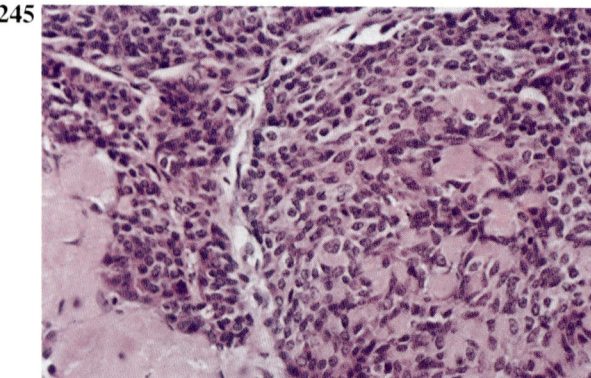

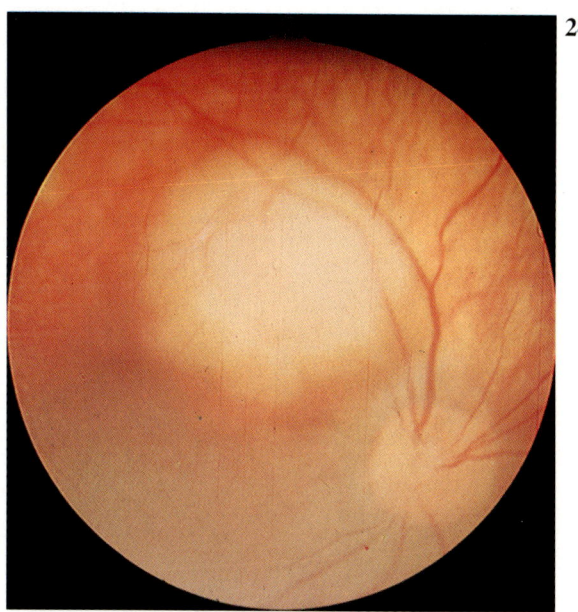

246 A young child presented with a squint, and routine ophthalmoscopic examination shows the following lesion.

a) What is the diagnosis? b) How should it be managed?

247 a) What is the diagnosis of this young girl who presented with hypochromic anaemia?
b) What are the complications of this condition?

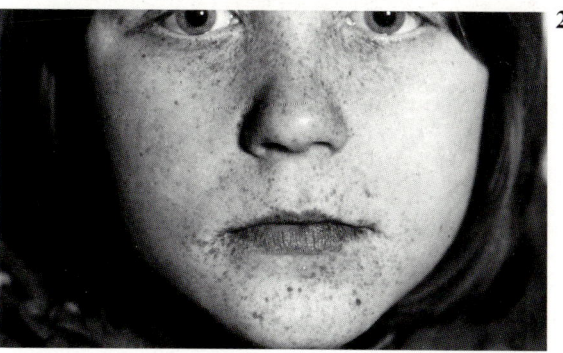

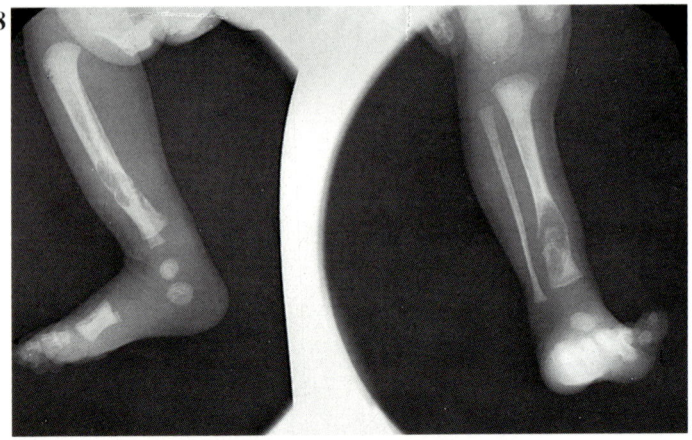

248 This is osteomyelitis of the tibia. Which of the following are characteristic of this syndrome?
a) Early X-ray changes.
b) Severe generalised toxicity.
c) Association with septic arthritis.
d) It is most common in post-term infants.
e) Associated shin swelling.

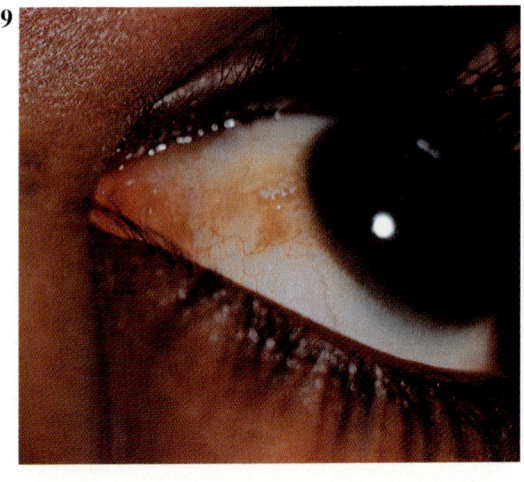

249 a) What is the small lesion close to the limbus?
b) Is this the common site for it?

250 a) What are these lesions?
b) How are they produced?
c) What is the clinical picture?

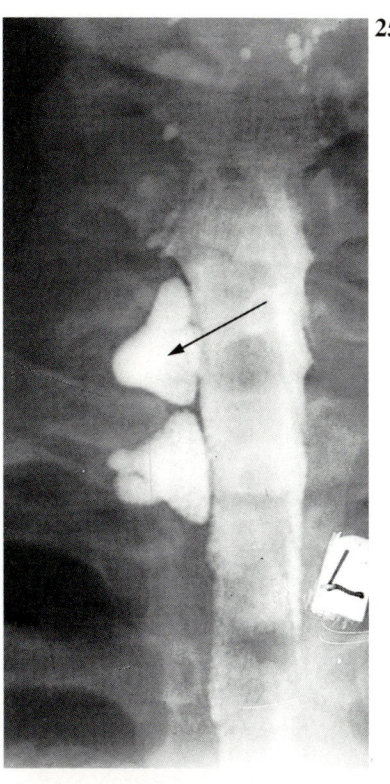

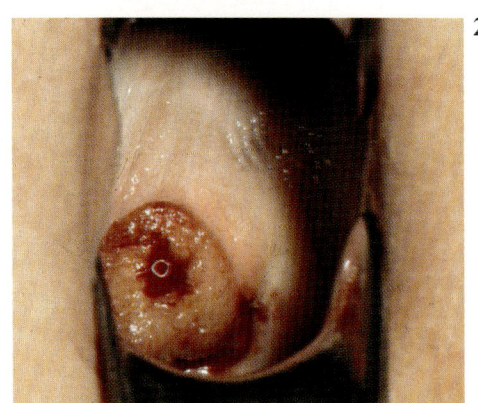

251 a) What are the likely symptoms?
b) How would you establish the diagnosis?
c) What methods of treatment are available?

252 A patient from the Turkana district of Kenya presented with an enlarged liver. X-rays revealed calcified shadows and at operation cysts were removed. What is the diagnosis?

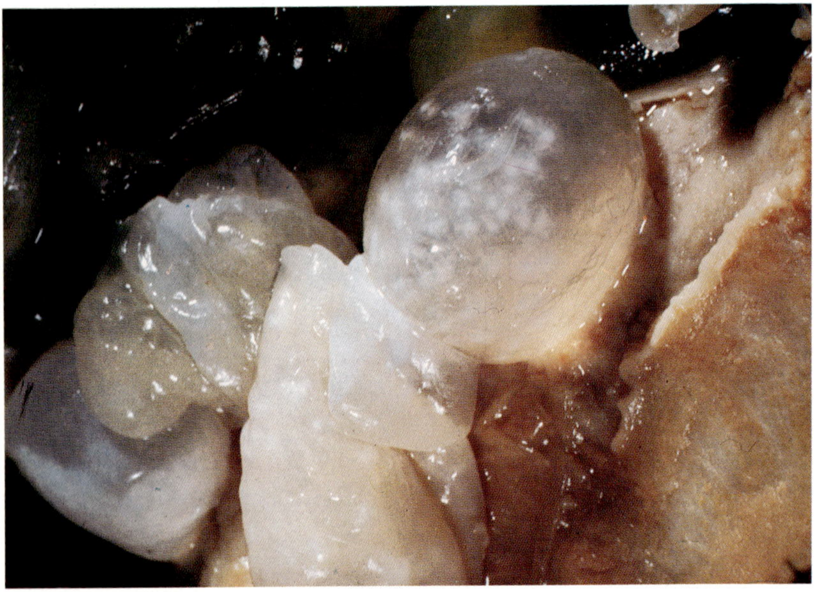

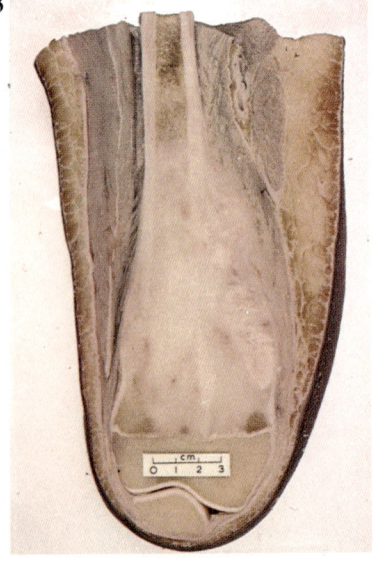

253 A hemisected amputation specimen from the lower limb of a 14-year-old boy.

a) What is this diagnosis?
b) Are any aetiological factors known?

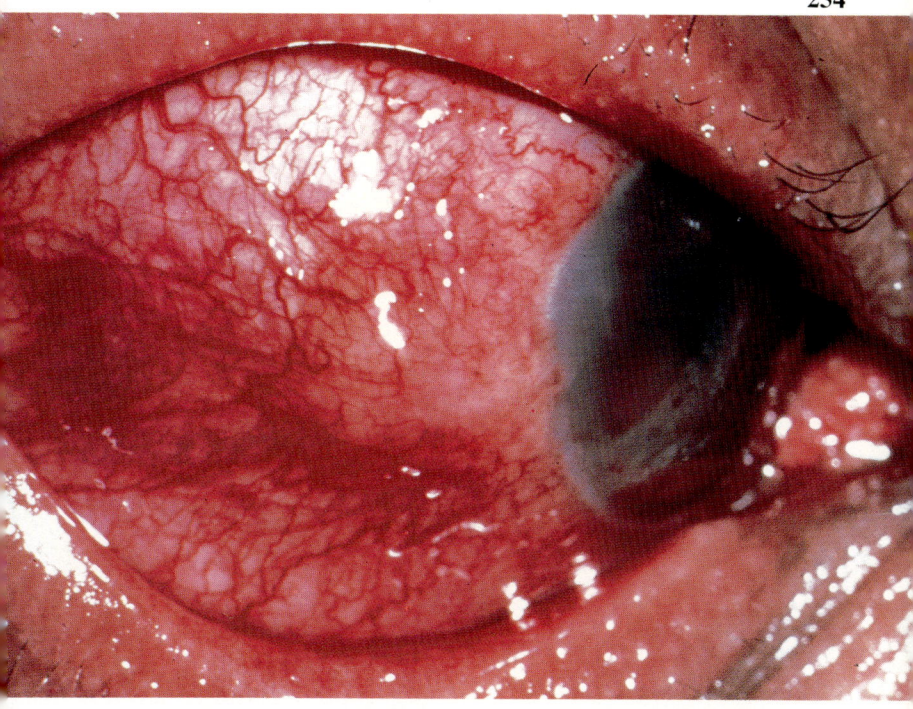

254 Intense scleritis adjacent to scleral nodule suggests which disease?

a) Marginal staph. ulcer of the cornea?
b) Rheumatoid arthritis?
c) Leprosy?
d) Allergic papulosis?

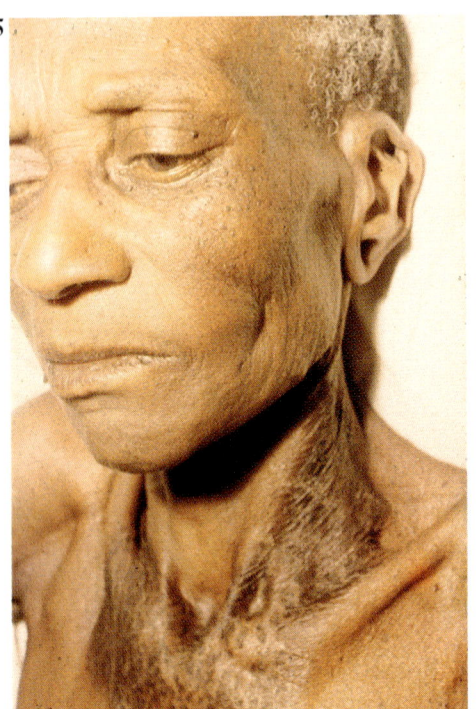

255
a) What aponym is associated with this lesion?
b) What is this disease?
c) What is its treatment?

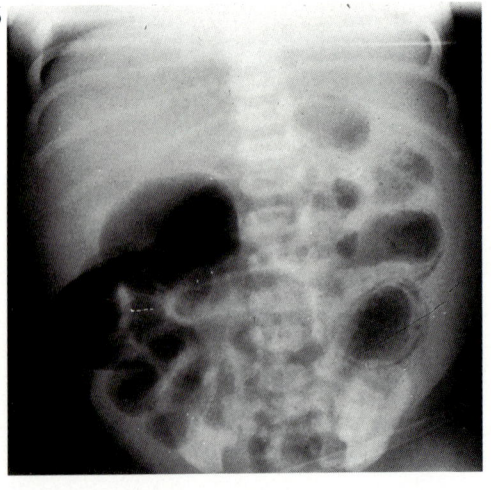

256 A 5-day-old premature infant develops abdominal distension and bilious vomiting.

a) What does the X-ray show?
b) What is the diagnosis?
c) What is the treatment?

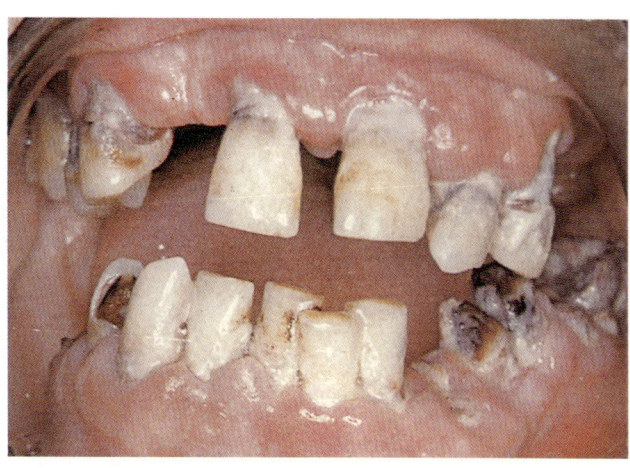

257 This is the oral presentation of a nutritional deficiency—swollen, fragile gingivae with evidence of dental neglect.

a) What is this likely to be?
b) In what type of patient does it classically occur in European conditions?
c) In what other groups of patients does it also occur?

258 What does the face of this 5-year-old girl demonstrate?

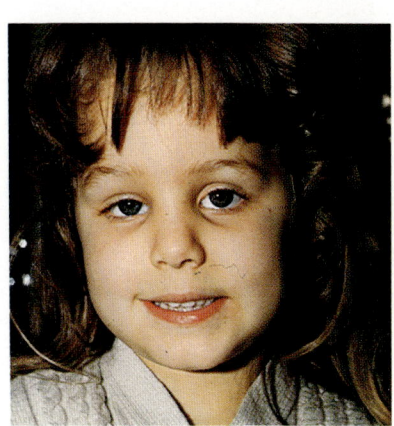
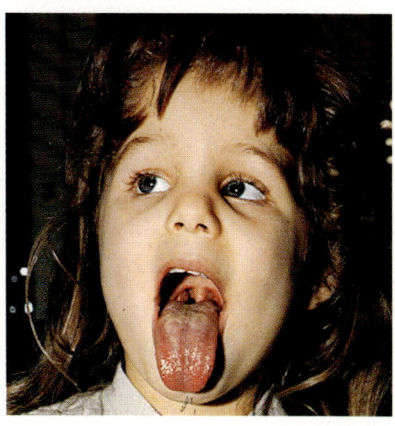

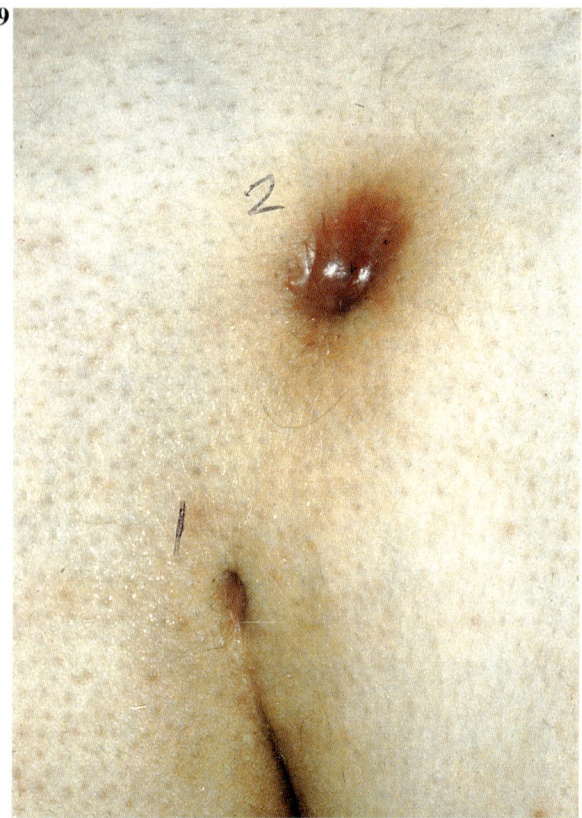

259 The internatal cleft is the commonest site for this sinus.

a) What is it called?
b) What lines the sinus tract?
c) What else does the sinus contain?

260 a) What are the abnormal features of this retina?
b) Give two possible diagnoses. How would you differentiate between them on the basis of functional examination?

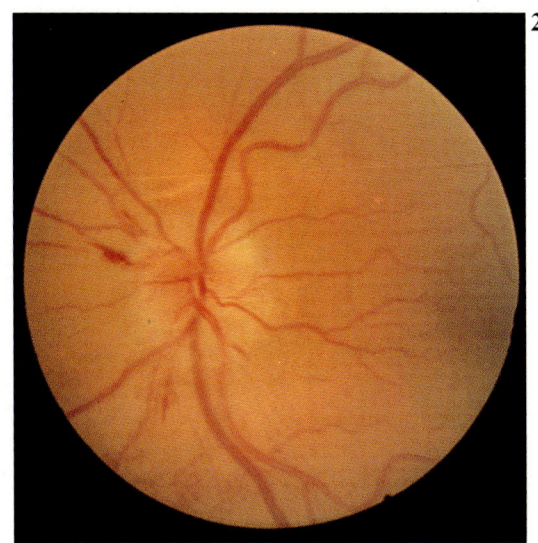

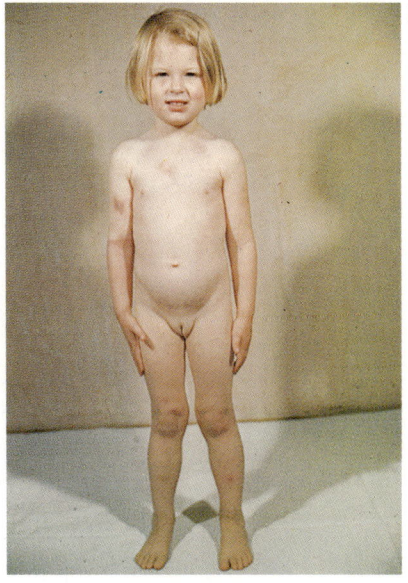

261 The 5-year-old girl's face and body is covered with large bruises. Since the age of two years she has had intermittent epistaxis and bruising. Name the condition and underlying pathology.

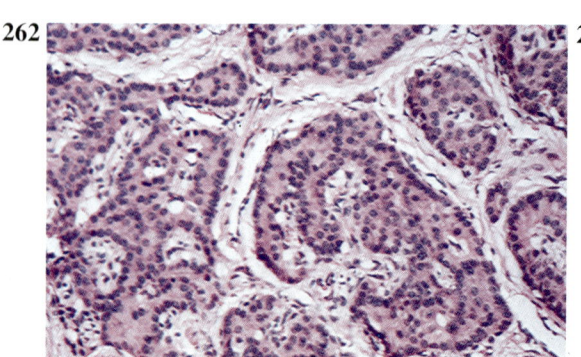

262 Photomicrograph of a tumour removed from the pancreas of a 33-year-old man who gave a history of recurrent episodes of coma over a 5-year period. (*H&E × 90.*)

a) What is the tumour and what is the clinical syndrome?
b) What other syndromes may be associated with tumours of similar origin?

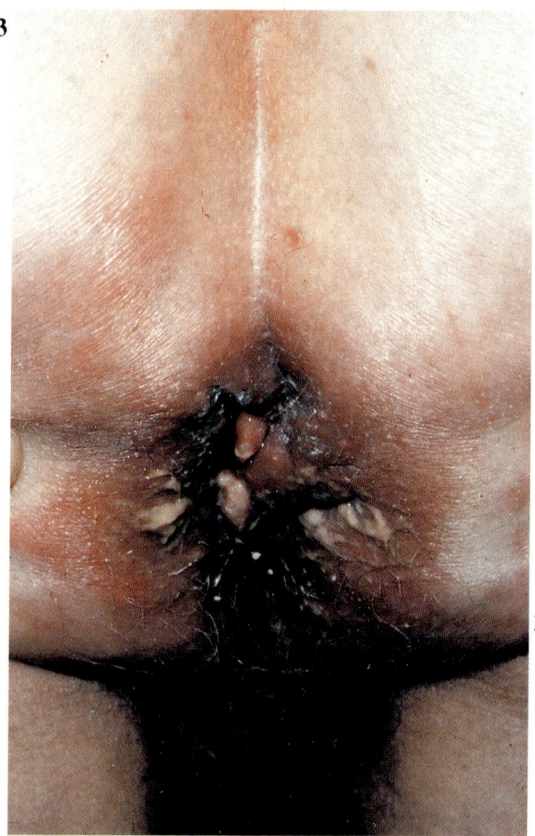

263 a) What condition is seen here and by what descriptive term is it also known?
b) In which disease is it most likely to occur?

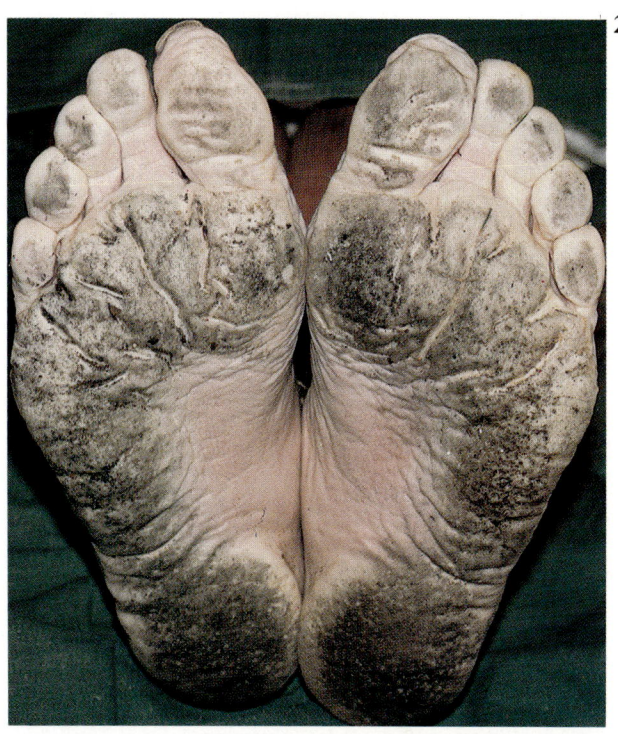

264 This old man wore wet boots for 4 days in a cold climate. This condition is most likely caused by:

a) Sub zero temperatures.
b) Prolonged wearing of soaking boots in temperatures just above freezing.
c) Fungal infection.

265

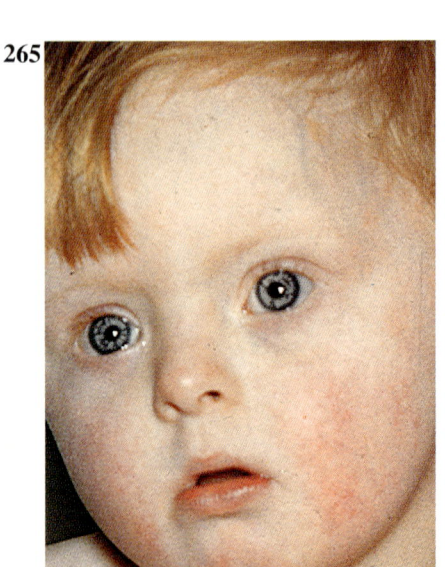

265 What do you note in the child's eyes?

266 At post-mortem a seven-week-old child was found to have these irregular areas of calcification in the lateral ventricles. What is the most likely cause?

266

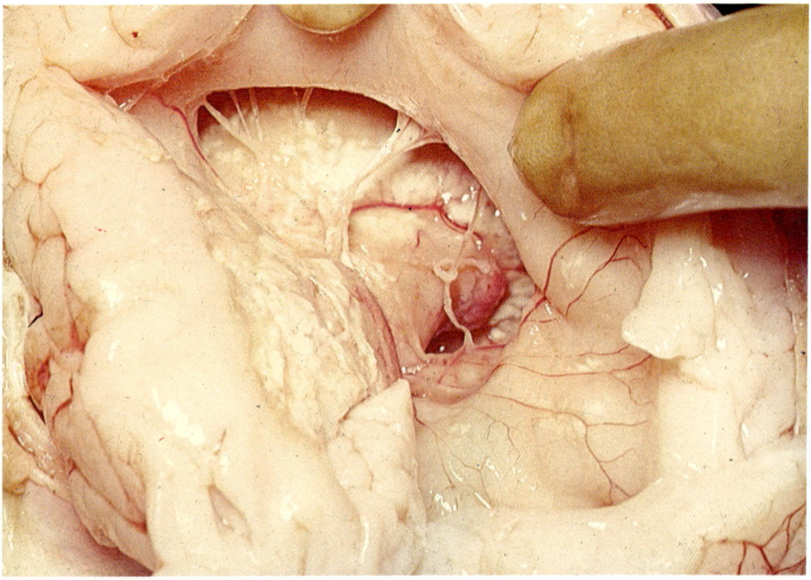

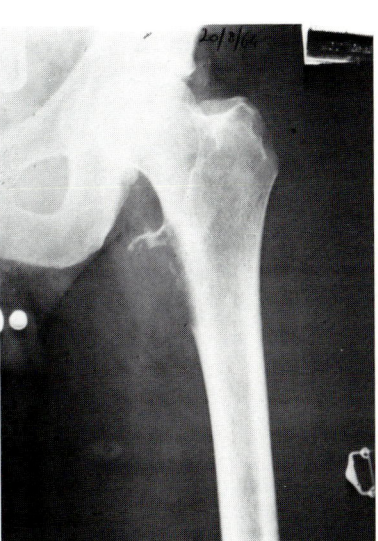
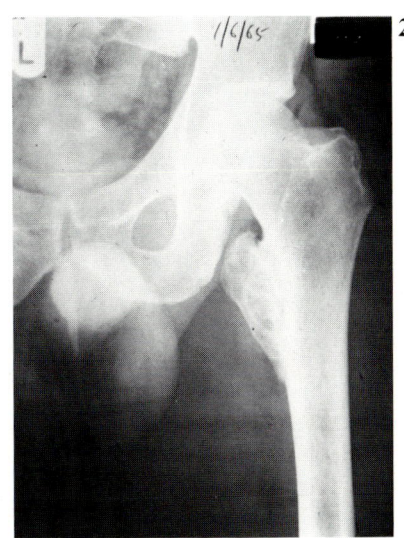

267 Radiographs of left femur before and after nephrectomy.

    a) What abnormality is present before nephrectomy?
    b) What has occurred after nephrectomy?
    c) For what reason was the kidney removed?

268 a) What is this mucosal condition?
    b) What aetiological factors may be involved?
    c) What is the prognosis of such a lesion?

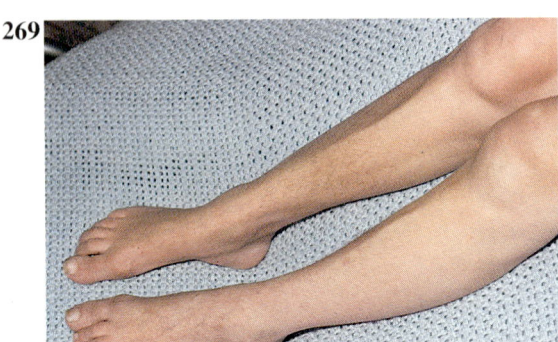

269 This 40-year-old woman had complained of cramps and then of weakness in the legs for 12 months. Her reflexes—once brisk—were unobtainable and she was unable to walk. Sensation, bladder control and the upper limbs were intact.

a) What is the abnormality illustrated?
b) What is the most likely cause?

270 Lacerations of the small intestine are often difficult to identify, even during surgery. One very likely location is:

a) At the junction of jejunum and ileum?
b) 50 cm from the ileocaecal valve?
c) Around Treitz' angle?

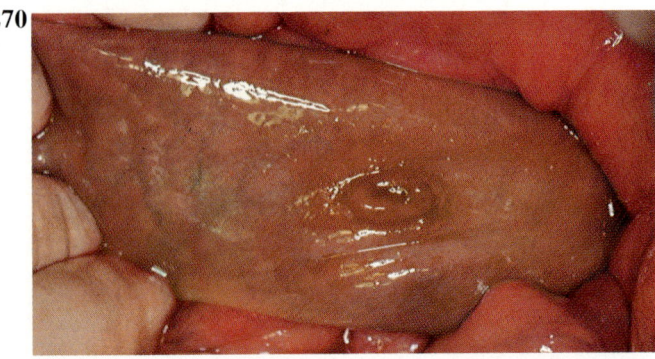

271 Identify the 6 nucleated cells shown from this bone-marrow aspirate. By what features do you recognise them?

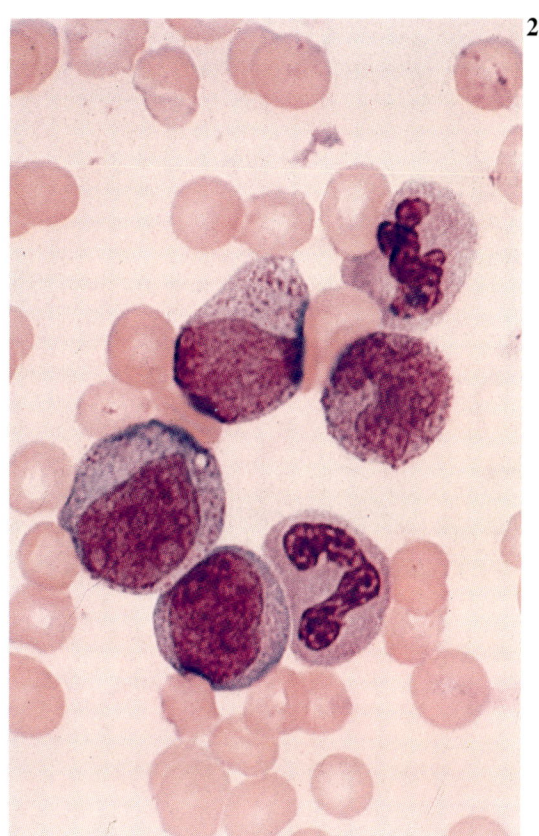

272 This is a painless, slowly growing firm lump in the palate.

a) What is the most likely diagnosis?
b) Might this be a dangerous lesion?
c) What treatment might be advised?

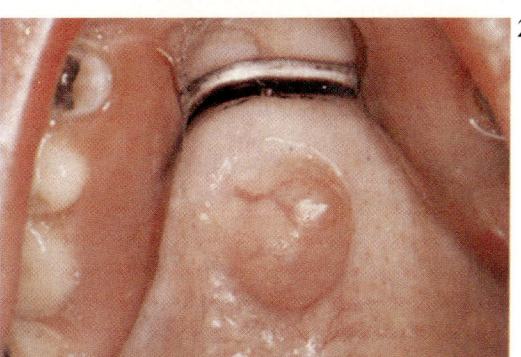

273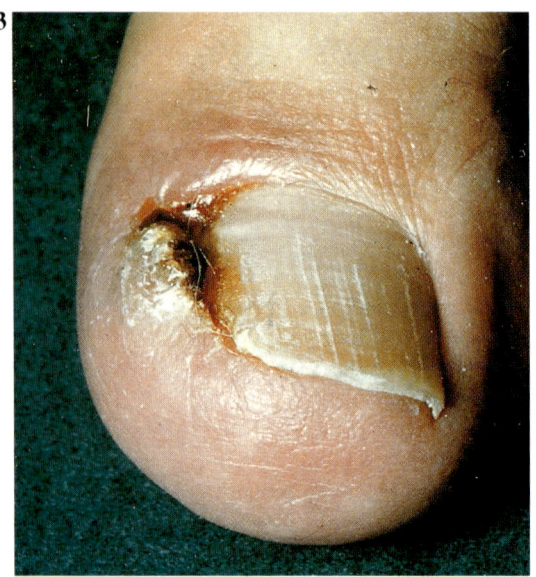

273 a) What is this condition called?
b) What factors predispose to its development?
c) What surgical procedures are used in its treatment?

274 What is abnormal in the vulvar aspect?

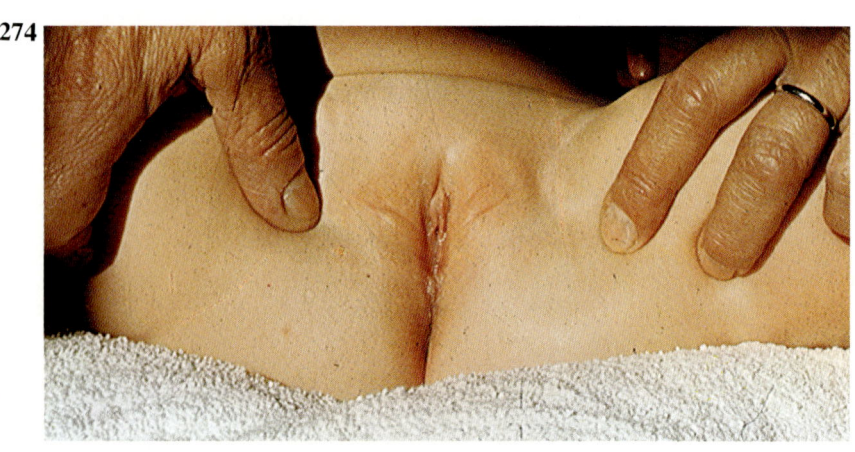

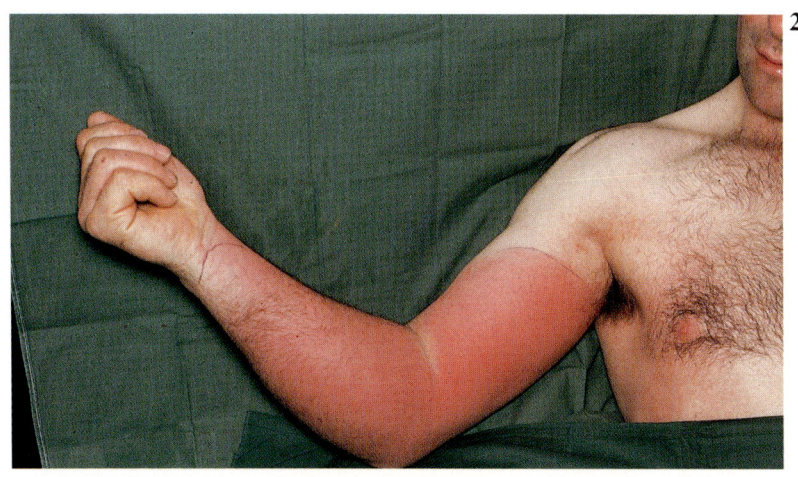

275 This condition:

  a) Always leads to pus formation.
  b) May resolve completely with appropriate antibiotics and rest.
  c) Is always caused by *staphylococcus aureus*.

276 a) Name and describe this condition.
  b) With which congenital defect is it most commonly associated?
  c) What treatment would you recommend?

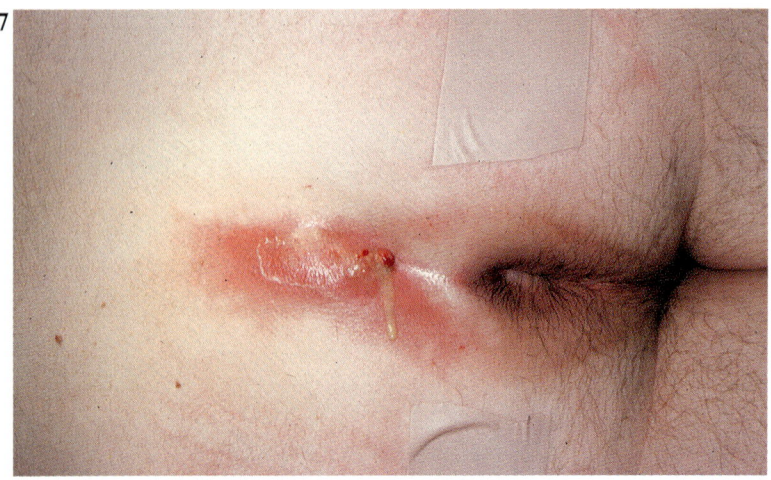

277 This condition is a:

a) Perianal abscess.
b) Pilonidal abscess.
c) May lead to the formation of fistula in ano.

278 IVU of patient with hypertension.

a) What is the abnormality?
b) What is the underlying cause?

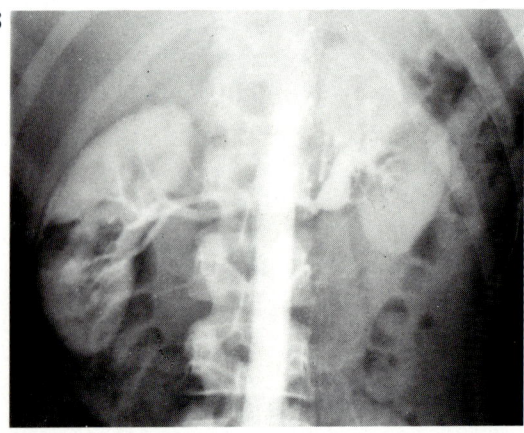

279 a) What abnormalities are visible on this illustration?
b) What other abnormalities might be present?
c) What is the diagnosis?

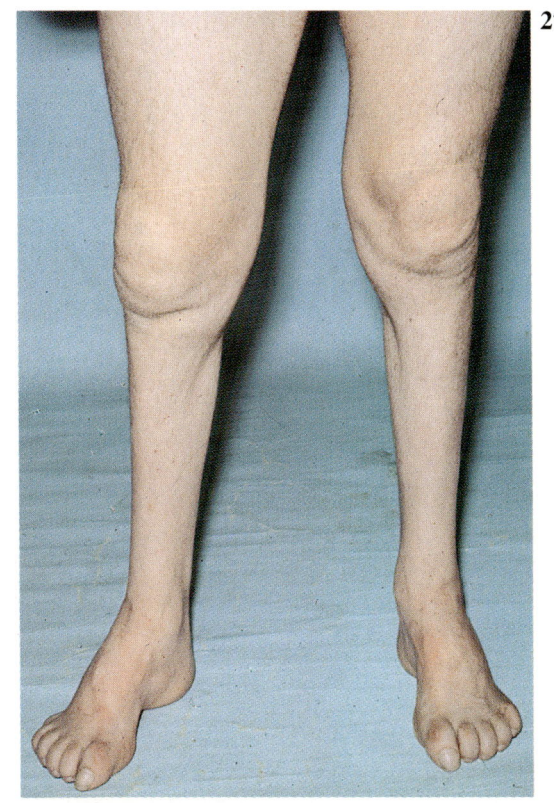

280 One of the following complications is not associated with the infraclavicular approach to entral venous cannulation:

a) Recurrent laryngeal nerve paralysis.
b) Cerebral fat embolism.
c) Chylothorax.

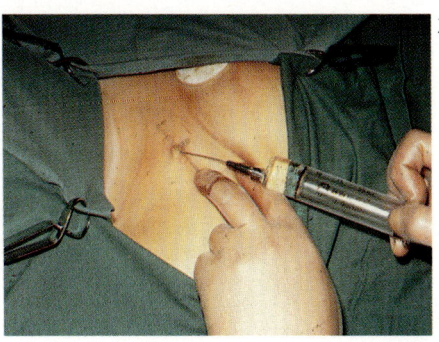

281

281 This is the appearance of juvenile papillomatosis of the larynx. What are the predisposing factors of this disease?

282 a) What nucleated cells are shown in this bone marrow smear?
b) What is the diagnosis?

282

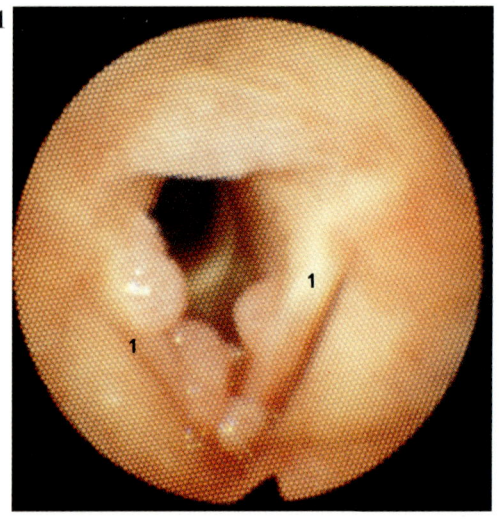

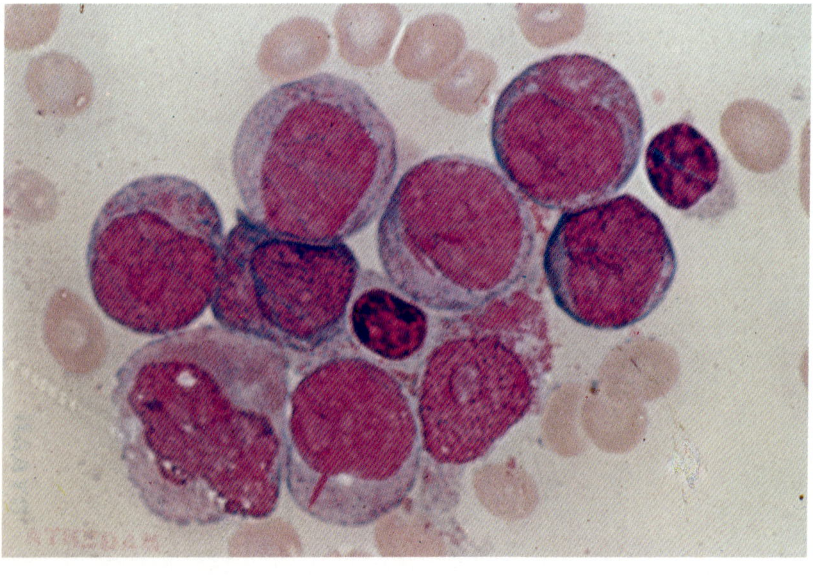

283 This is an X-ray barium enema of a patient from South America complaining of chronic constipation. What is the diagnosis?

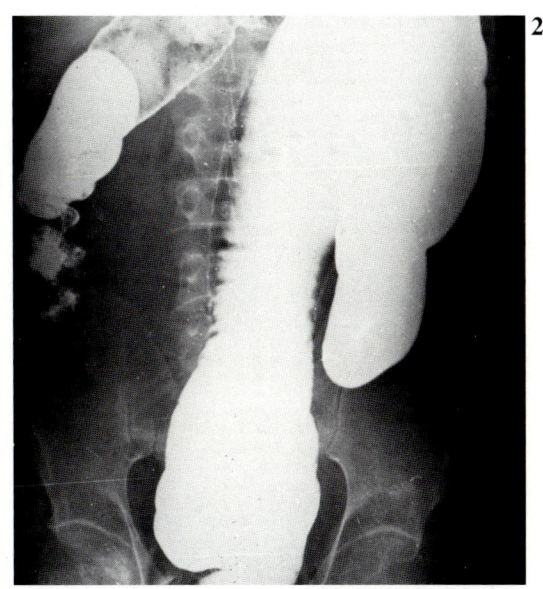

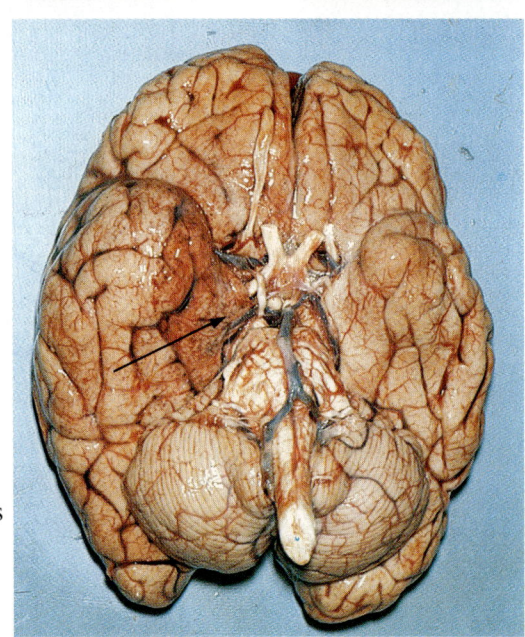

284 a) What does this slide show?
b) What are the symptoms of this condition?
c) How is the diagnosis confirmed?

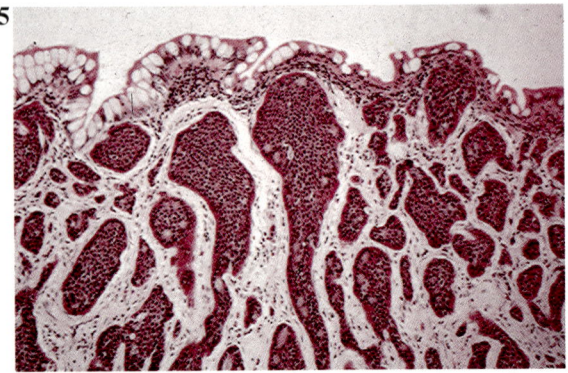

285 Photomicrograph of an ileal tumour excised from a 32-year-old woman. ($H\&E \times 90$.)

a) What is the neoplasm?
b) From what cells do such tumours arise?
c) With what systemic manifestations may the tumour be associated?

286 This typically cheesy infiltration, exclusively powdered over the iris surface in a patient who has anaesthetic nodules on the skin, suggests a uveitis syndrome involving what infection?

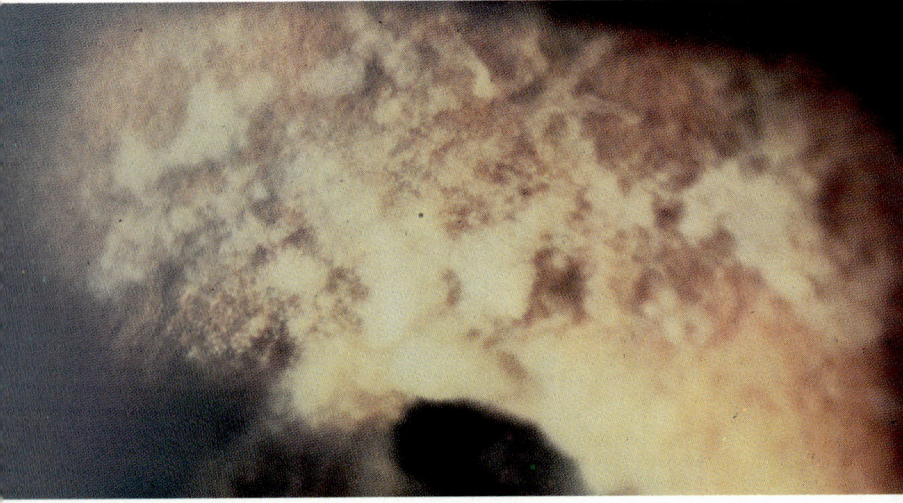

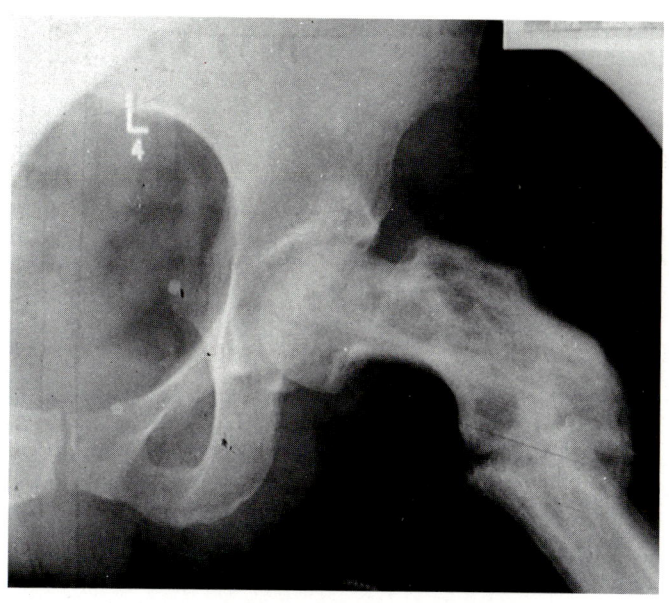

287 What two conditions does this X-ray show?

288 An opened left atrium and ventricle. Name the condition illustrated and when it may occur.

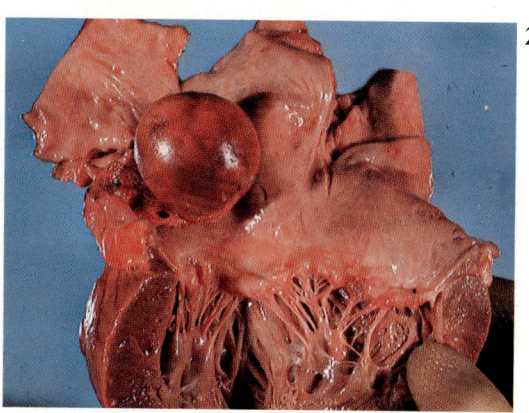

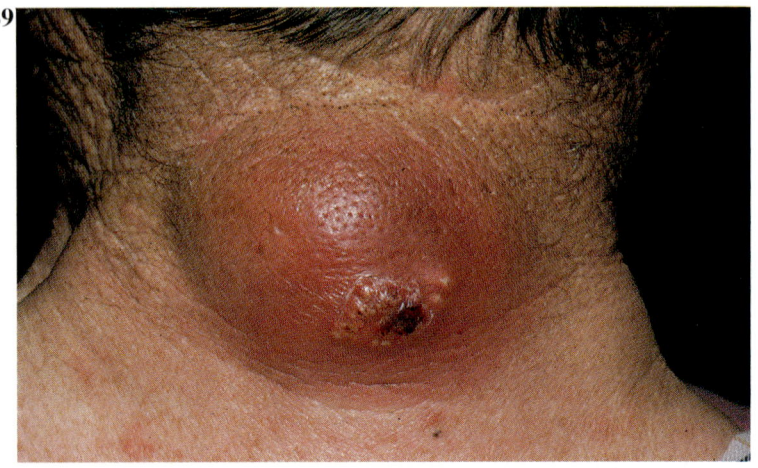

289 This man had a long history of swelling on the back of his neck. He gave a short history of increasing pain. The most likely diagnosis is:

a) A carbuncle.
b) An infected sebaceous cyst.
c) Sarcoma.

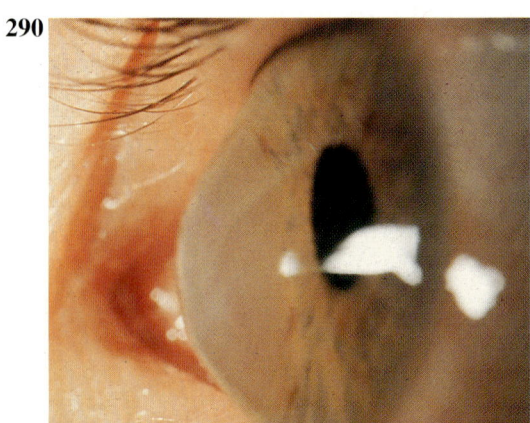

290 This eye condition may occur in isolation, but it is commonly associated with eczema, asthma or hay fever. What is it called and how is it managed?

291
a) What is the diagnosis?
b) What is the recurrence risk if the prenatal and perinatal period was normal?
c) What will the CT scan show?

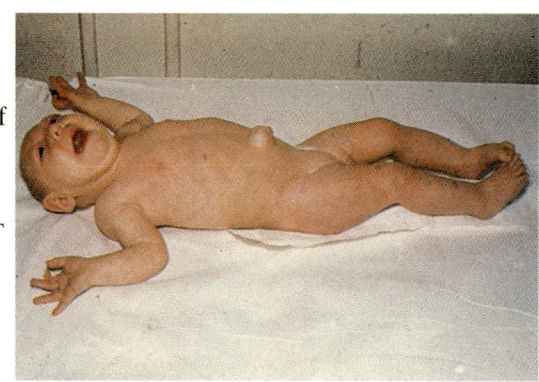

292 An endoscopic view with fibre-optic gastroscope that shows:

a) Vertebral osteophyte impression in the oesophagus?
b) A voluminous tumour of the stomach at the cardia?
c) Bulging of the mucosa through the pylorus?

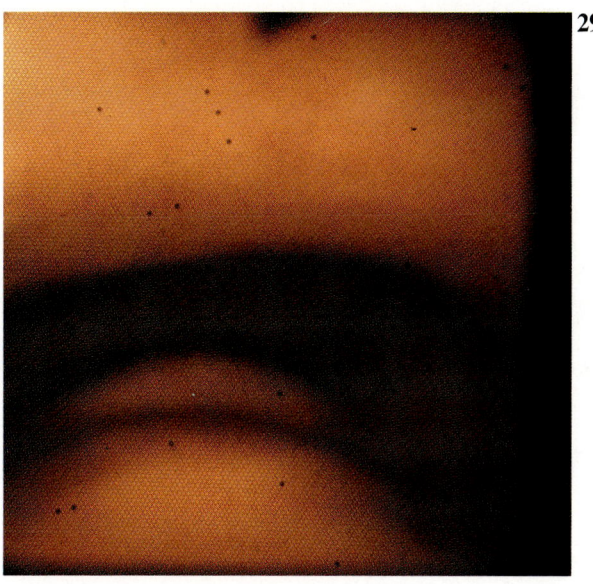

293 Patient with uveitis and striking facial profile demonstrating the resorption of the nasal cartilage. This is suggestive of what disease?

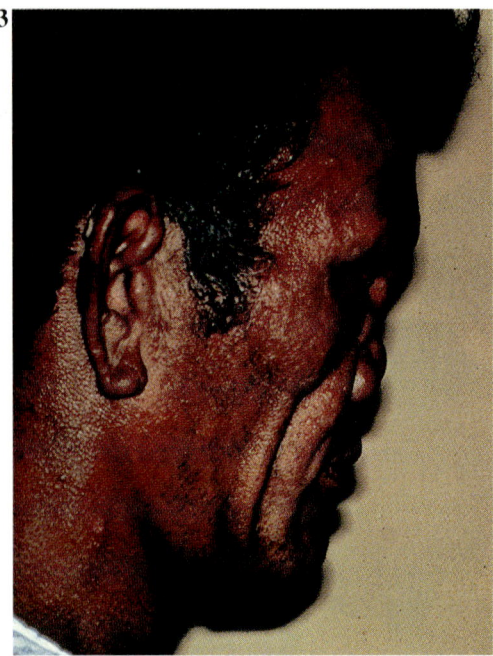

294 a) What name is given to these chronic lesions at the angles of the mouth?
b) What is the most likely cause?

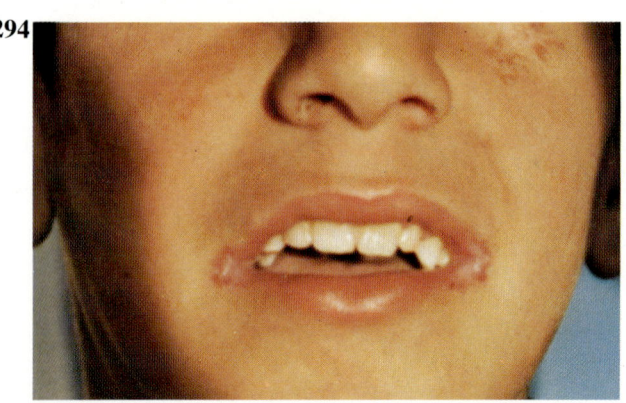

295 This followed a fist fight injury between two adult males. The most likely diagnosis is:

a) Suppurative tenosynovitis.
b) Septic arthritis from penetration of the metacarpophalangeal joint.
c) Orf.

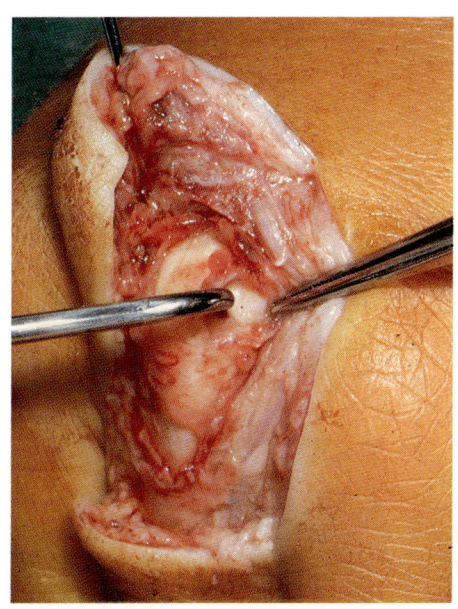

296 This renal tumour is:

a) Benign?
b) Malignant?
c) Of renal tubular origin?
d) Of pelvic urothelial origin?
e) Associated with a poor prognosis?

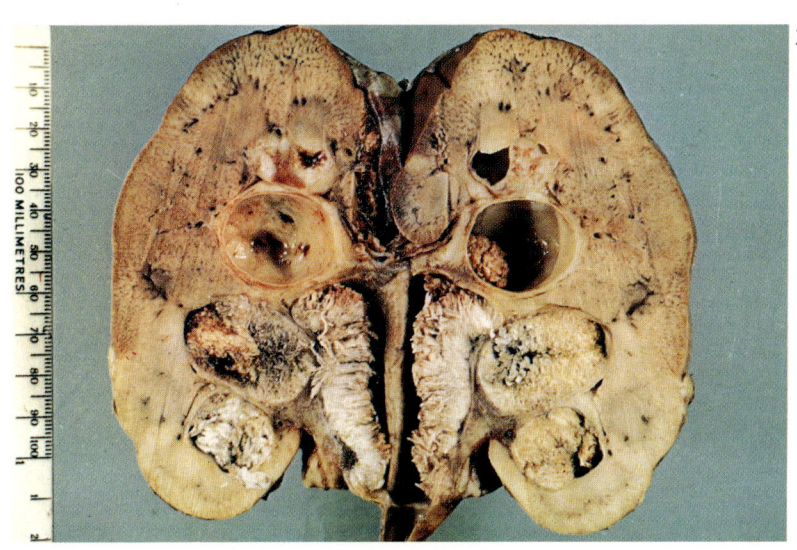

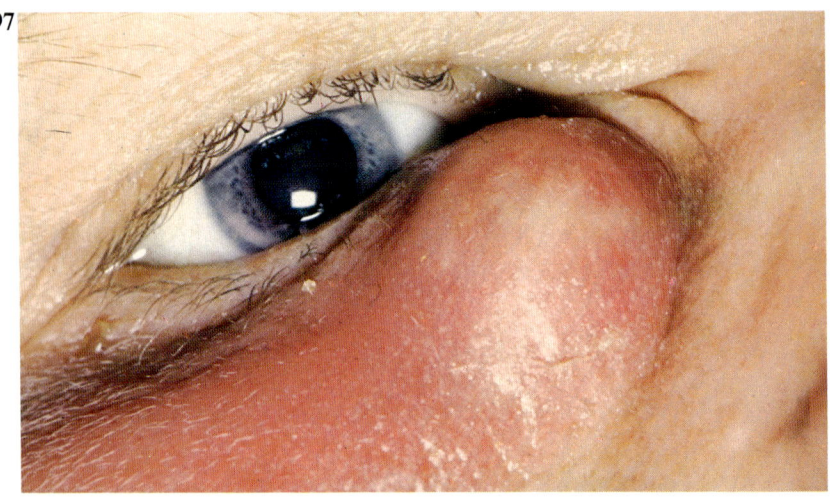

297 The patient complains of a running eye on this side for some months with the sudden appearance of a painful infected swelling.

a) What are the physical signs?
b) What is the diagnosis?
c) How should it be managed?

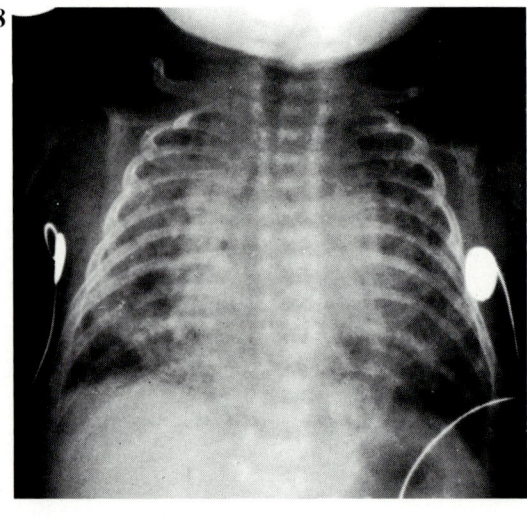

298 a) What is this condition?
b) Name two associated factors.

299 a) What cells are shown in this bone marrow aspirate and what cytological features do they manifest?
b) What is the diagnosis?

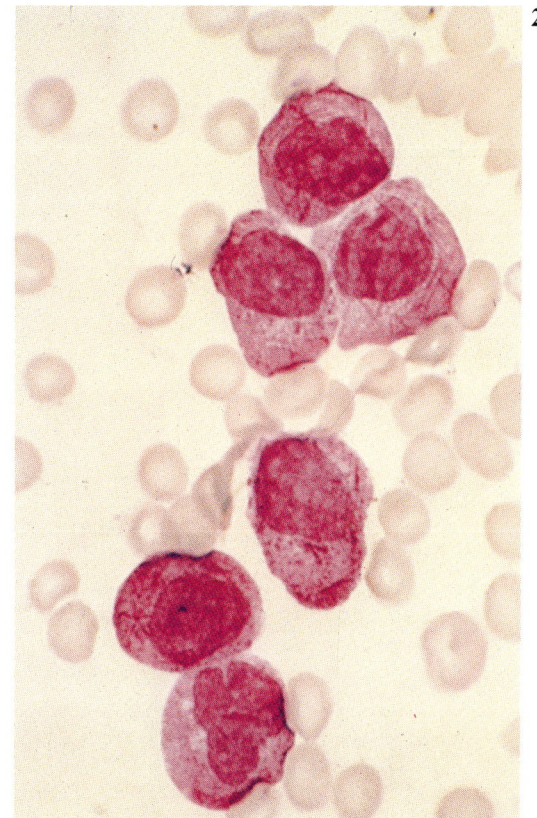

300 a) What is the probable diagnosis?
b) Name the radiological abnormalities.
c) What are the characteristic biochemical abnormalities?
d) What is the likely cause of painful arthritis affecting the large joint in this condition?

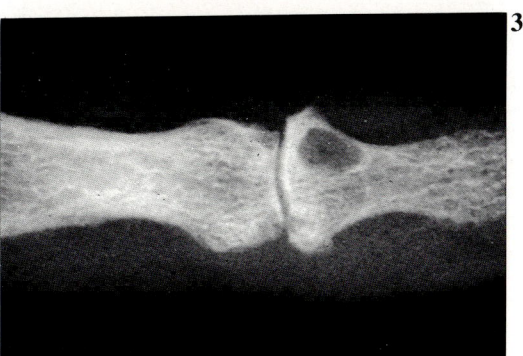

301

301
a) What is the matter with this patient?
b) Where is the lesion?
c) What are the most common causes?

302 This patient has presented with a painful eye, and fluorescein has been instilled. What is the condition?

a) Corneal abrasion.
b) Hyphaema.
c) Iridodialysis.

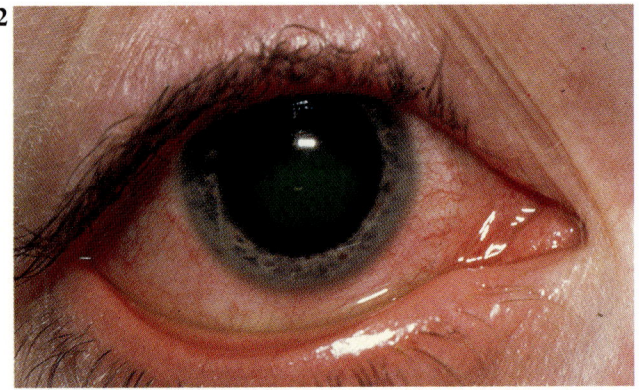

303 This picture shows several abdominal viscera as seen during:

a) A thoracotomy?
b) A laparotomy?
c) A vaginal hysterectomy?

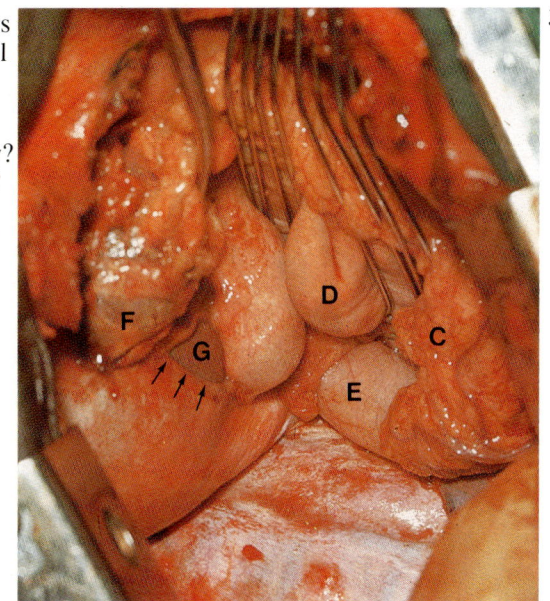

304 a) What do you notice?
b) If the child has a tracheo-oesophageal fistula and vertebral anomalies, what is the diagnosis?
c) Is it genetic?

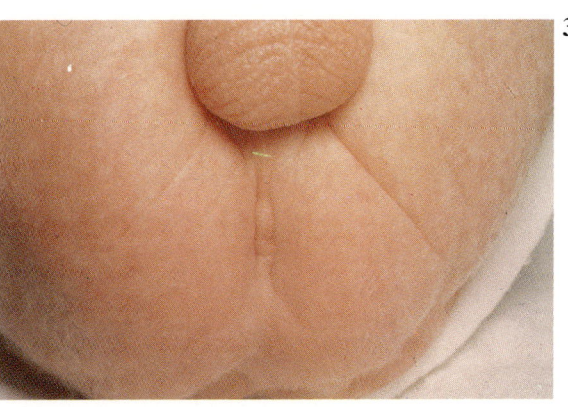

167

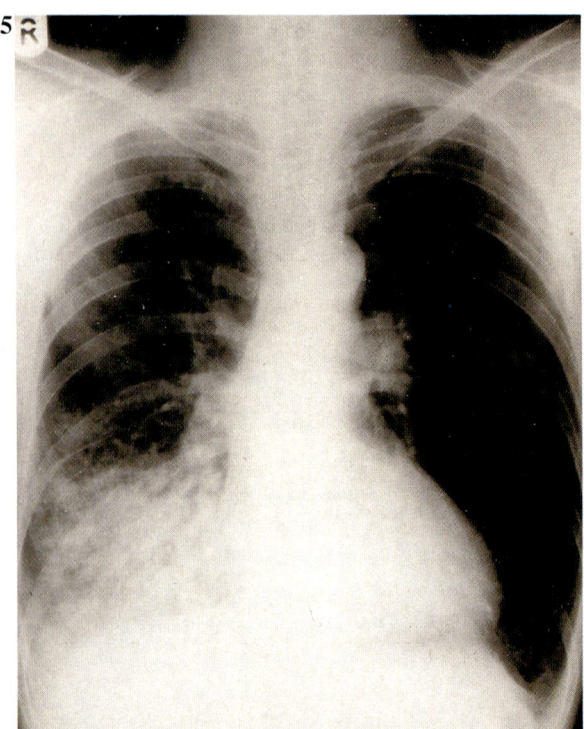

305 This chest radiograph was taken 48 hours following elective cholecystectomy.

a) What abnormality is shown?
b) How does this condition arise?

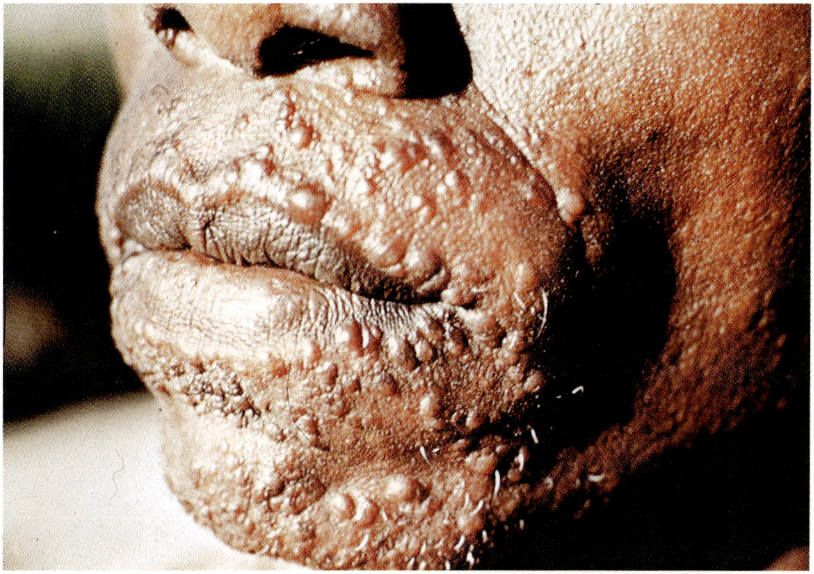

306 An Indian patient presented with these dermal lesions. He had been treated 3 years previously for visceral leishmaniasis. What is the diagnosis?

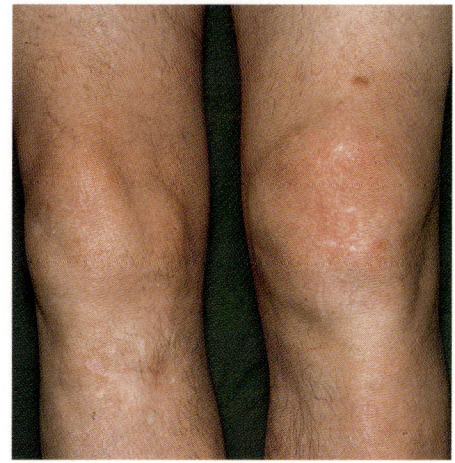

307 This patient suffered a transverse, separated fracture of the patella.

a) He will not be able to walk.
b) He will not be able to bend his knee.
c) He will not be able to extend his knee.

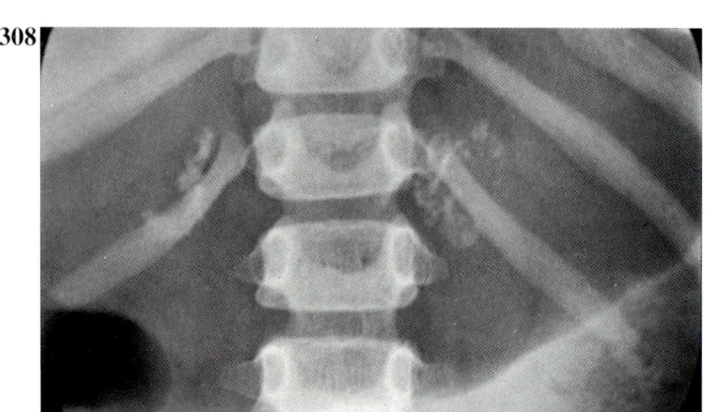

308 What does the radiograph show?

309 The complications of this penetrating wound of the perineum include:

a) Pilonidal abscess.
b) Damage to the bladder and urethra.
c) Ischaemic legs.

310 This lady presented with asthma, and her nasal enlargement was due to polyps. What syndrome should you suspect?

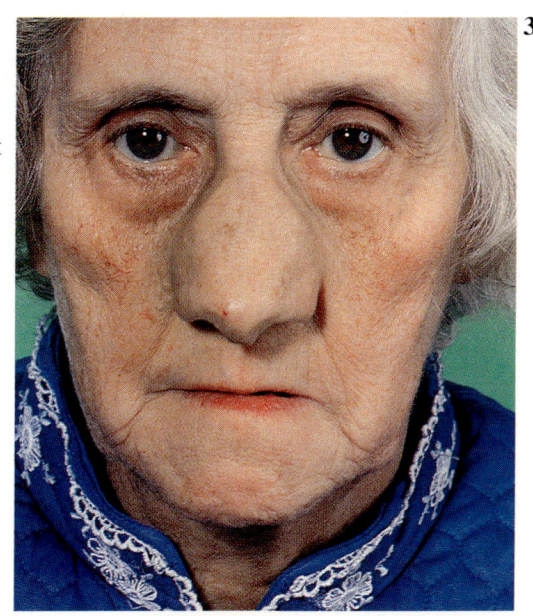

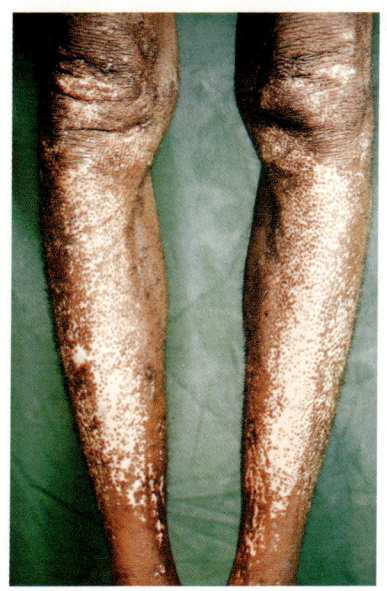

311 This patient from Upper Volta was found to have on examination de-pigmentation of both shins. What is the diagnosis?

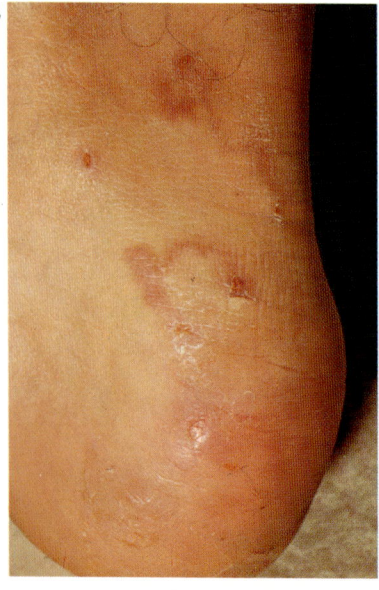

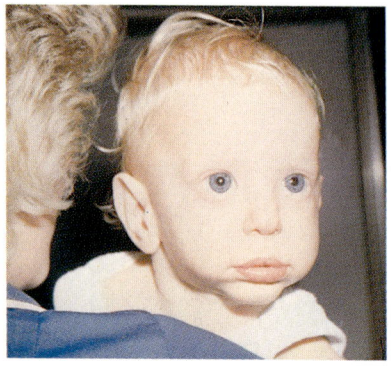

313 a) What is the diagnosis?
b) What biochemical abnormality might be found?
c) What cardiological finding is possible?

312 This lady had been sunbathing on a beach in West Africa with most of her body in direct contact with the sand. She presented with these lesions which were itchy. What is the diagnosis?

314 Photomicrograph of a biopsy from the nipple of a 46-year-old woman. (*H&E × 220.*)

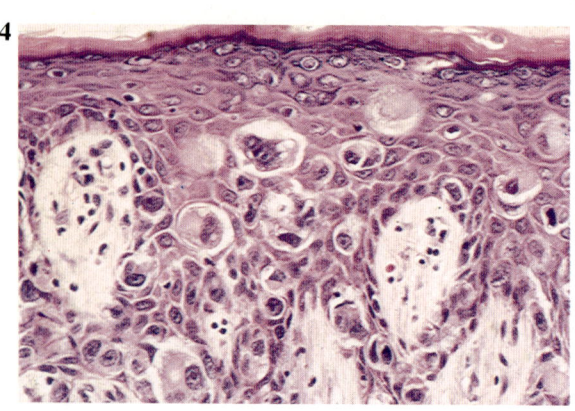

a) What is the diagnosis?
b) What are the microscopic features of the lesion?
c) What is its clinical significance?
d) In what other anatomical sites does the condition occur?

315 This aspect should evoke:
  a) Pneumoperitoneum?
  b) Haemopneumothorax?
  c) Rupture of diaphragm?

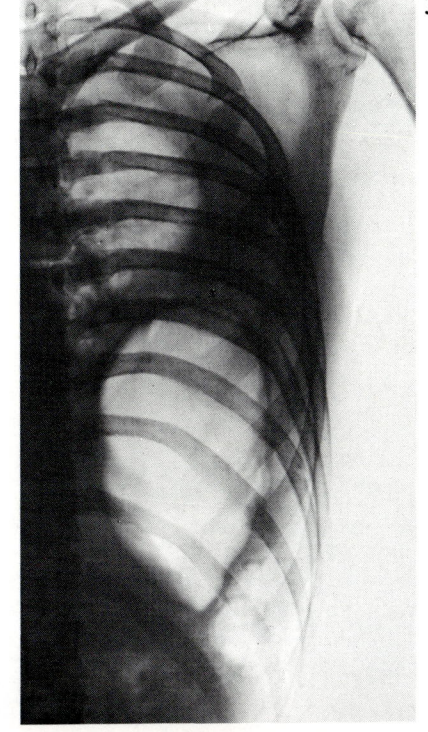

316
  a) What might be the cause of the staining of these teeth?
  b) The teeth are hypoplastic and carious. Is this due to the same factors as the staining?
  c) What age range might be at risk?

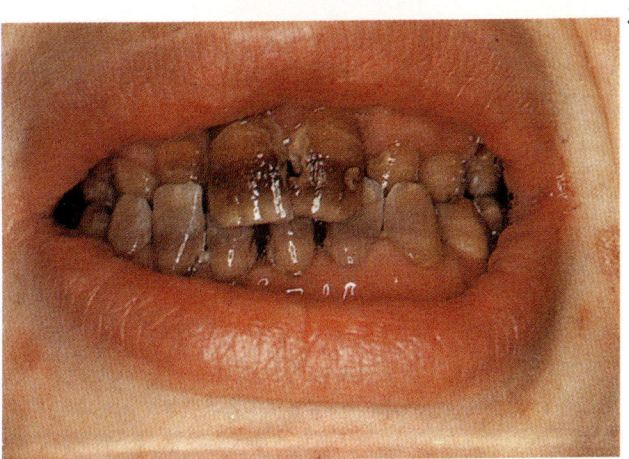

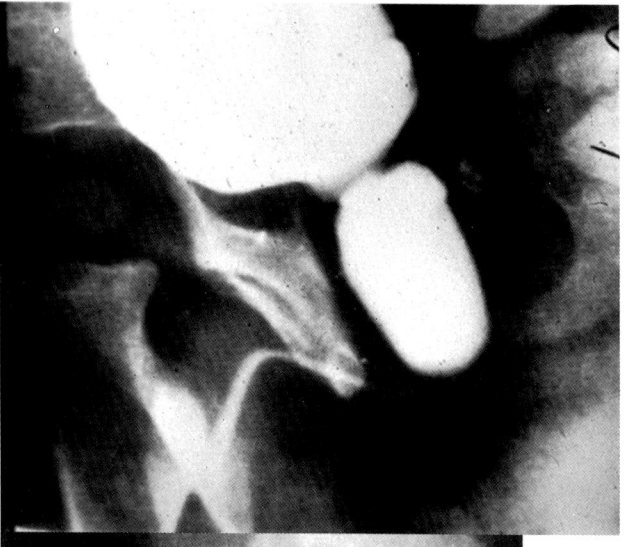

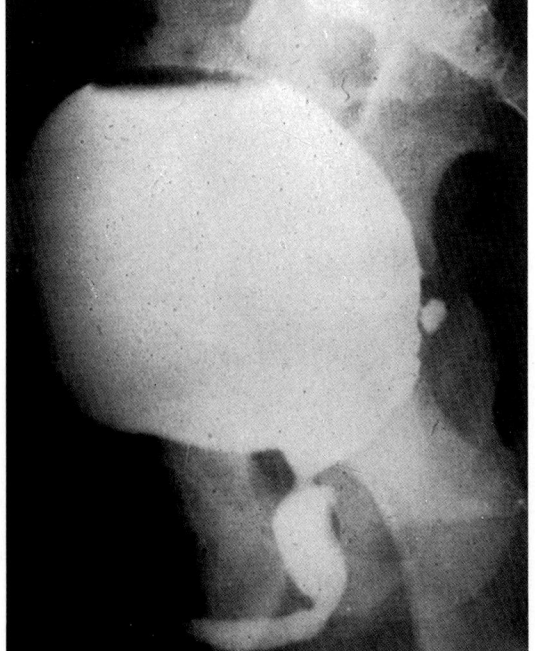

317 a) Name three abnormalities on this micturating cystourethrogram.
b) What is the likely aetiology?

318

319

318 Giant follicles presenting under the upper lid of an adolescent patient suggests what allergic disease?

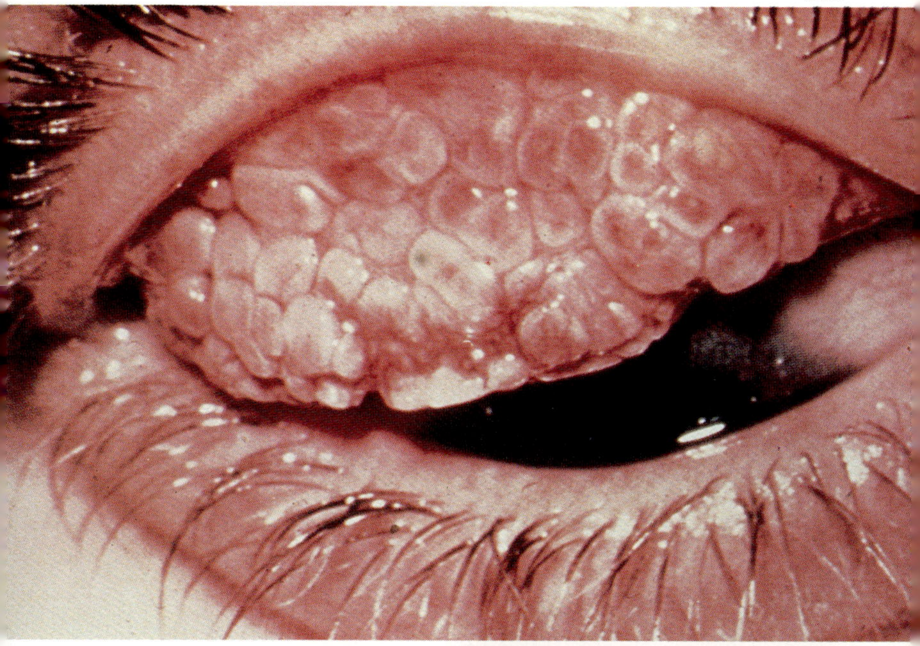

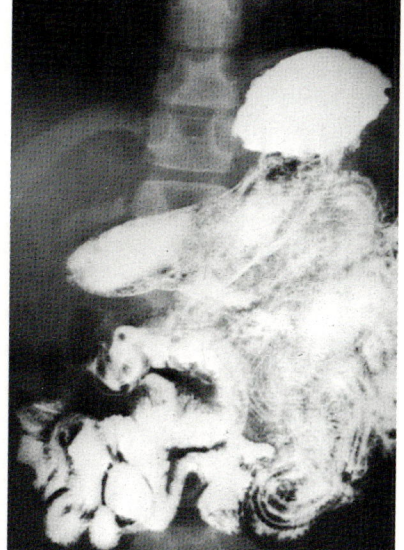

319 An Indian child presented with sub-acute intestinal obstruction and a barium meal revealed the following filling defects. What is the diagnosis?

320

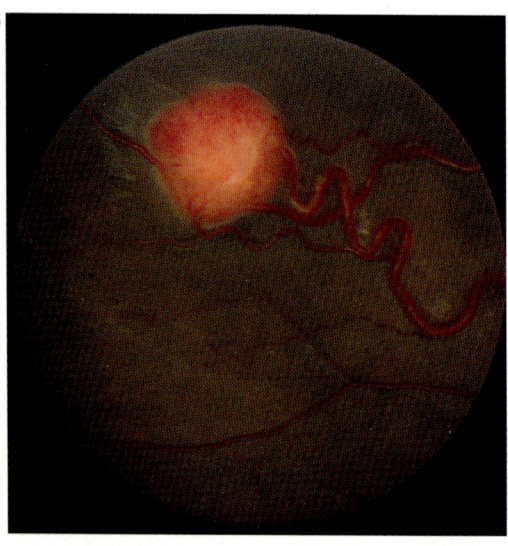

320 a) Name the retinal abnormality.
b) The CT scan showed an abnormality in the cerebellum and the patient also had polycythaemia. What is the diagnosis?
c) What is the cause of the polycythaemia?

321 Which of the following are true of this picture?

a) Drooping of the eyelid is caused by upper motor neurone lesion of the sixth cranial nerve?
b) The lesion may be in cervical sympathetic chain?
c) The patient has entropion?
d) Sometimes occurs with CA bronchus?
e) This is a typical appearance of posterior cerebral infarction?

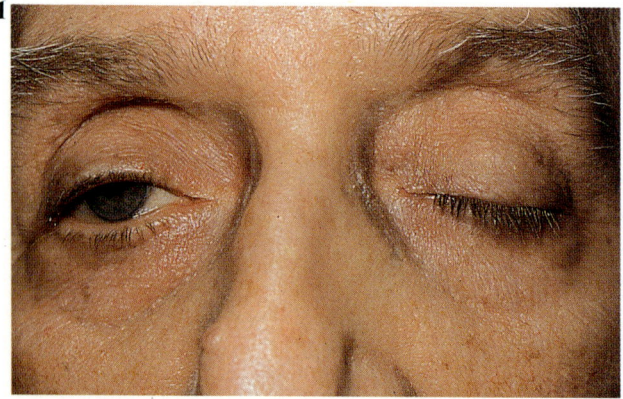

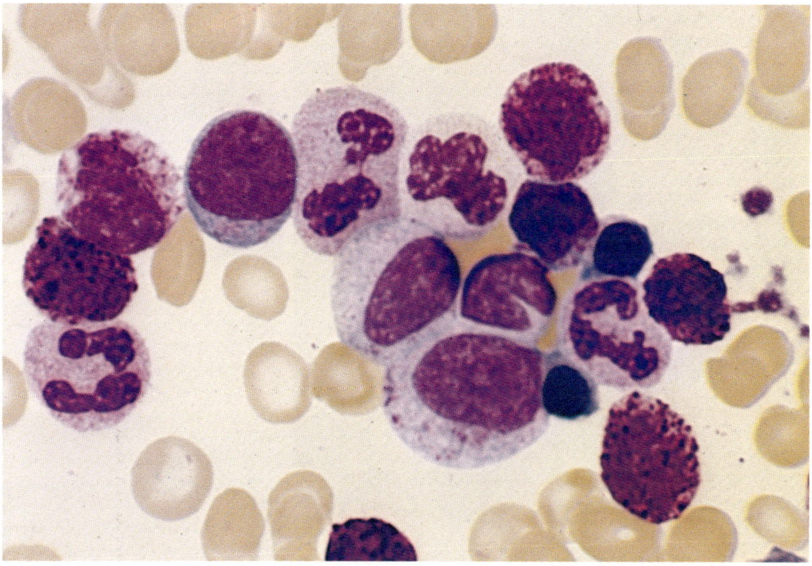

322 This is an area from the tail of a peripheral blood smear from a patient with a high leucocyte count.

a) What cells are shown?
b) What is the likely diagnosis?
c) How would you confirm it?

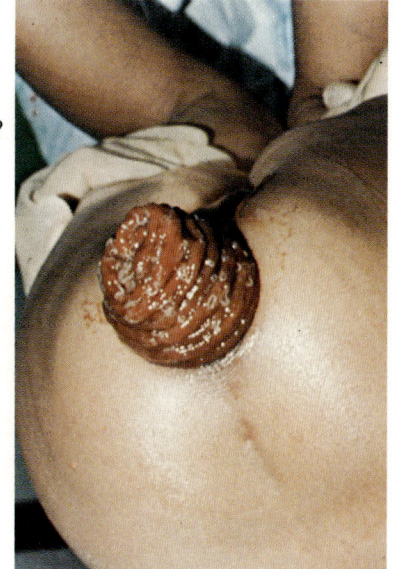

323 A Malaysian aboriginal infant was found to have this rectal prolapse and worms could be seen on the mucosa. What is the diagnosis?

324 This infection is sited in:

a) Bakers cyst.
b) Prepatellar bursa.
c) Semimembranosus bursa.

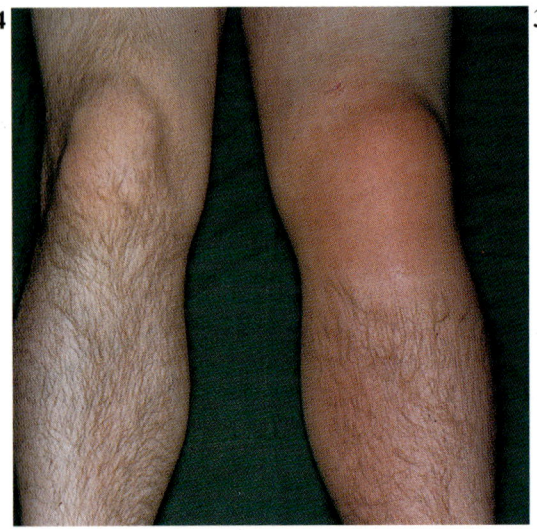

325 This patient was febrile and vomited violently five days prior to this presentation. What is the cause of it?

a) Typical pityriasis versicolor.
b) Artefacts of skin scratching.
c) A possible intrathoracic empyema.

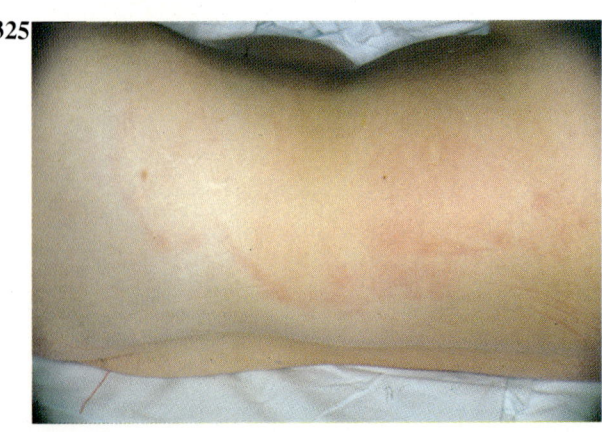

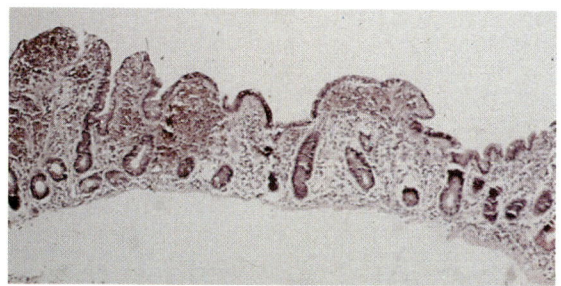

326 This patient had a normal jejunal biopsy just 6 hours before this abnormal result was obtained. What's the explanation, and what abnormalities are seen here?

327 This fundoscopic examination is showing:

    a) Intentional laser burning.
    b) Toxoplasmosis of the adult.
    c) Fat globules trapped in retinal vessels.

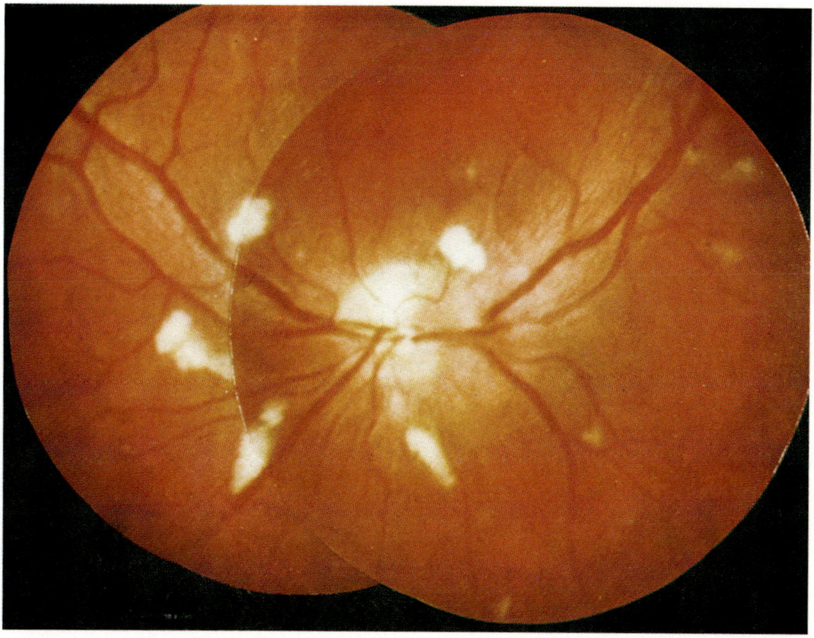

328 This rash in a child followed a streptococcal infection. What is the diagnosis?

329 This appearance of the right hand of a patient with a right dislocated shoulder should lead to a suspicion of:

a) A circumflex nerve neurapraxia.
b) Axillary vein compression.
c) Axillary artery spasm or compression.

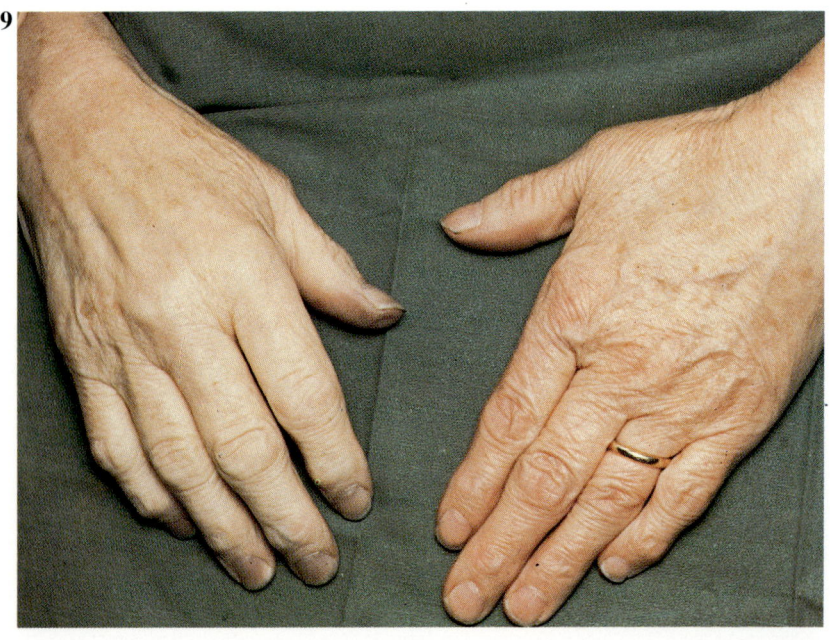

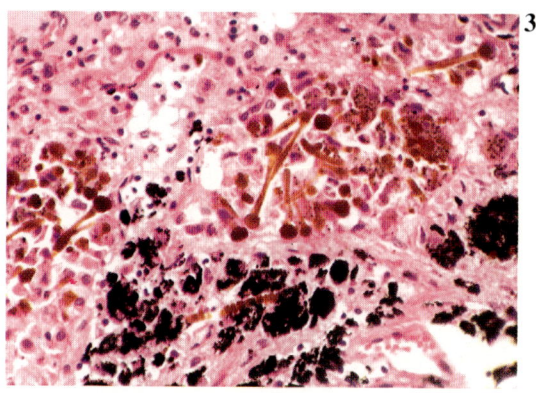

330 A photomicrograph of a section of lung tissue. (*H&E × 220.*)

a) What are the significant structures in the section?
b) With what lesions may their presence be associated?

331 An opened aortic valve with extensive commissural adhesions (arrowed). Name the disease.

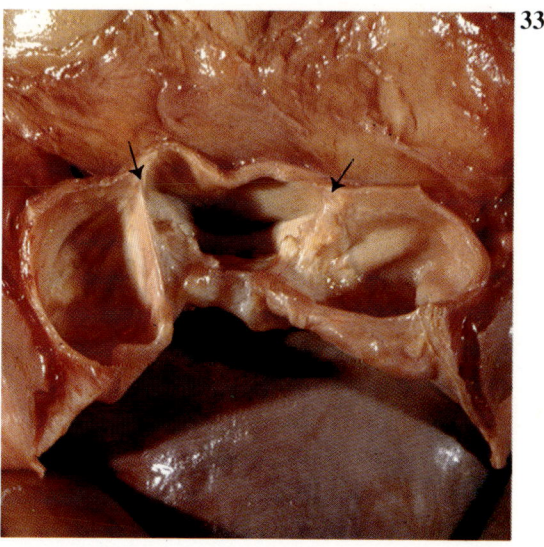

332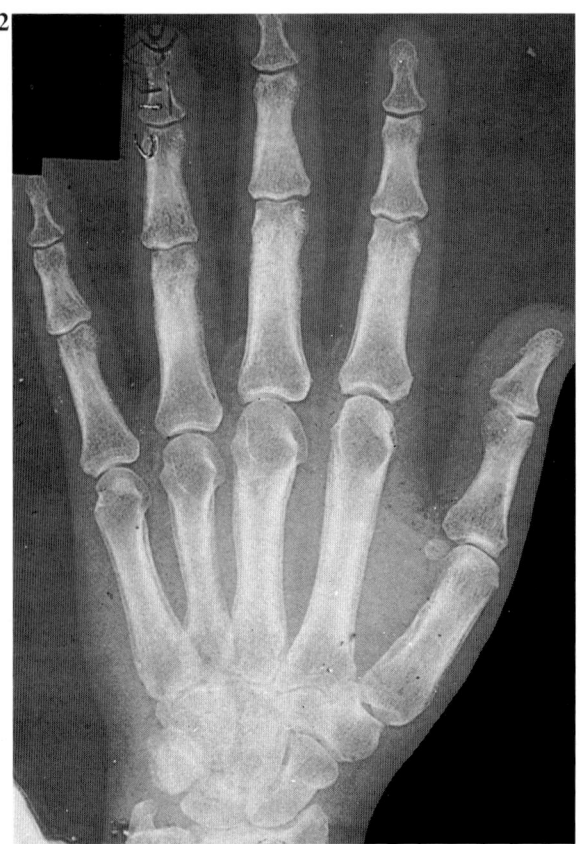

332 What abnormal features does this X-ray show?

333

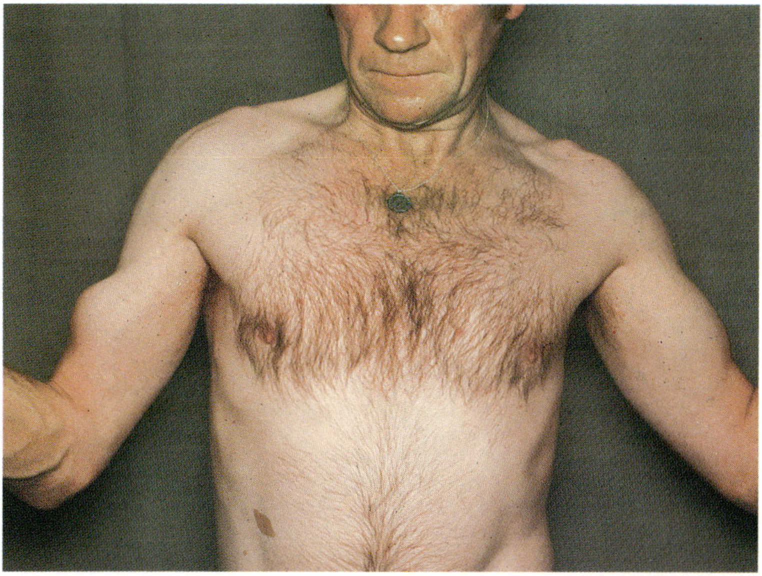

333 The appearance of this man's upper right arm can arise from:

a) A ruptured short tendon of the biceps?
b) A ruptured long tendon of the biceps?
c) A ruptured deltoid?

334

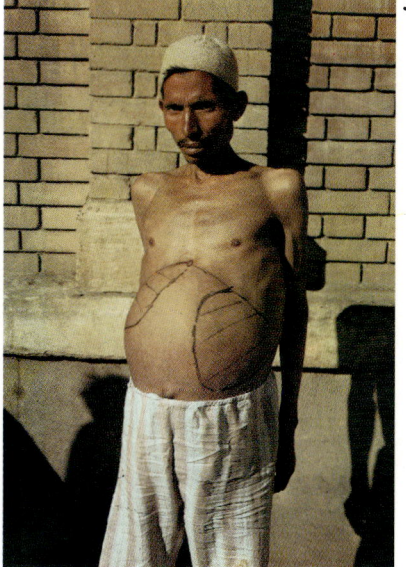

334 This Egyptian farmer presented with hepatomegaly, splenomegaly and ascites. What is the most likely diagnosis?

335 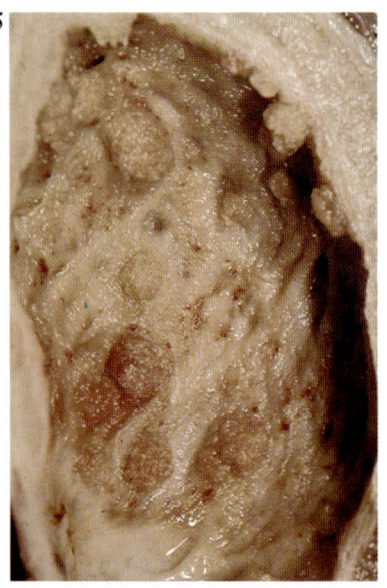 This photograph shows the interior of an opened cystectomy specimen from a 58-year-old man.

a) What is the diagnosis?
b) Enumerate possible aetiological factors.

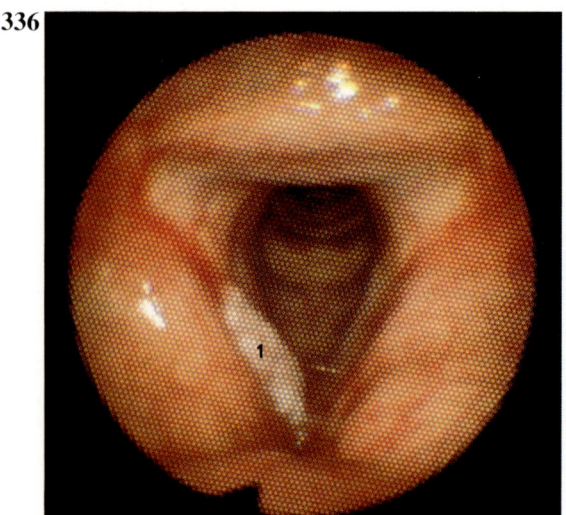

336 a) What is this lesion affecting the right vocal cord?
b) What are the pre-disposing factors, and how does the disease present?

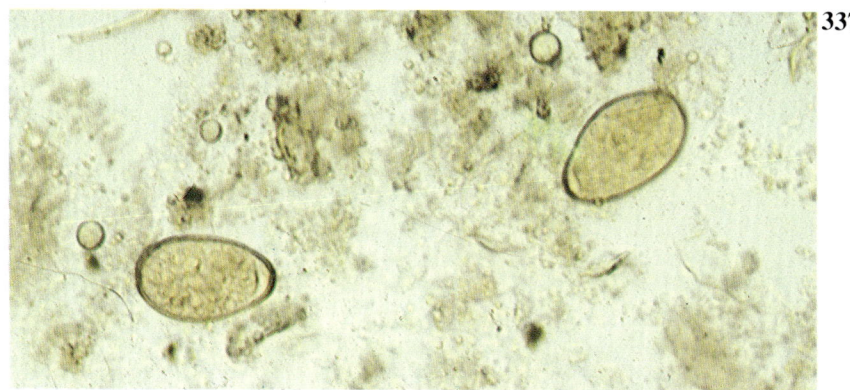

337 These eggs were found in the sputum of a patient from Thailand who complained of haemoptysis. What is the diagnosis?

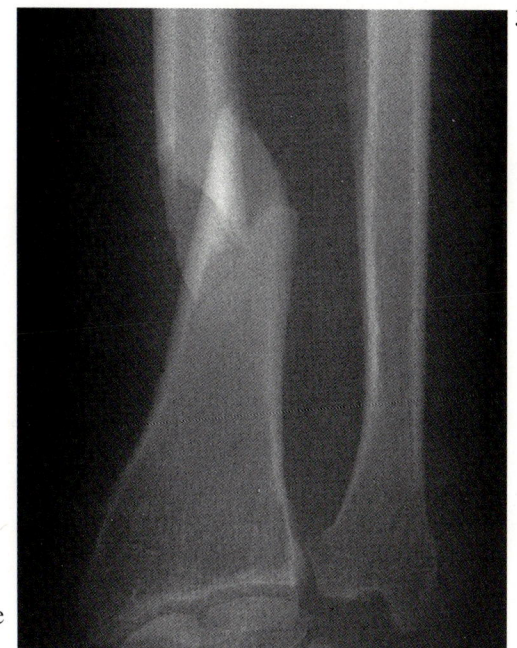

338 This injury is associated with:

a) Dislocation of the inferior radio-ulnar joint?
b) Dislocation of the superior radio-ulnar joint?
c) A fracture of the olecranon?

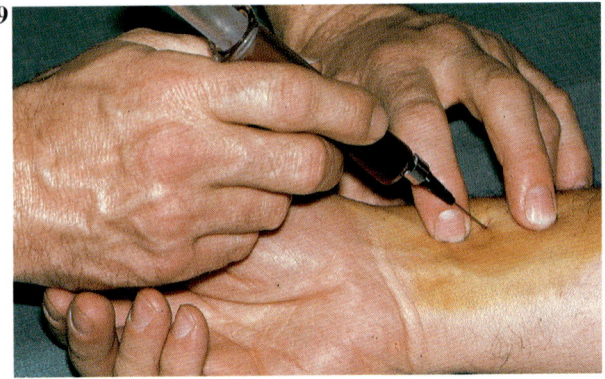

339 This procedure provides useful data in:

a) Iron poisoning?
b) Salicylate poisoning?
c) Cyanide poisoning?

340 Describe the cells in this peripheral blood field. What is the diagnosis and what other almost pathognomonic feature do the abnormal cells show?

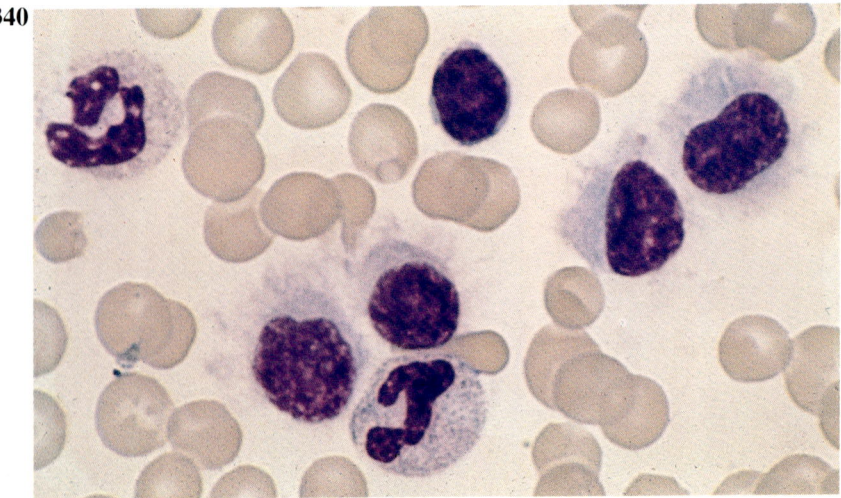

341 Typical externally quiet-appearing white eye, which has a dense white cataract in the pupil and iridocyclitis noted on slit lamp examination in a child who has had a fever or a short-lasting rash and joint pain, suggest what disease.

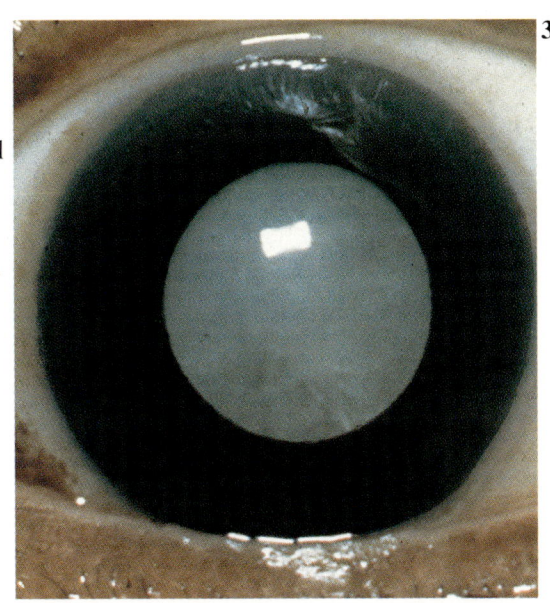

342 The most likely cause of a unilateral fixed dilated pupil in a conscious patient after injury is:

a) Extra dural haemorrhage.
b) Trauma to globe or reflex arc to the iris.
c) Sixth cranial nerve damage.

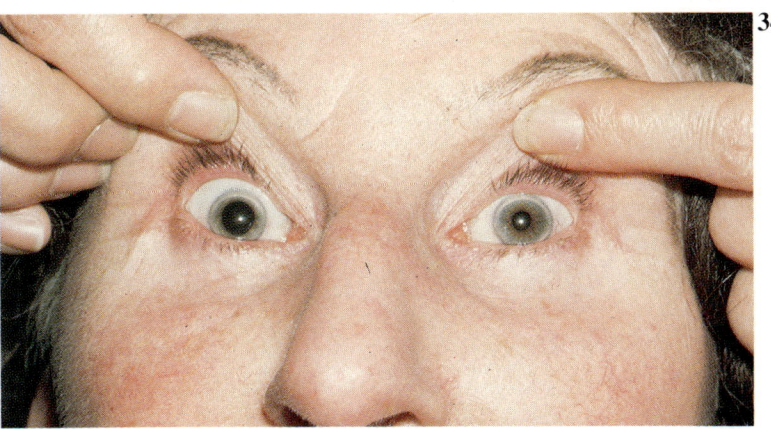

343
a) What is this lesion called?
b) In which patients is it most likely to occur?
c) Which organisms commonly cause it?

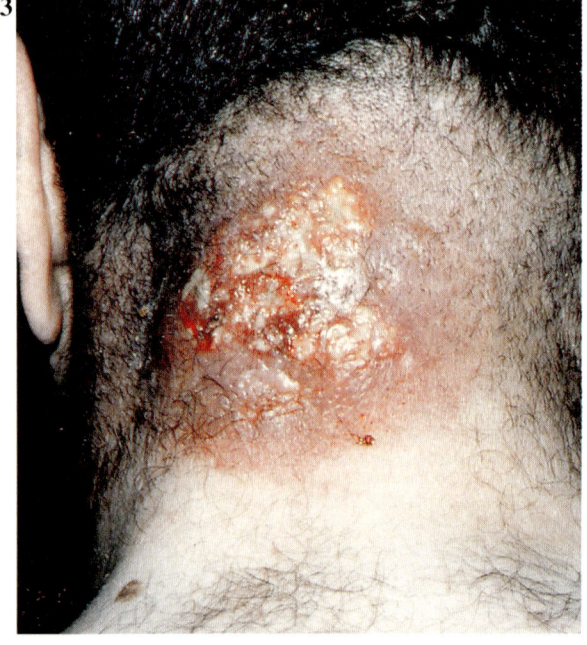

344 Section of the bladder wall from a 45-year-old Egyptian male. Cystectomy was performed for squamous-cell carcinoma. (*H&E × 90*.)

a) What are the structures stained deep blue with haematoxylin?
b) How is the disease contracted? How does it spread?

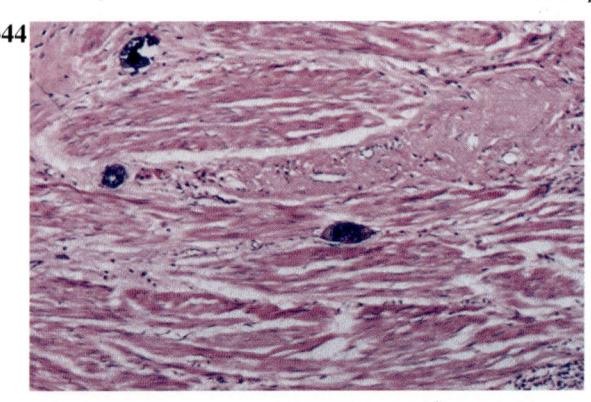

345 Why is this 17-year-old asthmatic so short?

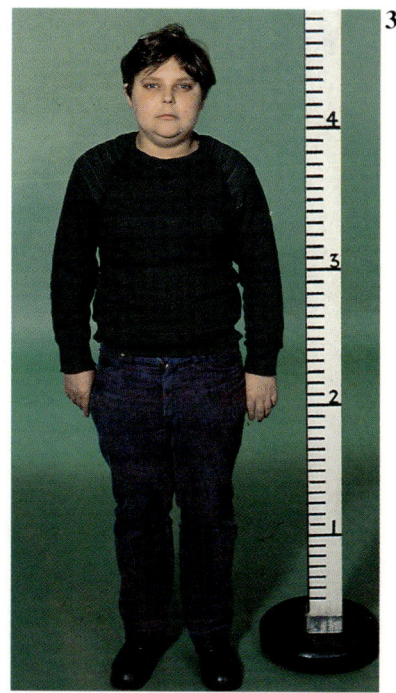

346 The Minnigerode's sign occurs in cases where:

a) A Levin tube mimicks air in soft tissues?
b) The oesophagus, either cervical or thoracic, has been wounded?

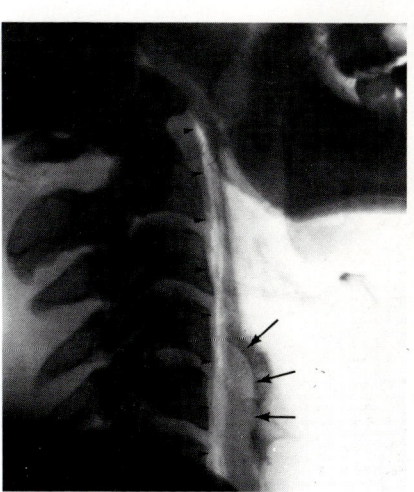
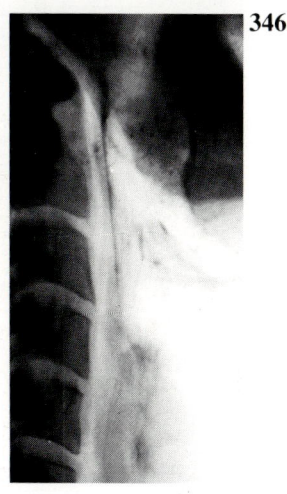

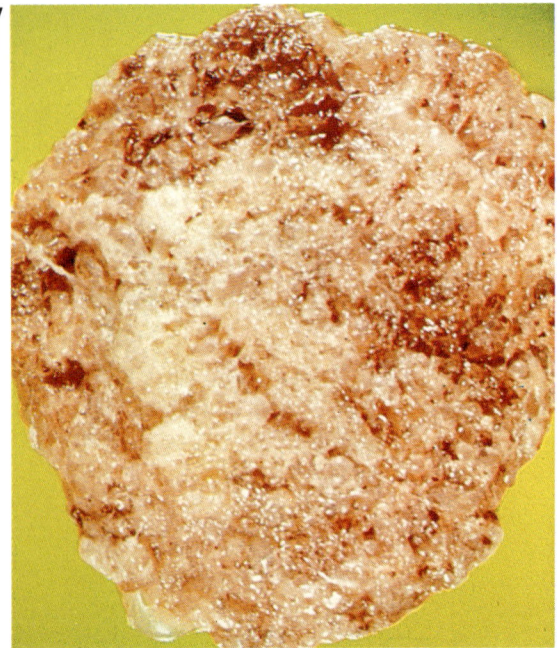

347 A patient passed this tissue when she aborted.
  a) What is the diagnosis?
  b) What biochemical test will confirm the diagnosis?
  c) What are the risks of this condition and what advice do you give to a patient?

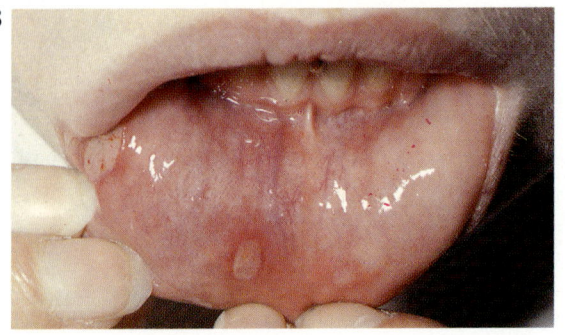

348 What is the diagnosis, and what's the cause?

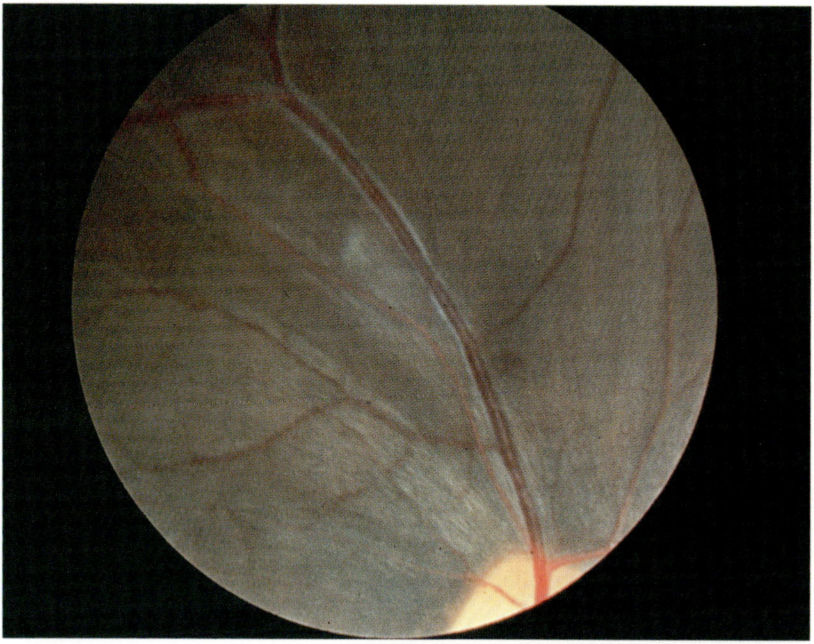

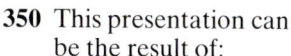

349 This perivasculitis in a 23-year-old patient suggests which diagnosis?

a) Sarcoidosis?
b) Tuberculosis?
c) Lupus erythematosus?
d) Syphilis?

350 This presentation can be the result of:

a) Spontaneous alopecia.
b) A bed sore.
c) A glucagonoma, necrolytic erythema.

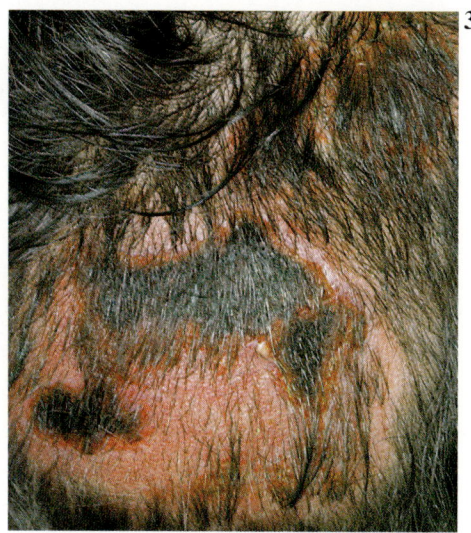

351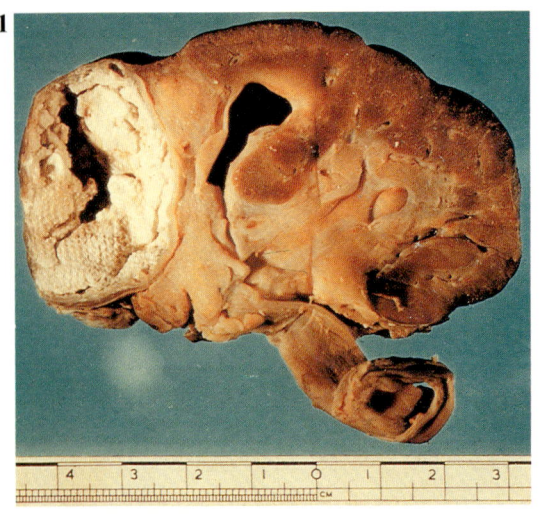

351 A cavitating lesion is seen in the upper pole of this kidney.
  a) What infective condition is shown?
  b) How does the infection reach the kidneys?

352 This appearance is an inversion strain film of the ankle is due to:

  a) A rupture of the deltoid ligament?
  b) A rupture of the lateral ligament?
  c) A rupture of the Achilles tendon?

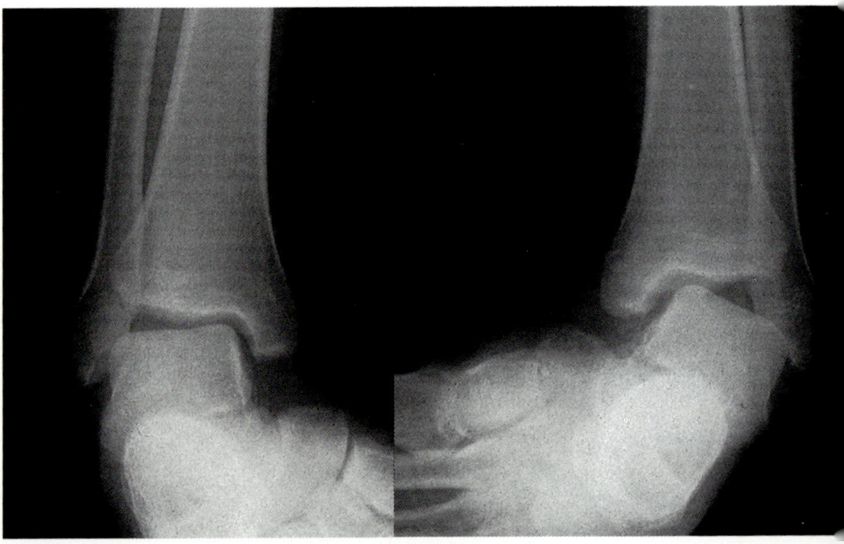

353 This nail-bed injury, caused by crushing, should be treated by:

a) Antibiotics to prevent infection of the haematoma.
b) Trephining the nail, to release the haematoma.
c) Relocation of the nail.

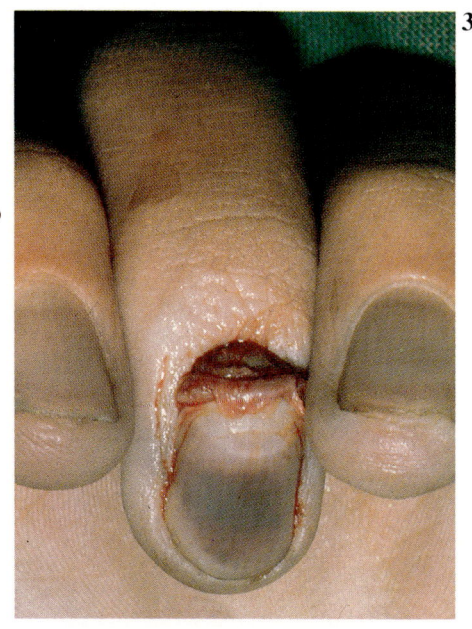

354 What is the name given to this inflammatory condition of the roots of the teeth and alveolar bone?

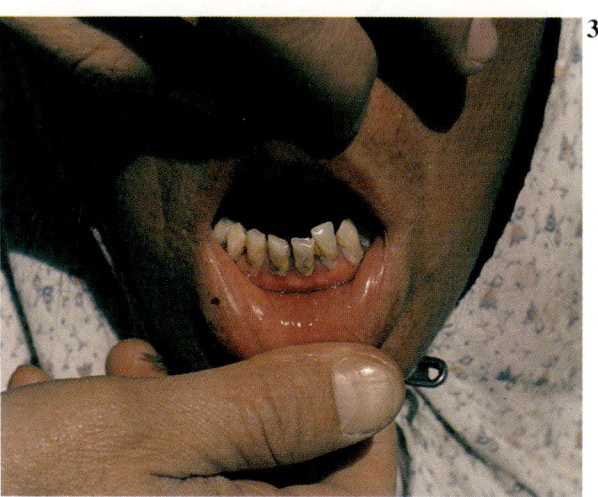

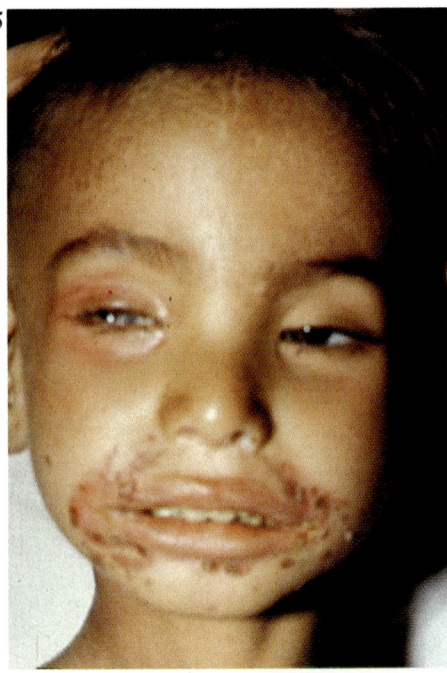

355 This young child had an inherited disorder characterized by a generalized psoriasiform dermatitis, hair loss, diarrhoea and growth retardation.

a) What is the condition?
b) What is the treatment?

356 a) What cells are found in this bone-marrow aspirate and comment on the cytological features shown.
b) What is the possible diagnosis?

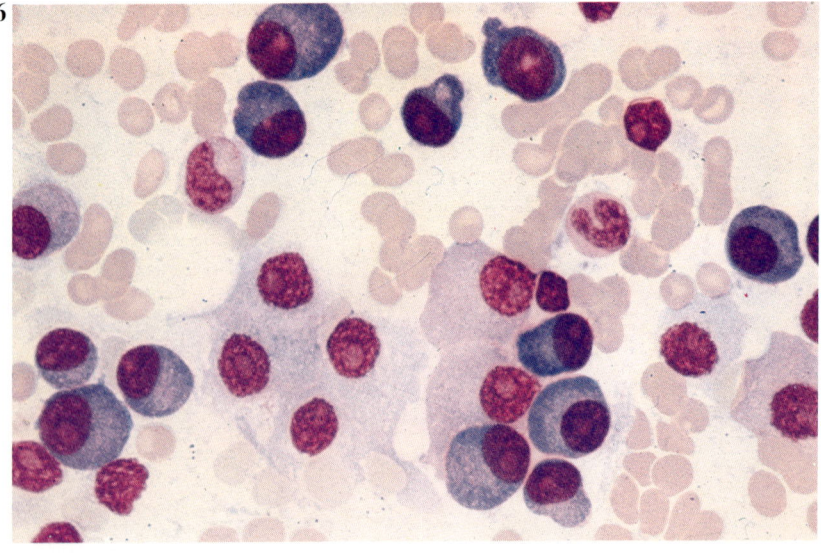

357 Focal haemorrhage and necrotizing vasculitis associated with a reactivating retinitis as seen here inferior to the two previously active lesions of inflammation, suggests what disease process which reactivates in the retina in a satellite location?

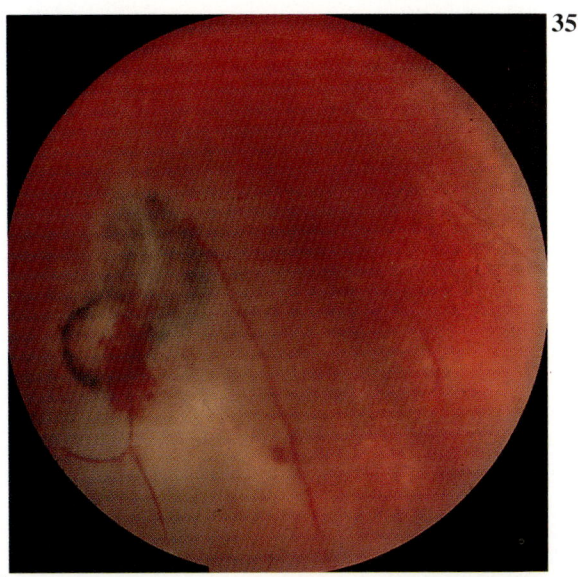

358 Photomicrograph of a tumour excised from the parotid salivary gland of a 30-year-old man. (*H&E × 90.*)

a) What histological features are shown?
b) What is the diagnosis?
c) In what other situations may tumours of this type occur?

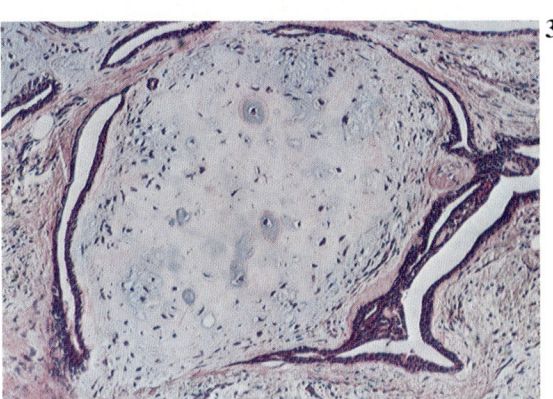

359
a) What is the diagnosis?
b) What are the two obvious signs here?

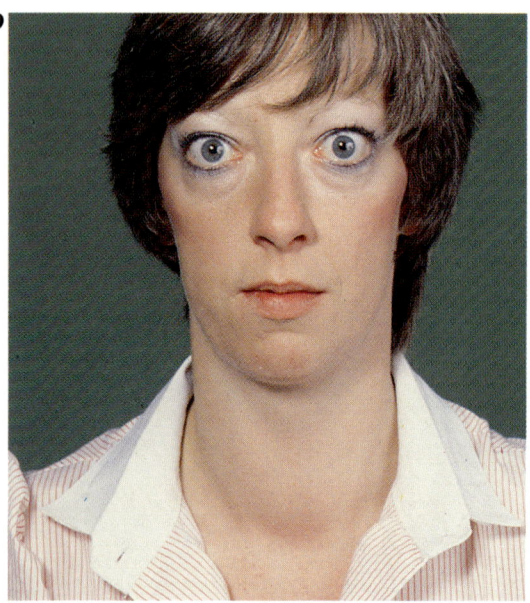

360 The cut surface of a hemisected orchidectomy specimen from a 27-year-old man.

a) What is the most likely diagnosis?
b) What is the prognosis?
c) In what other situations do morphologically identical neoplasms arise?

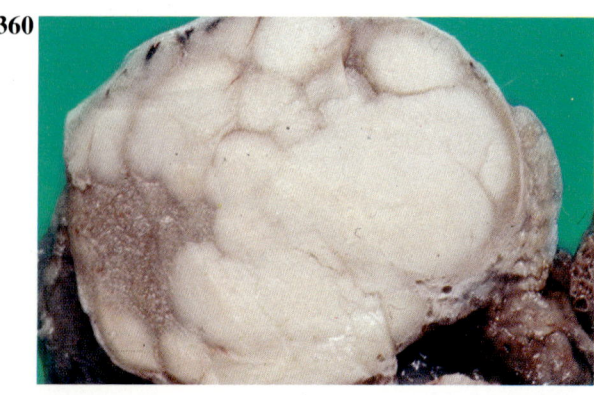

361 This injury:

a) Often leads to osteoarthrosis if not reduced accurately?
b) May be complicated by DeQuervain's syndrome?
c) Results from avulsion of the adductor pollicis insertion?

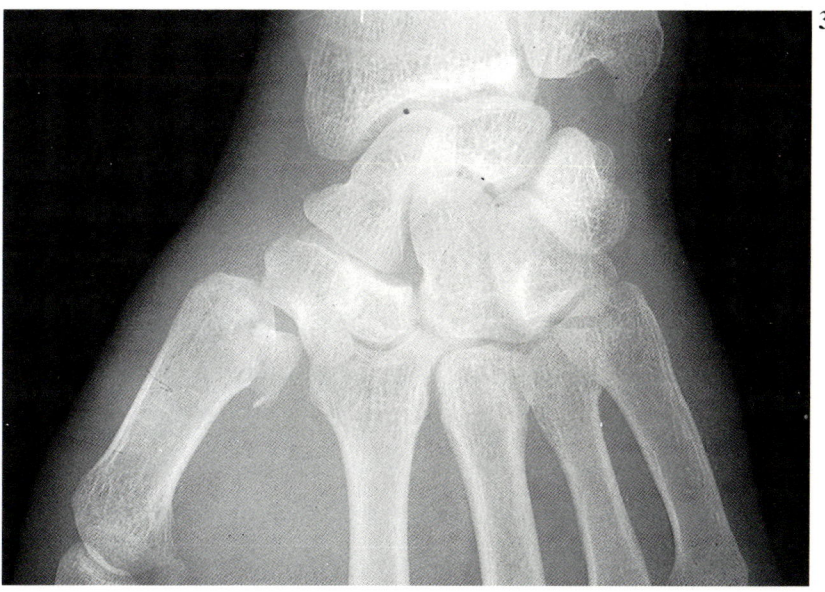

362 This diabetic patient has developed a common complication.

a) Name this condition.
b) Which factors predispose to its development in patients with diabetes mellitus?

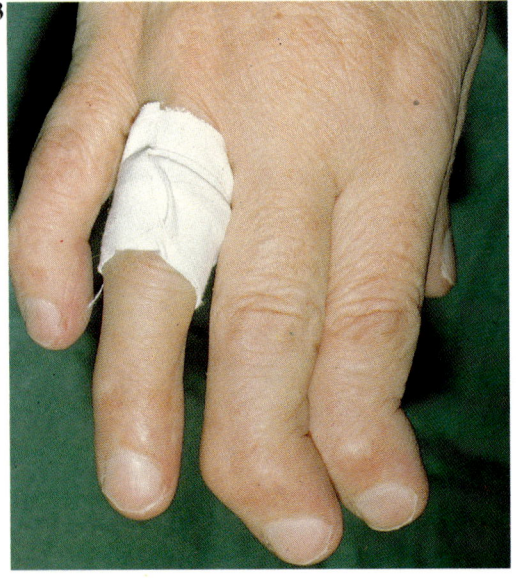

363 The diagnosis here is:
a) Trigger finger?
b) Avulsion of the flexor digitorum profundus tendon?
c) Mallet finger?

364 Photomicrograph of an anterior mediastinal tumour from a 63-year-old woman. (*H&E × 220.*)

a) What is the tumour?
b) What condition may be associated with neoplasms of this type?

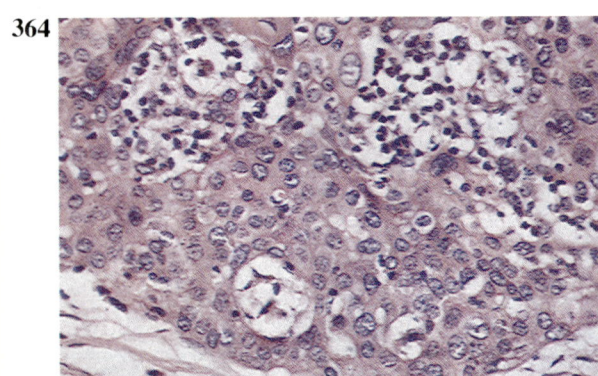

365 This child has a photosensitive dermatitis due to an inherited disorder characterized also by cerebellar ataxia and aminoaciduria.

a) What is the condition?
b) What is the cause?
c) What is the treatment?

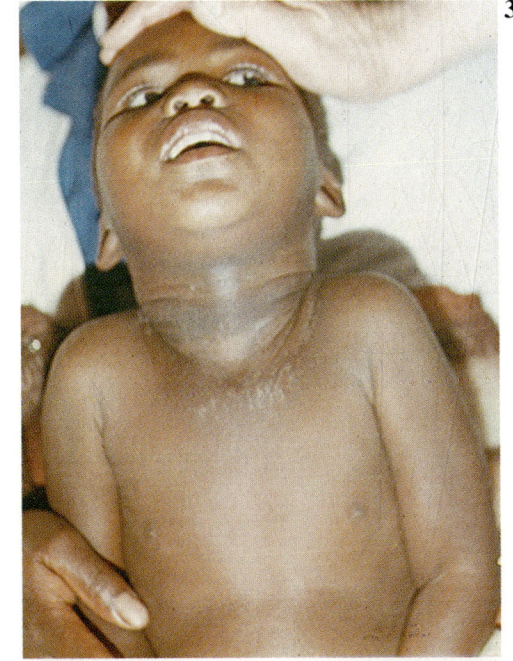

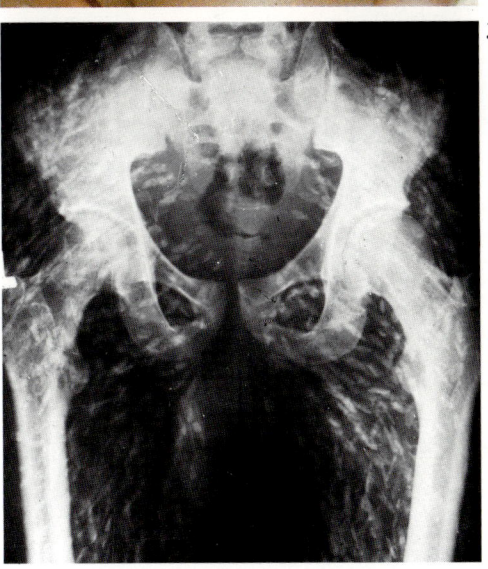

366 X-ray of the soft tissues of the pelvis and thighs revealed these numerous calcified shadows in a pork-eating West Irian. What is the diagnosis?

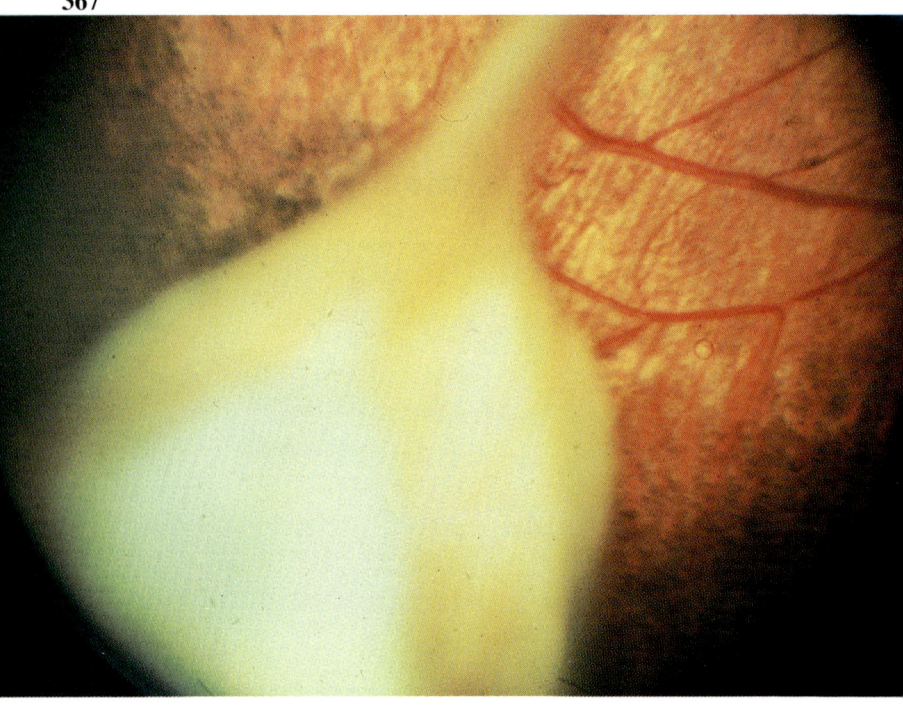

367 This 3-year-old child was noted to have this abscess in, and over, the retina and is associated with pica. While retinoblastoma needs to be ruled out what is the likely aetiology for this retinal abscess?

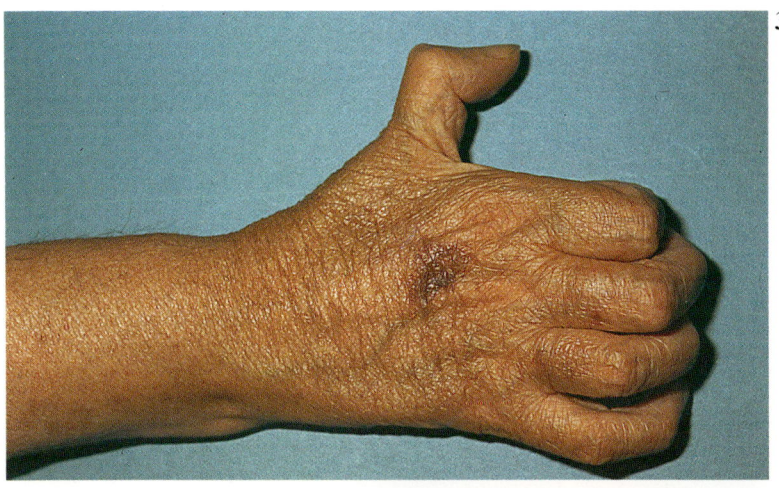

368 This picture of the hand shows:

a) Advanced rheumatoid arthritis?
b) Osteoarthritis?
c) Gout?
d) Claw-hand deformity?
e) Ulnar nerve palsy?

369 In this incised wound of the palm, the following structures are probably damaged:

a) The ulnar digital nerves.
b) Flexor digitorum profundus and sublimis to the index and middle fingers.
c) The radial nerve to the hand.

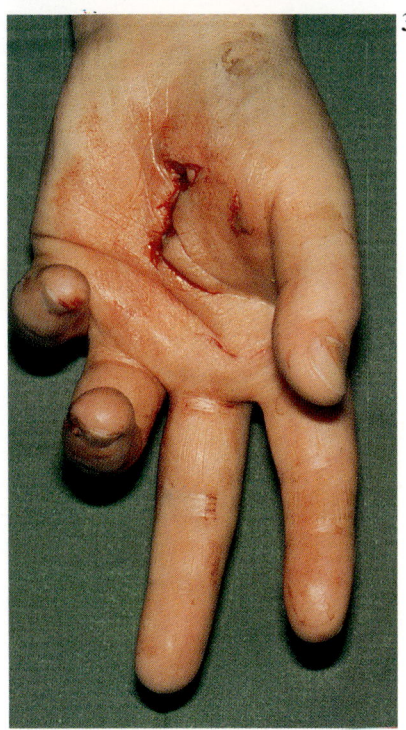

370 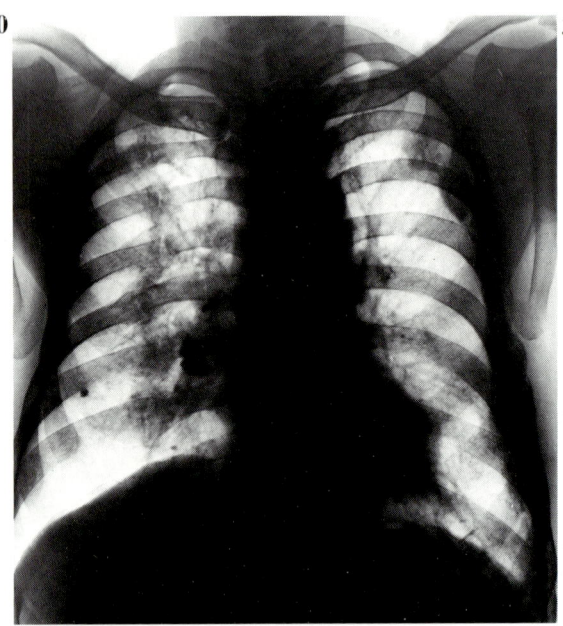 The typical aspect of:

a) Blastomycosis of the lung?
b) Post-traumatic pseudarthroses of the ribs?
c) Metastatic prostatic carcinoma?

371 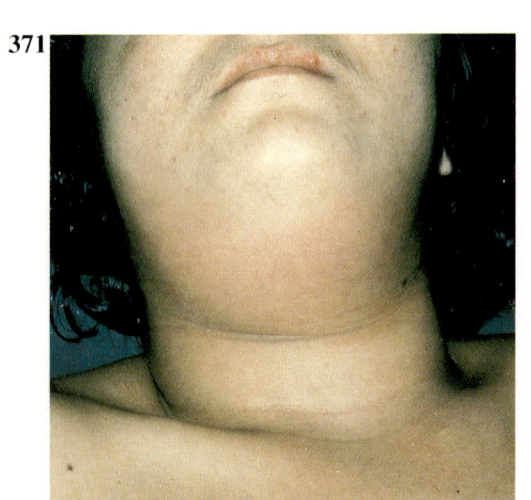 This patient developed a tender swelling in the upper part of her neck and complained of pain, dysphagia and dyspnoea. She had recently undergone a molar extraction.

a) What is the condition called?
b) Which type of organisms are usually causative?
c) What fatal complication may occur?

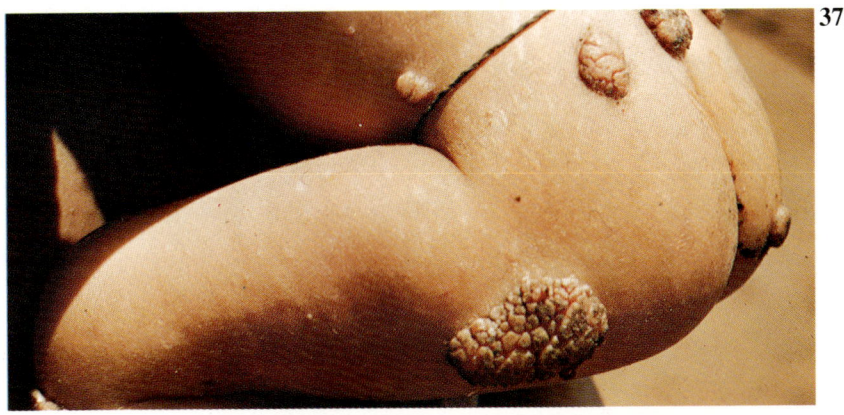

372 This child presented with these florid lesions. What is the diagnosis?

373 This patient presented with a vitreous haemorrhage in the eye and all of his vision was obscured by this haemorrhage. One can see the aetiologic explanation for this vitreous haemorrhage as a teardrop-shaped lesion in between the two blood vessels in the retina. What is it?

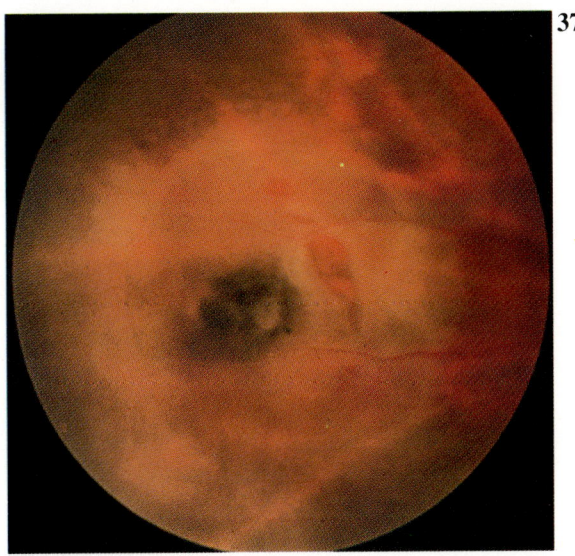

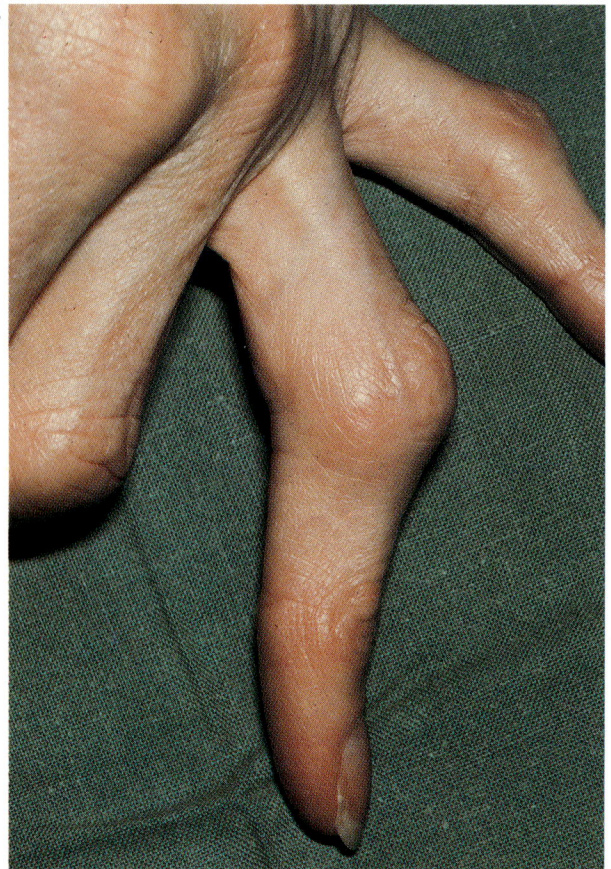

374 This deformity is caused by:

a) Division of the flexor digitorum sublimis?
b) Dupuytren's contracture?
c) Damage to the middle slip of the extensor tendon at the proximal interphalangeal joint?

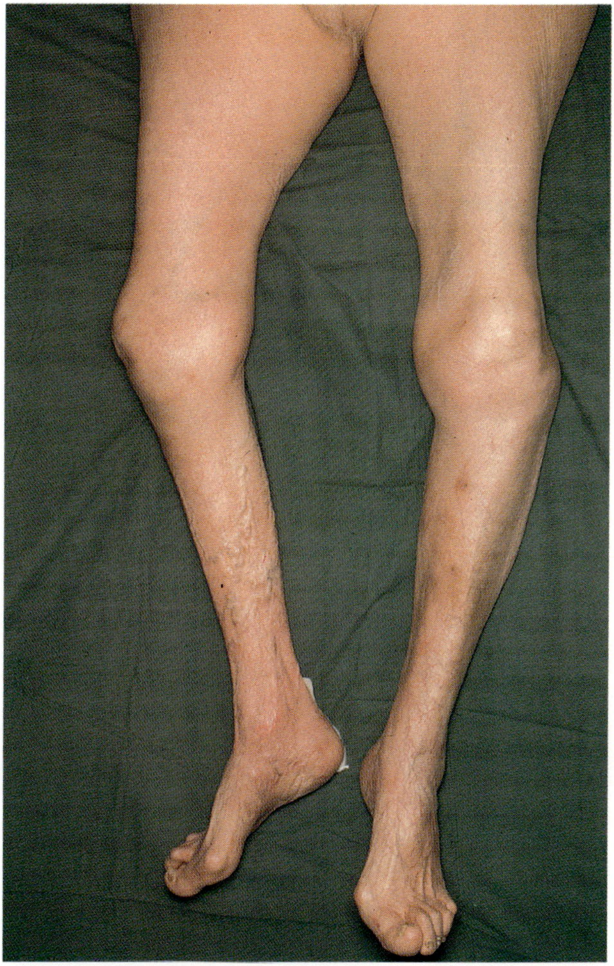

375 This painful deformity in an elderly woman is most likely due to:

  a) A dislocated hip?
  b) A fractured neck of the femur?
  c) A fractured pelvis?

376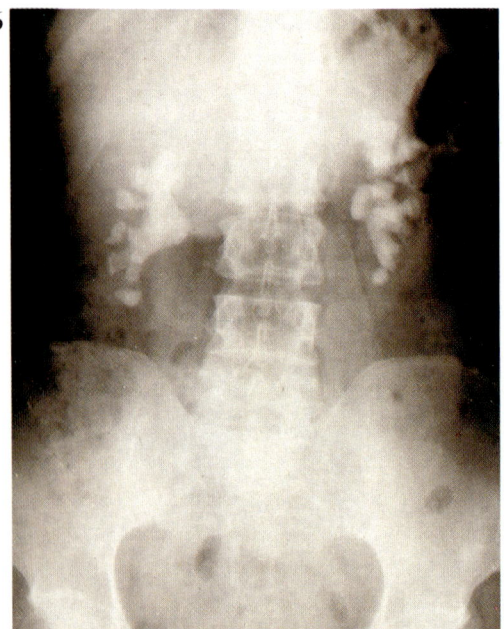
a) What type of renal calculi are shown on this plain abdominal radiograph?
b) What is their composition?

377 What does this picture show?

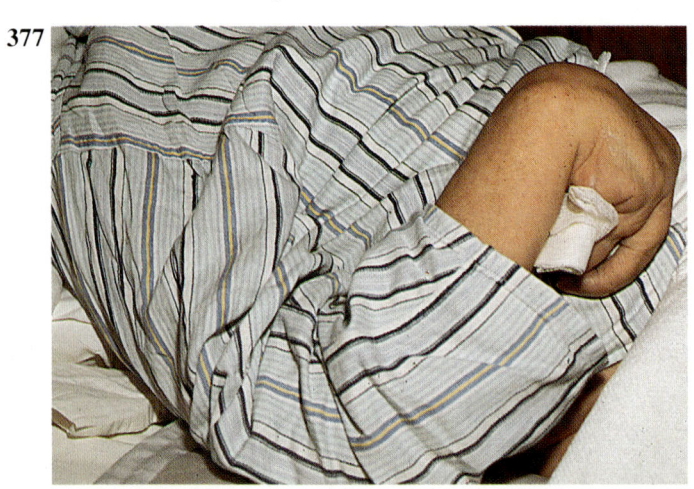

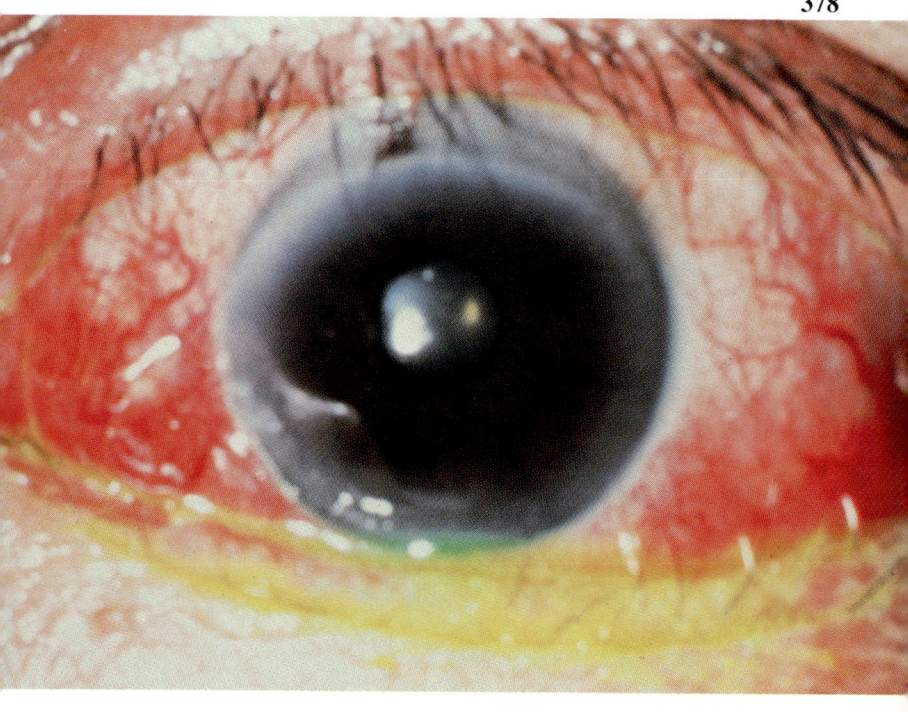

378 This undulating string-like finding in the anterior chamber of this patient who acquired an infection from a horse suggests what type of acquired infection which is most usually seen, but not always, in patients who have been to the tropics?

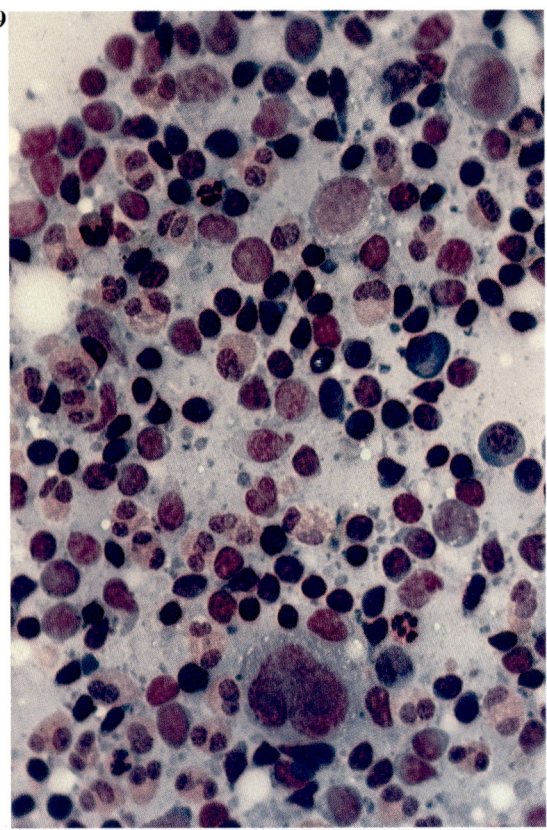

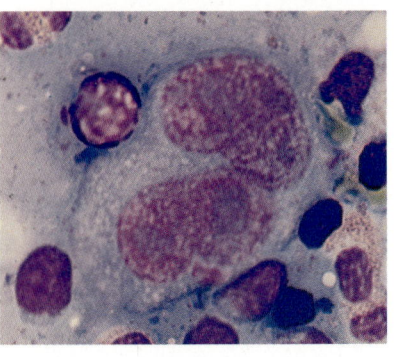

379 This field (above) is a low power view from an imprint made from the cut surface of a biopsied lymph node. A high-power view of one area is shown on the left.

a) Describe the cytological features.
b) What diagnosis do they suggest?

380 This man felt a sudden painful snap in his lower calf. He has:

a) A ruptured Achilles tendon?
b) A ruptured plantaris muscle?
c) A rupture of the gastrocnemius?

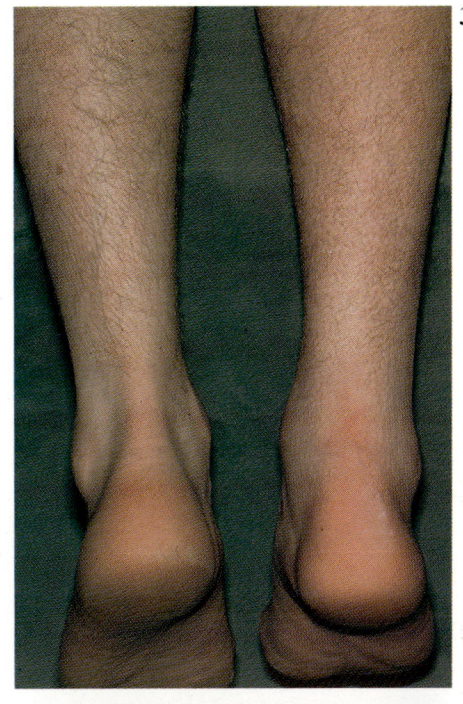

381 Intravenous pyelography revealed the following lesions in an Egyptian farmer. What is the diagnosis?

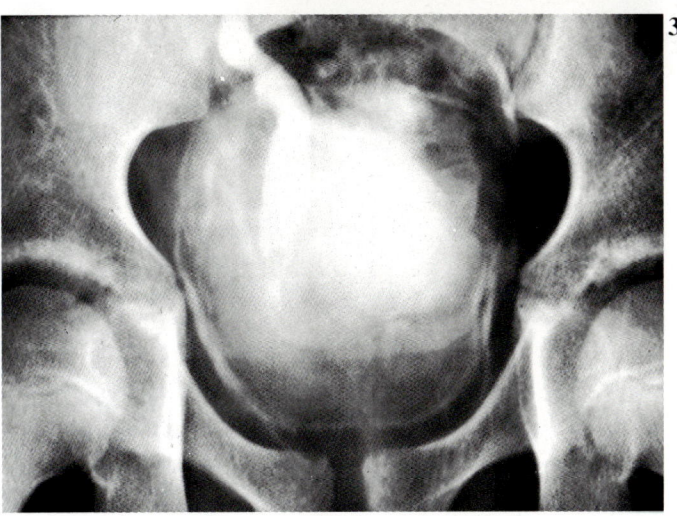

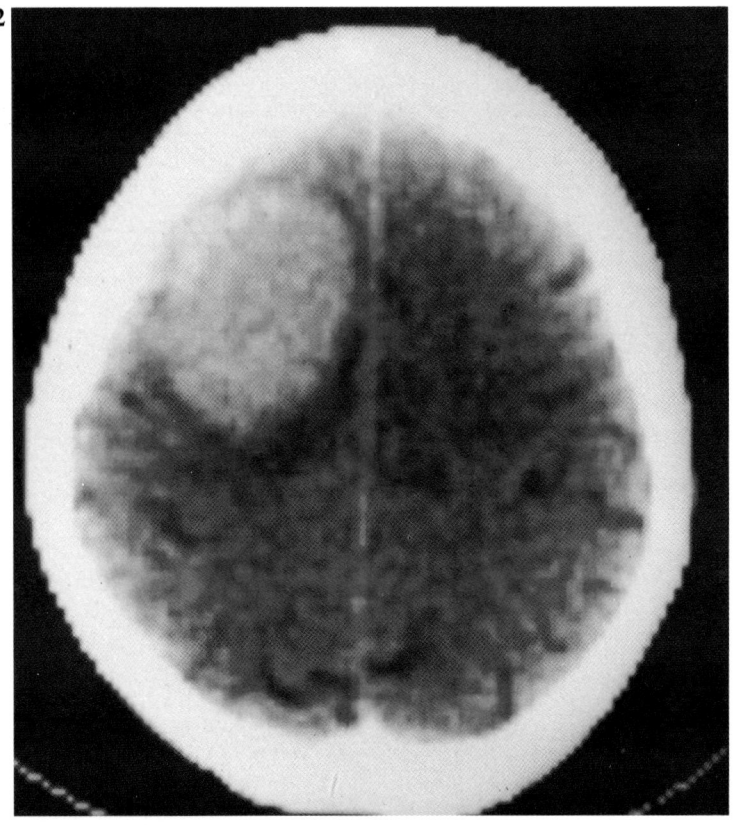

382 What does this CT scan of the brain show?

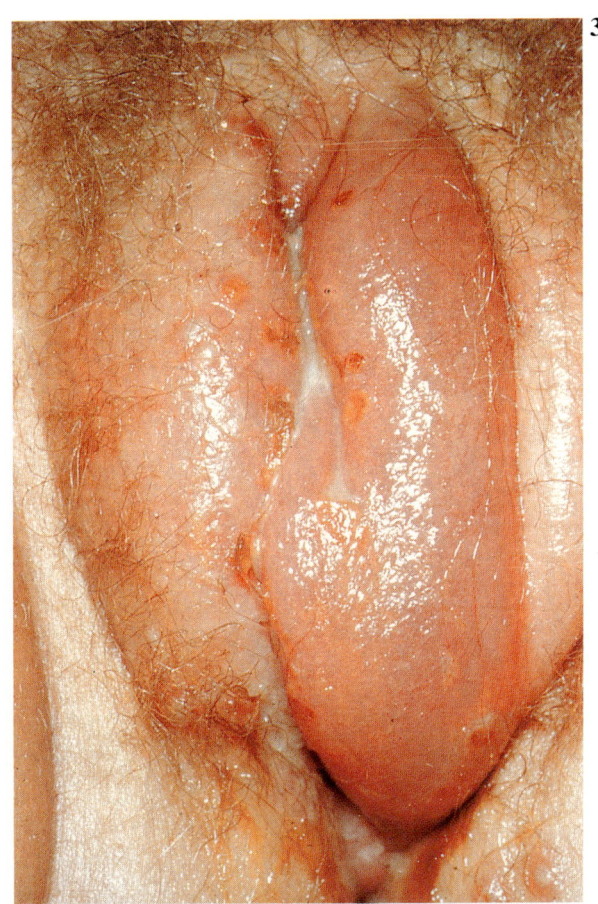

383 This patient presented with marked oedema and erythema of the left labium majus.

a) What is the diagnosis?
b) Which organisms are usually responsible?

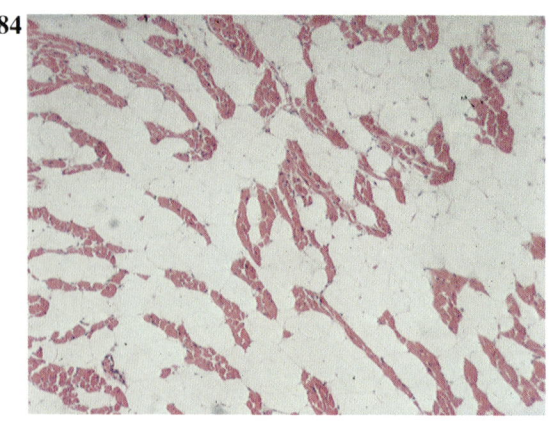

384 Section of the abnormal myocardium of a right ventricle. Name the condition.

385 Why are there prominent telangiectasia overlying both the true and the false vocal cords?

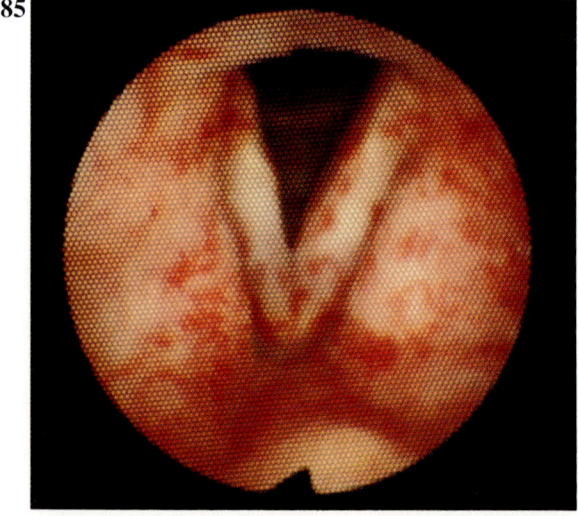

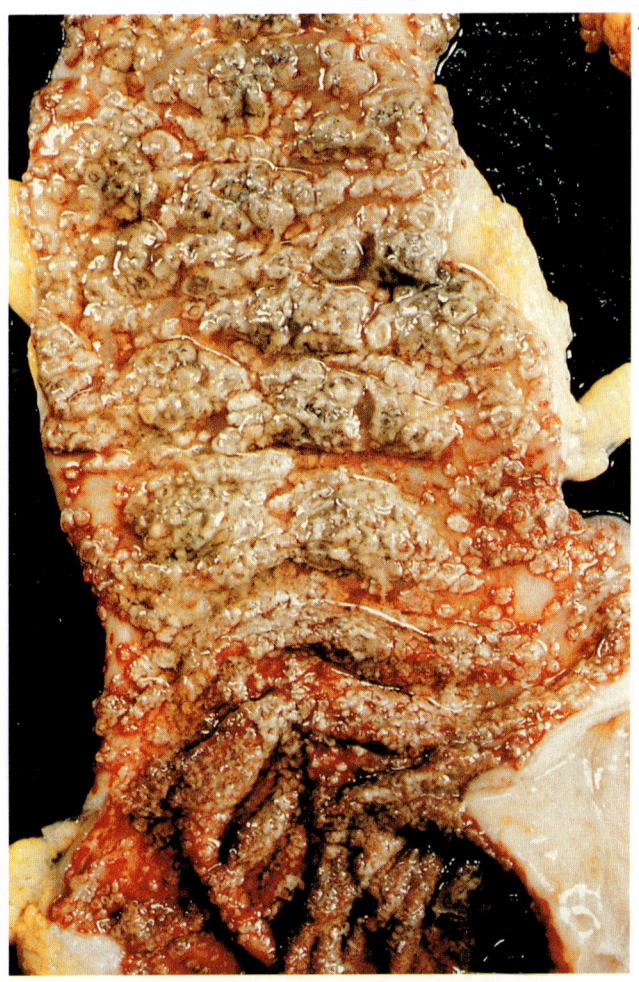

386 This specimen of the large intestine was removed at post-mortem from a patient who died following a severe pneumonia treated by several courses of broad-spectrum antibiotics. He developed marked diarrhoea before he died.

a) From what condition was he suffering?
b) Name the causative organism.

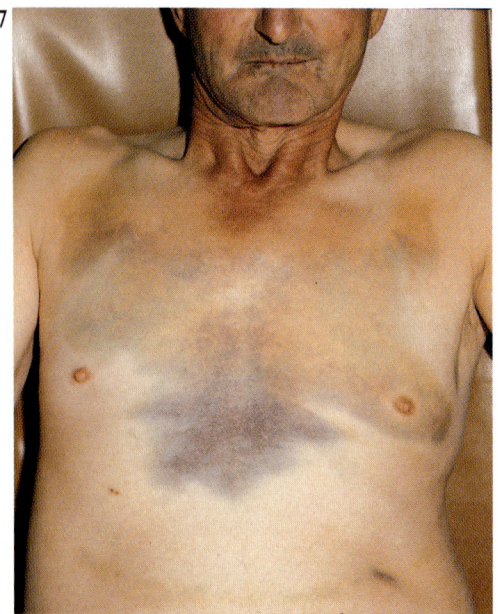

387 This is a patient presenting with:
   a) A lip melanoma and anterior thoracic spread?
   b) A probable heart contusion by the steering wheel?
   c) A Laennec's cirrhosis and vascular 'spontaneous' rupture?

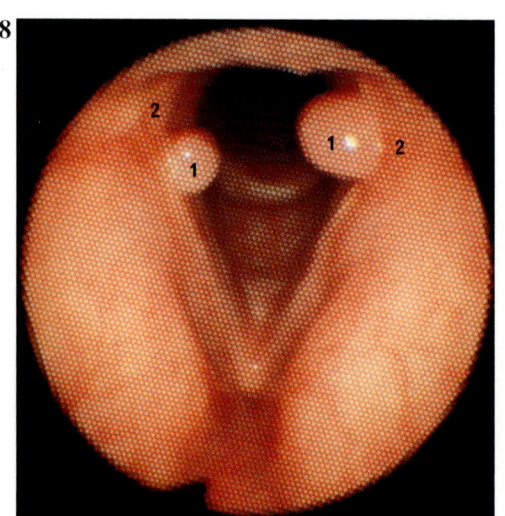

388 Why might this patient have spent 3 weeks on an intensive care unit?

389 What abnormality is shown on this erect lateral chest radiograph?

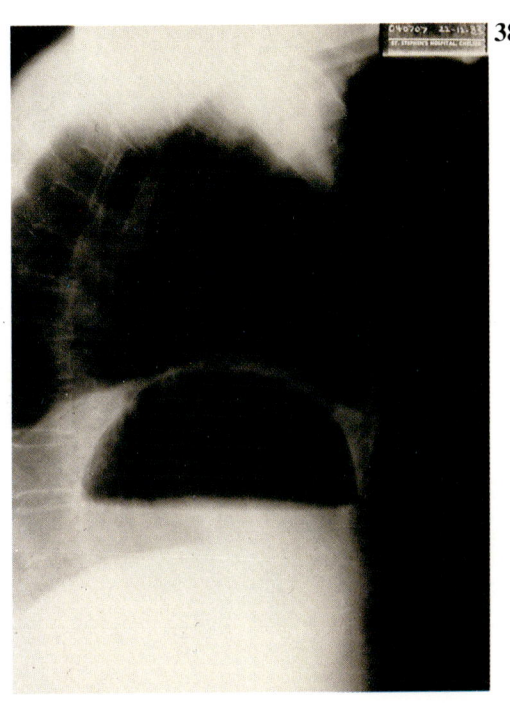

390 The bifurcation of the pulmonary artery opened at post-mortem of a patient who died suddenly.

a) Why did the patient die suddenly?
b) Name the primary disease.

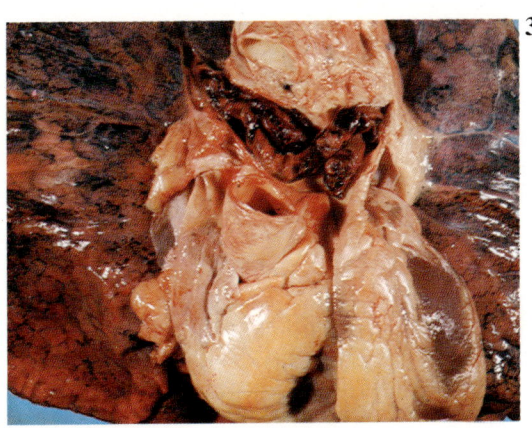

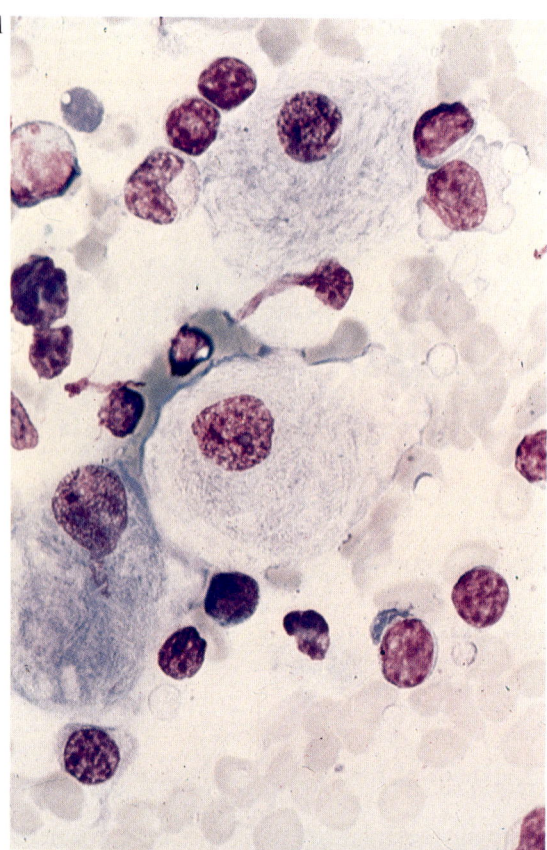

391 a) What cells are shown in this splenic imprint?
b) What diagnosis is likely?

392 This child is said to have 'fallen when scootering'. What does her presentation show?

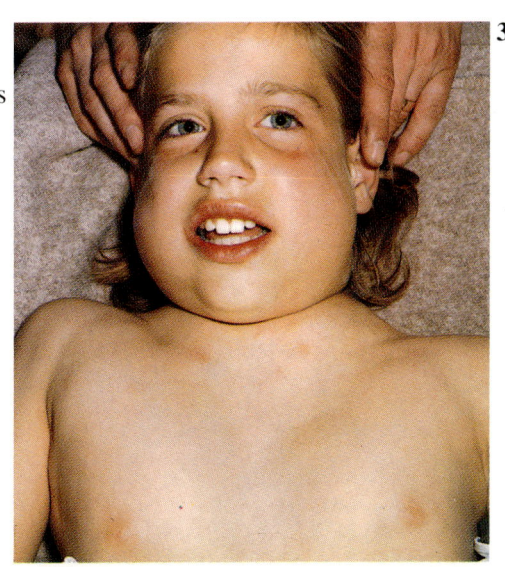

393 This girl has a fluctuant swelling beneath the anterior border of her left sternomastoid muscle.

a) What is the diagnosis?
b) From which structure does this lesion arise?

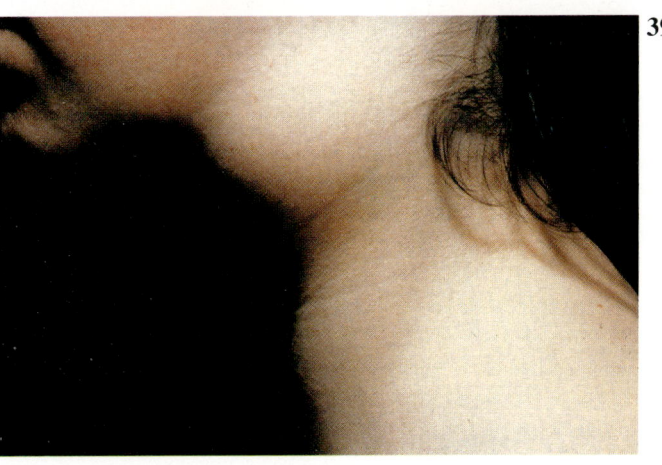

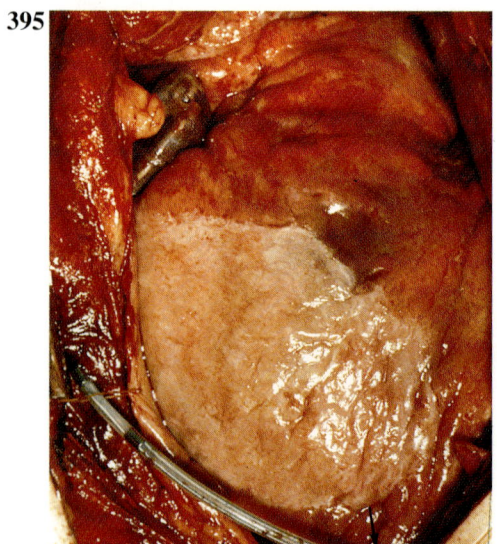

394 This patient has recently undergone total cystectomy.

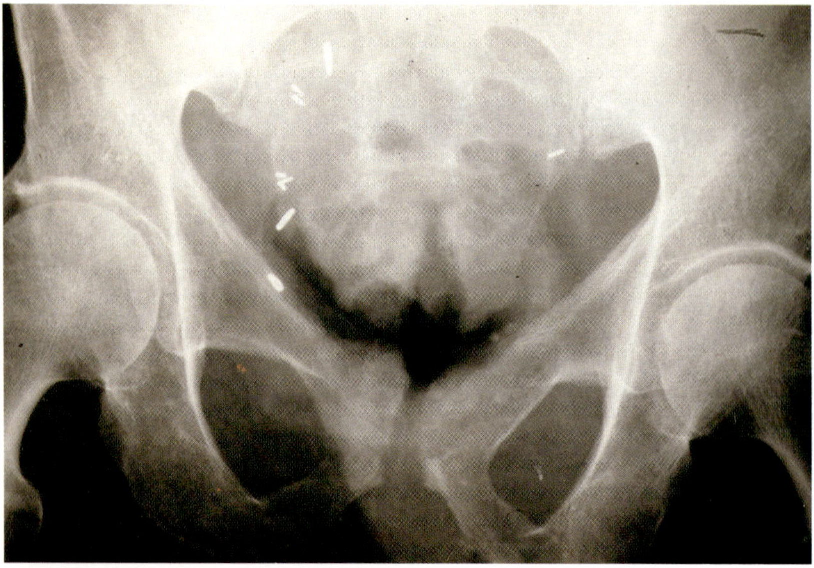

a) What rare complication has developed?
b) Describe the characteristic radiological features.

395 Perforation of the right heart from an electrode of a pace-maker often results in:

a) Hiccoughing by direct diaphragmatic stimulation; the photograph was taken during surgery?
b) Death by tamponade; the photograph was taken at autopsy?

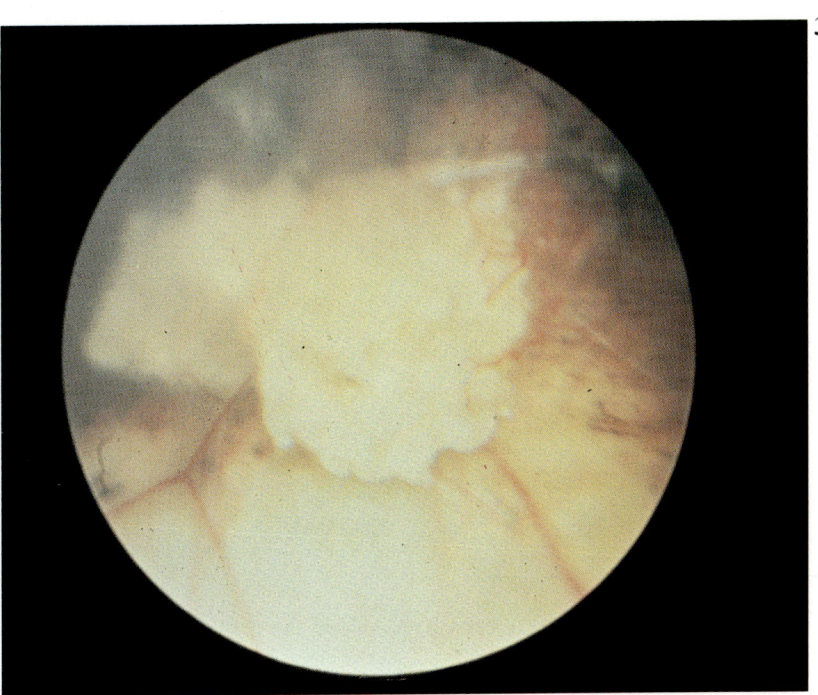

396 This 19-year-old man was refused entrance into the United States coast guard because he was noted to have an 'inflammation of the retina'. His other eye had been enucleated as a 2-year-old child because of a 'tumour'. What does this crumbly non-active lesion suggest?

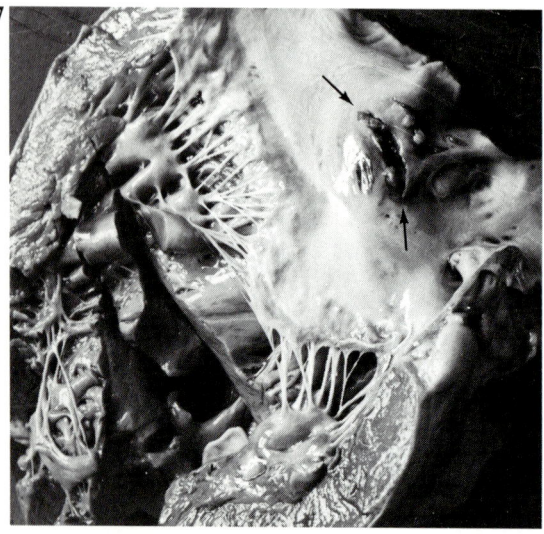

397 An atrial septal defect seen at autopsy and possibly due to:

a) Coronary arterial disease?
b) A road accident?
c) Swan–Ganz catheter misplacement?

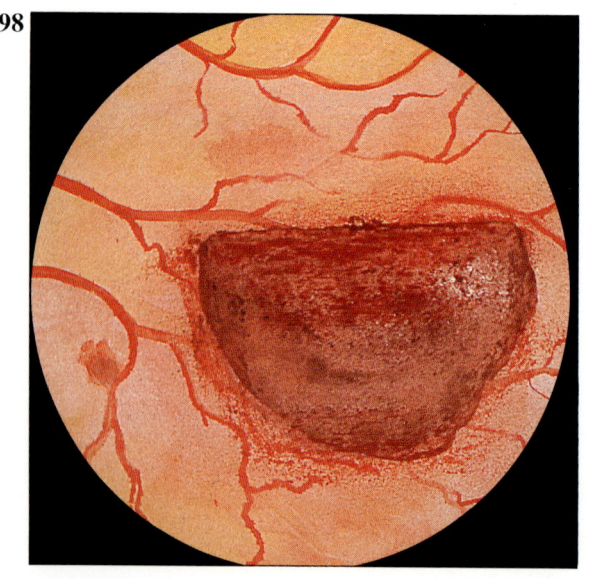

398 What does this ophthalmoscopic view of the fundus show?

a) Cherry red spot?
b) Hypertensive fundus?
c) Foreign body in the eye?
d) Sub-hyaloid haemorrhage?
e) Melanoma?

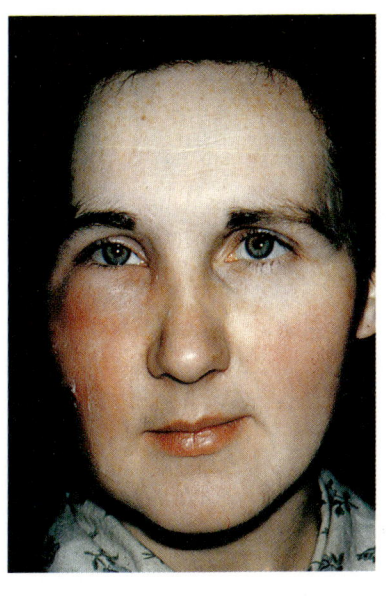
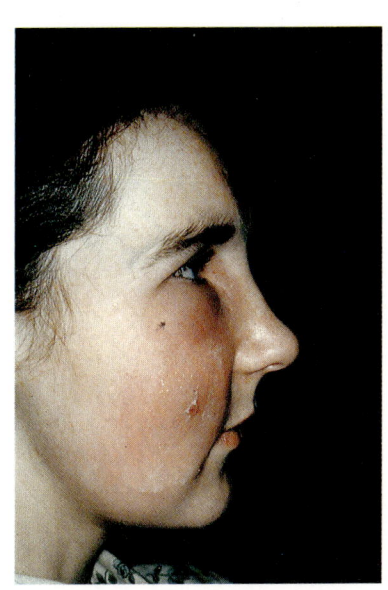

399 a) What infective condition is seen in this patient?
b) What serious complication may develop?

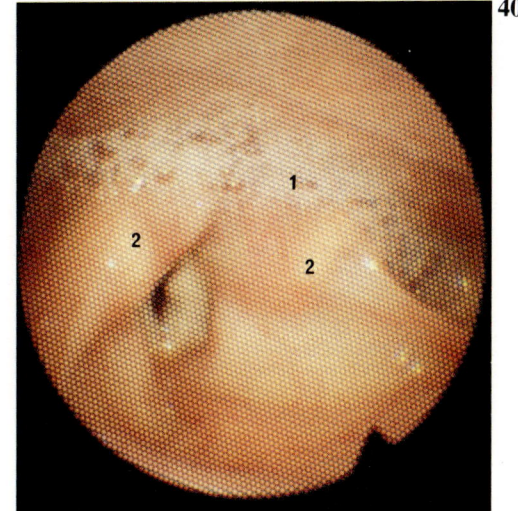

400 This sign of pooling of saliva (1) in the hypopharynx is typical of which disorders?

Answers

1. Calcinosis circumscripta; one of a group of collagen diseases with well-known clinical features but obscure aetiology.
   co

2. a) Imperforate hymen although the membrane is not strictly the hymen.
   b) The treatment is a cruciate incision of the membrane and nothing else, as there is a great risk of ascending infection of the genital tract and subsequent sterility.
   clgy

3. b), c) and d). The X-ray shows an enlarged pituitary fossa in a case of acromegaly.
   gm

4. a) Herpes hominis type 1 (type 2 in a small proportion of patients).
   b) From Erythema multiforme. If there has been a recurrence this diagnosis becomes much more likely.
   c) There is an approximately 50 per cent chance of subsequent recurrent facial herpes.
   om

5. b).
   ent

6. a) Adreno-genital syndrome which is a familial disease transmitted by a recessive gene through either the maternal or paternal side. The cause of the disease is an inherent error in the adrenal cortex, which is unable to complete the normal biosynthesis, whereby progesterone is converted to corticol. Typically, the metabolic change is broken at the hydroxyprogesterone stage, but there are several levels at which arrest occurs and therefore there are several variations. As a consequence, there is an excess of nearly all adrenal cortical hormones, including androgens.
   b) The diagnosis can be made antenatally in affected families by amniocentesis when high levels of hydroxyprogesterone and androgens will be detected.
   c) The ovaries, tubes, uterus and vagina are basically unaffected, so pregnancy is possible after appropriate corticosteroid therapy. Surgery is often required to produce more normal external genitalia.
   clgy

7. a) Acute crepitating extensor tenosynovitis.
   b) The condition presents as pain, swelling, and crepitus on the dorsum of the lower forearm associated with movement of the wrist. The patient in unable to continue normal activity in sport, typically rowing and canoeing. It is an acute over-use injury.
   c) It can now effectively be treated by decompression under local anaesthetic of the fascial envelope of abductor pollicis longus and extensor pollicis brevis which will allow virtually immediate return to normal activity.
   is

8. Sequence of erythroid cells, from proerythroblast with large size, relatively smooth nuclear staining and deep cytoplasmic basophilia, through early, intermediate and late normoblasts, with increasingly coarse nuclear structure, decreasing size and cytoplasmic basophilia and increasing pink polychromatic staining reflecting rising haemoglobin content, to non-nucleated red cells.
   hacy

9. a) Retinitis pigmentosa. Scattered areas of pigment in the fundus

show typical 'bone corpuscle' configuration, characteristic of this form of retinal pigmentary degeneration. The optic disc is pale and the retinal vessels are attenuated.
b) Laurence–Moon–Biedl syndrome.
c) Polydactylia.
esd

10 Myositis ossificans progressiva—a rare disease which usually manifests itself first in the neck and shoulder girdle.
co

11 a) Right hydronephrosis.
b) Aberrant lower polar vessel with upper ureter hooked over it.
ur

12 a) Acromegaly.
b) Coarse features: broad nose, deep skin creases, increased soft tissue thickness, goitre.
c) Diabetes; hypertension; cardiomegaly and heart failure.
d) Diagnosis may be confirmed by demonstrating an increased Growth Hormone level which is not suppressed during a glucose tolerance test.
end

13 a) Topagnosia or contralateral visual neglect.
b) The right parieto-occipital region.
c) Inability to appreciate simultaneous visual or tactile stimuli on both sides, and to locate those on the affected side accurately. With more severe lesions, loss of awareness of the affected limbs, or inability to appreciate that they are weak (anosagnosia). Inability to find the way around even in familiar surroundings.
cn

14 Rupture of the synovial membrane of the knee joint.
rh

15 a) and b).
ud

16 b), c) and e).
gm

17 Ring stages of *Plasmodium falciparum*, the causative agent of malignant tertian malaria. In severe cases numerous ring forms are usually seen.
tmp

18 c) Blood issuing from the urethra is very suggestive of a urethral tear in cases of fracture of the anterior part of the pelvic ring. The patient should not be catheterized, nor allowed to try to micturate. The help of a general or genitourinary surgeon should be sought immediately.
ae

19 a) An 'allergic' type of nasal polyp, originating from the ethmoidal sinuses.
b) Cystic fibrosis.
feurt

20 b) 'Large-for-dates' or 'heavy-for-dates' infants are prone to major congenital abnormalities.
nb

21 'Tapir mouth'. The pouting lips are due to weakness of the orbicularis oris and oculi muscles. The patient suffers from facioscapulohumeral dystrophy (Déjérine myopathy).
co

22 a) Monilial vulvo-vaginitis, for which there are several remedes, but nowadays Nystatin is one of the treatments of choice.
b) It is more common in diabetic patients, in pregnancy, associated with glycosuria and following the administration of oral broad spectrum antibiotics.
clgy

23 Inability to extend the knee may be due to locking as a result of a meniscus tear in a twisting injury of the knee but this is not always the case. Many patients are unable fully to extend the knee after injury due to protective spasm in the hamstring muscles. Muscles go into spasm during the last few degrees of extension to prevent full extension of the irritable knee. It is very easy to misdiagnose such a knee as 'locked' if a patient is only examined in supine lying because the true cause of the inability to extend the knee is not apparent. When the patient is turned onto his face and the knee extended the tight bulging of the muscle as it goes into spasm is readily demonstrable and easily diagnosed. In these cases treatment must be directed to the relief of secondary hamstring spasm as well as to the primary injury in the knee.
is

24 c) Crises in sickle-cell anaemia may cause intravascular thrombosis and if this happens in the cerebral circulation, then the patient may develop cerebral infarction.
st

25 a) The injury is a fracture of the anterior fossa of the skull.
b) The posterior limit of the subconjunctival haemorrhage cannot be visualised.
c) Effective child restraints for rear seat passengers will reduce the severity of injury in the event of an accident.
psd

26 Sucking cushions, pads of fat tissiue between the fibres of the masseter muscle. They remain unaltered by weight loss. They prevent the indrawing of the cheeks during sucking.
pd

27 Paget's sarcoma of the humerus. Approximately 1 per cent of cases of Paget's disease of bone may advance to develop a sarcoma of variable cell type.
co

28 Tonic neck reflex, one of the automatic reflexes of the newborn due to primitive neuro-muscular response to stimulation. Sudden turning of the neck produces extension of the limbs in the direction of the turn and flexion on the opposite side. With normal development this fades out within the first trimester.
pd

29 d).
ent

30 a) Villous tumour (villus adenoma) of the rectum.
b) In addition to bleeding, there may be symptoms resulting from fluid and electrolyte loss: dehydration, hypokalaemia, hyponatraemia, pre-renal azotaemia and circulatory collapse. Invasive carcinoma frequently develops.
th

31 a) The physical signs are congested eye with the redness maximal at the junction of the cornea and the sclera, an oval dilated fixed pupil and loss of the corneal reflex due to corneal oedema.
b) The treatment is immediate referral for intensive local therapy with a miotic—pilocarpine or eserine, for example—with subsequent surgery, that is, a peripheral iridectomy. It must be remembered that the other eye is also at risk for a similar attack at any time.
od

32 a) Cancrum oris, noma and infective gangrene of the mouth.
b) Organisms invariably present are *Fusobacterium fusiformis* and

Borrelia vincenti.
nd

33 a) Erythema marginatum or rheumatic erythema.
b) It results from sensitisation to *Streptococcus pyogenes.*
c) It is associated with subacute rheumatic fever.
ind

34 a) Female *Anopheles* biting.
b) Malaria is transmitted by various species of *Anopheline* mosquitoes.
tmp

35 a) The cramped, tremulous script suggests a diagnosis of Parkinson's disease. In a patient from a psychiatric unit, the possibility of drug-induced Parkinsonism had to be considered, and recovery was in fact due to withdrawal of a phenothiazine.
b) Phenothiazines act by blocking dopamine receptors. Levodopa and allied drugs are therefore ineffective in this form of Parkinsonism, but atropine-like drugs are still effective.
c) A benign or essential tremor—which is worse when the limb is in use— is relieved by alcohol and is often familial. The tremulous writing differs from that seen in Parkinson's disease in that the script is of normal size.
cn

36 Hypertrophied lymphoid tissue (nasopharyngeal tonsil, adenoids) (1) is almost obstructing the choana and is abutting against the inferior turbinate (2), the middle turbinate (3) and the posterior edge of the nasal septum (4).
feurt

37 a) Trisomy 18.
b) Small jaw, low set ears, and a prominent occiput.
cg

38 a) Acute lymphangitis.
b) *Streptococcus pyogenes.*
c) Acute lymphadenitis.

39 a) Sebaceous glands of the labia with black domed secretion. Similar to Cock's peculiar tumour in which septic ulceration of a neglected sebaceous cyst may simulate an epithelioma.
b) The treatment of choice is excision and the lesion may occur in any site of the body where there are sebaceous glands.
clgy

40 Morquio–Brailsford disease is the best-known of a group of serious skeletal disorders characterized by an inborn error of metabolism of mucopolysaccharide (MPS). He suffers from MPS 4.
co

41 Sugar baby. The term was first used in Jamaica where a high sugar, and consequently low protein, diet was held responsible. Oedema, low serum albumin and fatty liver are the main features, with absent or minimal skin changes.
nd

42 a) There is a 'salmon pink' swelling of the conjunctiva.
b) This is pathognomonic of a lymphoma but the lesion should be biopsied. A general examination should be undertaken as they may sometimes be associated with systemic lymphomatous deposits elsewhere, and the case should therefore be referred for specialist assessment.
ot

43 a) Gross trabeculation; 'fir-tree' bladder; left vesico-ureteric reflux.

b) Neuropathic disease such as multiple sclerosis.
ur

44 a), d) and e).
gm

45 Trichuriasis. The operculated egg of *Trichuris trichiuria* is diagnostic.
tmp

46 Secondary carcinoma.
cpa

47 c) Paronychia is caused by subcuticular or intracutaneous infection.
ae

48 Albright's syndrome. Polyostotic fibrous dysplasia associated with cutaneous pigmentation, generalized disorder of bone and sexual precocity (commoner in the female).
co

49 a) Ranula—a retention cyst in the floor of the mouth.
b) Caused by retention and/or extravasation of mucus from the sublingual or submandibular salivary glands.
c) Treatment is by marsupialization.
psd

50 e).
gm

51 a) Contact allergic dermatitis to nickel caused by metal found in earrings.
b) This affects 10 per cent of European women.
c) Avoidance of nickel containing jewellery should be advised.
d) Patch tests.
al

52 There is no resistance to leg extension and the popliteal angle (normally 90°) is absent due to abnormal hypotonia. The child is a case of Down's syndrome.
pd

53 a) The diagnosis is an hypopyon, that is, pus in the anterior chamber as is shown by the level of white fluid behind the cornea. Although it may arise spontaneously in some conditions, it should be borne in mind the patient may have previously been prescribed some eye drops which contain local steroids and would facilitate the growth of any organisms breaching the integrity of the cornea.
b) It is dangerous to prescribe local steroids, with or without an antiobiotic, unless adequate serial observation is made with a slit-lamp. Hypopyon ulcers are extremely serious as the infection may pass into the vitreous jelly inside the eye and a pan-ophthalmitis will result. Occasionally, an hypopyon may be seen as part of a systemic 'collagen disease'. All cases of hypopyon should be referred for urgent specialist treatment.
od

54 Chronic protein-energy malnutrition. It is seen not uncommonly in adults and older children and may appear during re-feeding of chronically under-nourished subjects.
nd

55 Uncertain! Sever's calcaneal apophysitis is a condition diagnosed clinically. It appears to be a response to repeated traction on the calcaneal apophysis in young people and to that extent is akin to Osgood–Schlatter's disease (anterior tibial tubercle epiphysitis). The patient complains of pain in the heel and is tender over the apophysis. Abnormal radiological appearnce of

the apophysis as in this case is gratifying but is not necessarily present in patients with clinical Sever's disease—some patients with abnormal apophysis on random X-ray have no history of discomfort nor any positive clinical signs!
is

56 a) One hour after admission, ECG documents episodes of ventricular tachycardia.
chtr 2

57 Dyschondroplasia—Ollier's disease.
co

58 b), c) and d).
bd

59 a) Localised myxoedema.
b) Graves' Disease; Autoimmune (Hashimoto's) thyroiditis.
c) Deposition of mucopolysaccharides.
d) High circulating levels of thyroid stimulating antibodies.
end

60 Loaiasis. The adult worm (*Loa loa*) can be extracted with fine forceps after anaesthetizing the conjunctiva.
tmp

61 a) The patient has left facial palsy, with inability to close the eye, show his teeth or contract the platysma on that side. The severity of the weakness suggests a lower motor neurone palsy.
b) (i) Ask the patient to wrinkle his brow—if this is a lower motor neurone palsy the left side will be paralysed.
(ii) Test for loss of taste and ask about hyperacousis—which may be present if a lesion in the petrous temporal bone has damaged the chorda tympani or the nerve to the stapedius.
(iii) Look in the ear for evidence of zoster or otitis media.
(iv) Look for papilloedema, nystagmus, loss of the corneal reflex, deafness or ataxia due to a tumour in the cerebello-pontine angle.
c) The need for tarsorrhaphy to protect the exposed cornea.
cn

62 e) This is a giant hairy naevus. Approximately 10 per cent of these develop into malignant melanomas.
nb

63 A large Bartholin's abscess of the left side which is obscuring the introitus. The operation of choice is marsupialization of the abscess.
clgy

64 Well-demarcated even-density spherical mass showing cyst of left kidney.
ur

65 a) Dermatitis herpetiformis.
b) Direct immunofluorescence of freshly frozen skin reveals deposit IgA in the dermal papillae. Jejunal biopsy should be performed as this condition is associated with subtotal villous atrophy.
c) Some patients with long-term involvement of the small bowel may develop lymphoma.
d) Most patients respond to Dapsone but a gluten-free diet should be encouraged.
al

66 c) Note the gross facial, upper limb and trunk petechiae.
ae

67 Measles. Cell-mediated immunity is markedly impaired, serum albumin falls dramatically, and xerophthalmia may be precipitated.
nd

68 None, except to illustrate the maxim that deformity is preferable to loss of function in the hand. This hand belongs to a black-belt judoka, himself a county champion who has had many injuries to the fingers including dislocations of inter-phalangeal joints and fractures. Happily the little finger has remained uninjured! Nevertheless hand function has been excellent because, in part due to the patient's own excellent motivation, treatment of his injuries has always been directed primarily to restoring proper function in the hand.
is

69 a) This is Scheuermann's disease or adolescent kyphoscoliosis.
b) It is associated with osteochrondritis of the spine. It produces deformity both in the dorsal spine, where it is most obvious as a kyphosis, and in the lumbar spine which is hyperlordotic. Among changes associated with this condition are elongation and compression of vertebral bodies which may be associated with chronic back pain in later life.
is

70 The patient has a complete cleft palate. The flexible rhinolaryngoscope has been passed into the nasal cavity through the palatal cleft and angled forwards towards the mouth.
feurt

71 Dengue haemorrhagic fever (DHF). During the last two decades, epidemics of DHF have occurred in S.E. Asia. In a recent epidemic in Cuba, similar cases have been seen for the first time in the Western hemisphere.
tmp

72 1. Pulmonary valve.
2. Aortic valve.
3. Atrial appendages.
4. Superior vena cava.
5. Right pulmonary veins.
6. Left pulmonary veins.
cpa

73 a) Lateral rectus palsy due to damage to the sixth cranial nerve.
b) The weakness usually improves rapidly and complete recovery takes place within a few weeks.
id

74 a) A left lower motor neurone facial palsy with a tarsorrhaphy, wasting of the left sternomastoid and weakness and wasting of the left side of the tongue. The patient is wearing a hearing aid on the left.
b) An extensive lesion on the left side of the brain stem—possibly a glomus jugulare tumour.
c) By looking for a vascular 'polyp' in the left external auditory meatus.
cn

75 All stages of asexual parasites, from young trophozoites to schizonts, appear in the peripheral circulation in benign tertian malaria due to *Plasmodium vivax*.
tmp

76 a) The physical signs are a row of opacities against a red reflex as seen with the ophthalmoscope. These opacities are extremely anterior and therefore must be in the lens.
b) The diagnosis is thus a cataract.
od

77 a) Toxic epidermal necrolysis, 'the scalded skin syndrome'.
b) Drug allergy, particularly sulphonamides.
c) Staphylococcal infection.
al

78 a) This is genu recurvatum or

hypermobility of the knee with hyperextension.
b) It is frequently found in hypermobile joint disease in juveniles. Flexibility of joint has been described as the one modality of physical fitness of which an athlete or sportsman can have too much. Hypermobile joints do not stand up well to the rigours of body-contact sport such as association or rugby football. Additionally in the knee hypermobility, i.e. hyperextensibility, is a potent factor in the development of chondromalacia patellae due to the fact that in full extension the patellar tends to lift out of the femoral groove thus reducing the restraining properties of the lateral femoral condylar ridge.

is

79 a) The X-ray shows a radio-opaque catheter curled up in the upper oesophagus. No air has entered the gastrointestinal tract.
b) The diagnosis is that of oesophageal atresia without a fistula.

psd

80 c) and e).

bd

81 b) A graft repair of the drum and reconstruction of the ossicles may be necessary in this case.

ae

82 a) Autoimmune (Hasimoto's) thyroiditis.
b) Measurement of serum TSH (thyrotrophin) and total or free thyroxine (T4).
c) Measurement of thyroid microsomal and thyroglobulin antibodies.
d) Hypothyroidism; pernicious anaemia.

end

83 a) Multicystic disease of both kidneys.
b) Unlike polycystic disease it does not progress to renal failure.

ur

84 Overstretching of ligaments after breach delivery with extended legs. Recovery will be complete after some days. Abnormality of the hip joint has to be excluded.

pd

85 There are three cells of the erythroid series, respectively early, intermediate and late megaloblasts, with the large size, the open chromatin nuclear network, and the premature haemoglobinisation characteristic of megaloblasts. There are two neutrophil polymorphs, one with two nuclear lobes and the second with five, and two earlier granulocyte precursors, one a neutrophil myelocyte and the second a neutrophil metamyelocyte. The eighth cell is a lymphocyte. In the absence of further information the likely diagnosis is megaloblastic anaemia, probably secondary to vitamin B12 or folate deficiency, although other causes of defective synthesis of nucleic acids are possible.

hacy

86 a) Cystic hygroma or lymphangioma.
b) The treatment consists of careful excision. The small cystic lesions tend to invaginate between the great blood vessels and nerves of the neck.
c) The danger of delayed treatment is sudden increase in size due either to haemorrhage, or infection, which can result in compression of the trachea with life-threatening respiratory distress.

psd

87 a) Hydrocephalus due to a colloid cyst in the third ventricle.

b) Headache (often paroxysmal), vomiting, ataxia, dementia and falls due to sudden loss of consciousness or weakness.
c) Dementia, papilloedema and an unsteady gait.
cn

88. a) Neurofibromatosis.
b) Pigmentation—café-au-lait spots.
c) Phaeochromocytoma.
end

89. A fish bone (1) is impacted in the base of the tongue (2). The epiglottis (3) and the larynx (4) can also be seen distally. The otalgia is referred via the glossopharyngeal nerve.
feurt

90. a) Onchocerciasis.
b) With a razor blade or a scalpel, a tiny piece of skin is snipped off and placed in a drop of saline on a microscope slide under a cover slip. After some minutes, actively-moving microfilariae of *Onchocerca volvulus* can be seen to emerge from the skin into the surrounding saline.

tmp

91. a) Incisional hernia.
b) Wound infection, abdominal distension, increasing age, obesity, use of absorbable sutures for wound closure and resuturing an abdominal dehiscence.

92. a) A 'cold' abscess arising from tuberculosis of the spine.
b) A radiograph of the dorsal spine should be performed to determine and localize the tuberculous infection.
co

93. Behçet's disease.
ud

94. a) These are changes on the articular aspect of the patella typical of chondromalacia patellae.
b) There is manifest degeneration of the articular cartilage but it is not certain to what extent this is responsible, if at all, for the production of the symptom of anterior knee pain. It may well be that this type of derangement is simply a reflection of a derangement of patello-femoral joint function which in some other way is responsible for the development of pain. Attempts to treat chondromalacia by a primary attack on the changes occurring in the articular cartilage tend to be on the whole disappointing.
is

95. a) The arteriogram shows displacement of the anterior cerebral artery to the left due to the presence of a crescenteric avascular mass between the vault and the right hemisphere. A fracture line runs obliquely across the left side of the skull.
b) An extradural haematoma due to rupture of the right middle meningeal artery.
c) Urgent referral for surgery.
cn

96. 'Horse-shoe' deformity.
'Adult-type' cystic disease.
rd

97. a) Pectus excavatum.
b) Operation is usually undertaken around the age of 5 years for cosmetic and psychological reasons.
psd

98. a) Addison's disease.
b) Yes.
c) Adrenal antibodies.
d) Chest and abdomen for evidence of tuberculosis.
end

99 a) Glaucoma.
b) Autosomal recessive.
nb

100 a).
ae

101 a) Neurofibromatosis.
b) Autosomal dominant.
c) Scoliosis and pseudoarthrosis of the tibia.
d) In about half of the cases.
cg

102 a) Gas in the soft tissue.
b) Gas gangrene (Clostridial myonecrosis).
c) *Clostridium perfringens* is the most important species; others which may be implicated include *C. septicum*, *C. histolyticum* and *C. sporogenes*.

103 a) The physical sign of note is the wide and deep cup in the optic disc. This sign almost certainly indicates some form of chronic glaucoma.
b) The patient should be referred for a specialist assessment, e.g. perimetry and tonometry.

Similarly, a patient with a difference in the cupping of the disc on each side may be suffering from some form of glaucoma and should be promptly referred.
od

104 Red blood cell.
Epithelial cell or podocyte.
Endothelial cell.
Mesangial cell.
rd

105 Tuberculous dactylitis.
co

106 Condylomata of the vulva, or carcinoma of the vulva. Despite the size of the lesion the regularity suggests condylomata, but obviously a biopsy would give the precise diagnosis.
clgy

107 *Dracunculus medinensis* or Guinea worm. Boiling of the water would have killed the intermediate host *Cyclops* harbouring the larvae. The success of the Water-Sanitation Decade could eradicate this infection.
tmp

108 a) The obvious physical sign is pallor of the inferior portion of the retina caused by a patch of thickening so that the choroid is not seen as clearly as that above. Inspection of the vessels shows a block of the central retinal artery. Thus this is a block of the lower branch of the central retinal artery. Sometimes the whole retinal artery can be blocked so the whole fundus presents the milky appearance and the ensuing visual loss is usually catastrophic and permamnent.
b) Causes are numerous but the one that should be considered first is temporal or giant-cell arteries in the elderly. If this condition is not diagnosed the other eye may well be affected and the patient may become permanently blind. Other causes are hypertension, arteriosclerosis, collagen disease and emboli.
od

109 a) The X-ray shows a left diaphragmatic hernia with a shift of the mediastinum to the right side (apparent dextrocardia).
b) A nasogastric tube should be passed to decompress the gastrointestinal tract. If this does not dramatically improve the infant's condition, mechanical ventilation via and endotracheal

tube is required. Repair of the hernia through the abdomen in order to correct the associated malrotation.
psd

110 a) Acute pseudomembranous candidiasis (thrush).
b) The surface layer wipes off easily, leaving a bleeding surface. The material removed can be directly stained to show fungal hyphae.
c) Thrush occurs only in the mouths of debilitated patients —anaemias, diabetes and other conditions may be precipitating factors and should be suspected.
om

111 Bilateral cephalhaematoma due to sub-periostal bleeding, divided by the firm attachment of the periosteum to the sagittal suture. Gradual resorption occurs.
pd

112 Leonine facies of a patient suffering from lepromatous leprosy.
co

113 a) Infantile spinal muscular atrophy (Werdnig–Hoffman disease).
b) Fasciculation.
c) 1 in 4.
cg

114 a) Angular cheilitis.
b) Loss of vertical face height, the result of inadequate dentures.
c) This may also occur in patients with anaemias, diabetes and other debilitating diseases—sometimes as an early sign.
om

115 a) Calcification in the articular cartilage.
b) Chondrocalcinosis.
rh

116 a) Coronary artery occlusion causing myocardial infarction.
b) Right coronary artery.
cpa

117 Prolapse of the urethral mucosa, urethral carbuncle, papilloma of the urethra, carcinoma of the urethra.
clgy

118 a) Syphilis. Herpes is unlikely to produce a crusted lesion which lasts for over two weeks. In older male patients in particular, the differential diagnosis of crusted lesions of the lip should include the possibility of carcinoma.
b) The lesion is likely to be highly infective.
c) The oral and perioral lesions of syphilis are usually described as painless.
om

119 a) Thrush.
b) *Candida albicans*, a yeast.
c) In infants, infection may be derived from the mother or from other infants as a result of cross-infection. In adults, the infection is usually endogenous and is found in dehydrated or debilitated patients or when the flora of the buccal cavity has been disturbed by antibiotic therapy. Chronic superficial and deep-seated infection may complicate disorders of immunity.
id

120 There is a left vocal cord palsy present. The left arytenoid cartilage (1) and ary-epiglottic fold (2) have prolapsed towards the midline. Left-sided vocal cord paralysis is four times more common than right-sided vocal cord paralysis because the left recurrent laryngeal nerve courses through the chest and

is likely to be involved in a bronchial carcinoma. The right recurrent laryngeal nerve lies within the neck only.
feurt

121 a) Burst abdomen (abdominal dehisence).
b) Increasing age, obesity, post-operative abdominal distension, advanced malignant disease, uraemia, jaundice, debility and malnutrition.

122 a) Adson's test.
b) Listening for a subclavian arterial bruit caused by partial obliteration of the artery by cervical rib pressure.
co

123 a) There is an area of increased pigmentation in the lower part of the conjunctiva deepening as it passes down into the fornix. Occasionally, it involves the upper part of the conjunctiva and even the backs of the lids and sometimes spreads onto the skin.
b) The diagnosis is a conjunctival melanosis.
c) No treatment is needed except observation as occasionally the condition can turn malignant, in which case the patches become heavily pigmented, thicker and more vascular. Such cases should be referred promptly for specialist treatment.
ot

124 a) Flattening of the thenar and hypothenar eminences indicates that there is gross wasting of the small muscles of the hand. There is also atrophy of the tips of the fingers, suggesting a diagnosis of leprosy.
b) Motor neurone disease, syringomyelia, peroneal (or distal spinal) muscular atrophy and compression of the deep terminal branch of the ulnar nerve in the palm.
c) Motor neurone disease and syringomyelia can both produce a bulbar palsy, fasciculation and a spastic paraplegia. In motor neurone disease, however, the arm reflexes are brisk and sensation is normal. In syringomyelia the arm reflexes are lost and scoliosis and a suspended dissociated sensory loss are found. Peroneal atrophy—which is familial—also produces a characteristic deformity of the legs. Compression of the palmar branch of the ulnar nerve spares the hypothenar mass. None of these conditions produces gross trophic changes.
cn

125 Aortic aneurysm involving the descending aorta and caused by arteriosclerosis. Note streaks of calcification in the muscle wall. The patient also had history of angina pectoris, hypertension, one previous stroke and features of early peripheral vascular disease. These various disorders indicate a generalized atheroma.
st

126 a) Median glossitis.
b) This is not a developmental lesion as at once thought, but is associated with candidal infection. Anti-fungals may be quite effective in reducing the extent of the lesion.
c) There is no evidence that this is a premalignant lesion (although it is often mistaken for a carcinoma at first sight). However, it may be difficult to eliminate completely by any means, medical or surgical.
om

127 b) There are several lacerations: the visible apical laceration is superficial but continues to bleed. Haemostasis.
chtr 2

128 b) & c) Osteoid osteomas are benign neoplasms of osteoblasts. A rounded focus of osteoid is present in a richly vascular connective tissue stroma.
bd

129 d).
nb

130 a) Prolapse of the uterus (Second degree, as the cervix protrudes through the introitus).
b) The dryness of the skin around the cervix suggests it has been protruding for some time.
c) The treatment of choice is surgical depending on other factors, a Manchester repair operation, or a vaginal hysterectomy and repair operation.
clgy

131 a) Turner's syndrome.
b) Primary amenorrhoea and lack of secondary sexual characteristics.
c) Increased carrying angle.
d) Chromosome analysis. The typical form of the syndrome is associated with deletion of one X chromosome (karyotype 45X0), but the incomplete forms and mosaics may be seen, in which case the patient may be chromatin positive.
end

132 a) Ectopia lentis (dislocated lens).
b) Marfan's syndrome.
c) Homocystinuria. In Marfan's syndrome the lens usually dislocates superiorly; in homocystinuria, inferiorly.
d) Dissecting aortic aneurysm; mitral valve disease.
esd

133 a) Pyostomatitis gangrenosum.
b) This is the oral equivalent of pyoderma gangrenosum, which may occur particularly in the ulcerative colitis but also in other gastrointestinal tract disorders.
c) Generalised stomatitis and oral ulceration resembling simple aphthous ulceration may occur in bowl diseases. Crohn's disease may extend to the oral cavity in a specific form resembling the condition in other parts of the gastrointestinal tract.
om

134 This the commonest site of rupture during the first week after a transmural myocardial infarct.
cpa

135 Tuberculoid leprosy.
tmp

136 a) Chloroquine.
b) Abnormal retinal pigment is arranged in a ring-like fashion in the macula—a 'bull's-eye macula'.
c) Irreversible loss of vision with a central scotoma.
esd

137 Formation of keloid scar.

138 a) Pyelonephritis.
b) By blood-borne or retrograde ureteric pathways.
rd

139 An early lesion of espundia due to *Leishmania braziliensis*. The lesions of mucocutaneous leishmaniasis are first evident as ulcers involving the mucocutaneous

areas of the mouth and nose.
tmp

140 a) Mallory-Weiss syndrome: 2nd day fibroscopic study. The patient suffered a single episode of haematemesis (followed by melaena) after drinking two glasses of beer. A longitudinal mucosal laceration of the right posterior wall begins 3.5 cm above the cardia. Here it is deep (viewed 3 cm above the cardia which is held open by insufflation).
chtr 2

141 a) Necrotising retinochoroiditis. White atrophic foci in the fundus are surrounded by pigment.
b) Toxoplasmosis.
esd

142 b), d) and e).
nb

143 b) The skull radiograph may be negative. Patients should be treated with prophylactic antibiotics because of the danger of meningitis.
ae

144 a) Loosening of femoral head prosthesis.
b) Staphylococcal infection.

145 Blue sclerae—a feature of osteogenesis imperfecta.
rh

146 a) Chickenpox virus pneumonia.
b) A widely used disseminated interstitial pneumonia with patchy haemorrhagic consolidation. The alveoli are filled with protein-rich fluid containign red cells and mononuclear cells. This pneumonia is caused by the chickenpox virus and not by secondary bacterial infection.
id

147 a) Lymphosarcoma.
b) Presentation may be with dyspnoea, cough, and symptoms of superior vena cava obstruction. May also present as an acute emergency with severe airway obstruction.
psd

148 a) A third nerve palsy and ophthalmoplegia.
b) This followed an attack of herpes zoster affecting the ophthalmic division of the fifth cranial nerve on the right. The upper eyelid is drooping and the patient is unable to look upwards. The conjunctiva on the affected side is markedly congested. There is pigmentation and scarring of the skin on the right side of the forehead and nose.
id

149 a) Systemic lupus erythematosus.
b) Pleuritis and/or pericarditis develop a haemolytic anaemia which can exacerbate these symptoms.
c) Antibodies to double stranded DNA, are found in over 80 per cent of patients.
al

150 c) The prolapse reaches a diameter of 3 cm, and here the temporarily strangulated gastric mucosa becomes cyanotic.
chtr 2

151 c) Osteophageal stenosis 16 months after a bleach burn. Intraparietal inflammation and submucosal hypervascularisation are clearly in evidence. Surgery at this stage often leads to iterative stenosis.
chtr 2

152 a) *Wuchereria bancrofti* can be an aetiological agent in the formation of hydrocoele.
b) The diagnosis can be confirmed by finding the parasite in the hydrocoele fluid and/or in the blood taken at night.
tmp

153 b), d) and e).
gm

154 a) This is a post-traumatic pseudocyst. Here it is seen through the lesser omentum. Derivation to the posterior stomach.
chtr 1

155 a) Eczema herpeticum.
b) Herpesvirus hominis.
id

156 a) Apart from a weakly staining myelocyte and two metamyelocytes the field consists chiefly of erythroid series, ranging from a proerythroblast through all stages of erythroblast maturation to late normoblasts and mature erythrocytes. The nucleated erythroid cells all contain free iron, mostly arranged as a continuous or almost continuous ring around the nucleus—they are 'ringed sideroblasts'.
b) This iron is chiefly concentrated in mitochondria and is most characteristically seen in primary acquired refractory sideroblastic anaemia—a myelodysplastic preleukaemic state. It occurs less commonly and less strikingly in secondary forms associated with exposure to isoniazid, cycloserine, alcohol and some other drugs, or as a component of other myeloproliferative or reactive erythroid states, or more rarely in some systemic autoimmune diseases. There is also an hereditary, sex-linked, form of sideroblastic anaemia.
hacy

157 a) Neural tube defects.
b) 1 in 30.
c) Aminocentesis and a good ultrasound should be offered.
cg

158 a) Thanatophoric dysplasia.
b) Very low.
c) Yes.
d) H-shaped vertebrae, short ribs and 'telephone-handle', bent femora.
cg

159 There are multiple plaques of *Candida albicans* (thrush). This may also occur in patients receiving broad-spectrum antibiotics or steroids, and in diabetics and other debilitating states.
feurt

160 Cortical narrowing.
A fine granularity of the cortical surface.
Increase in peri-pelvic fat.
Prominent muscular arteries.
rd

161 Uterine prolapse and rectal prolapse of which the latter is more marked. Both are benign conditions, and surgical repair of the respective lesions is the treatment of choice.
clgy

162 The X-ray skull shows enlargement of the sella turcica. The patient has a pituitary tumour causing acromegaly. Further investigations revealed that the patient had congestive cardiac failure, diabetes mellitus and osteoporosis, along with enlarged facial features and depression. Following a thorough medical assessment, treatment was initiated with bromocriptine.
st

163 e).
gm

164 a) Malignant hypertension.
b) Acute renal failure.
rd

165 a) Rubeosis iridis.
b) Adhesion of the abnormal blood vessels of the iris to the anterior lens capsule thereby forming posterior synechiae.
c) Ocular and particularly retinal ischaemia.
d) (i) Diabetes, central retinal vein occlusion, carotid stenosis; (ii) long–standing retinal detachment, chronic uveitis, intra-ocular tumour.
e) Neovascular glaucoma.
esd

166 *Borrelia duttoni*, the cause of thick-borne relapsing fever, which acquires its name from the typical relapsing nature of the fever. It only appears in the blood during the febrile episodes which are numerous and of short duration.
tmp

167 a) Cleidocranial dysplasia.
b) Autosomal dominant.
c) Nil.
cg

168 a) Giant pigmented hairy naevus.
b) No.
c) No. There is a small risk of melanomatous changes.
cg

169 Giant-cell tumour of bone occurring in its most typical site.
co

170 a) Herpetic vulvovaginitis.
b) This results from primary infection with *Herpesvirus hominis*.
c) The diagnosis may be confirmed by demonstrating a herpesvirus on electron microscopy, or by identifying the virus on tissue culture or primary human amnion cells or primary rabbit kidney cells, although many other cells are susceptible.
id

171 Nephrotic child with *Plasmodium malariae*. A close association has been established between quartan malaria and the nephrotic syndrome in children.
tmp

172 a) Cheiralgia paraesthetica.
b) Injury to the superficial terminal branch of the radial nerve, which runs over the styloid process of the radius.
c) Injury to the nerve at this point by tight wrist-watch straps, shopping-basket handles, cut-down drips, handcuffs, etc.
cn

173 a), b) and c).
gm

174 Snapping or subluxing peroneal tendons. This is a peculiar condition the cause of which is uncertain. The peroneal tendons ride out of their grooves on the posterior aspect of the lateral malleolus and dislocate or sublux onto the subcutaneous surface of the lower fibula. The condition can be quite disabling and requires treatment by surgical reconstruction of the peroneal tendon sheaths to bring the peronei back to their proper relationship with the malleolus below which (rather than over the side of which) they run to their insertions in the foot.
is

175 a) *Trypanosoma gambiense* or *rhodesiense*.
b) They are the causative organisms of African sleeping sickness.
tmp

176 a) Sprengel's shoulder.
b) A radiograph of the cervical spine should be done in all cases, because of its association with severe skeletal abnormality.
co

177 This is a typical ophthalmoscopic appearance of a small embolus seen as a refractile body filling the lumen of a branch of a retinal artery. This causes transient loss of vision. Also called amaurosis fugax, which is a type of transient cerebral ischaemic attack.
st

178 a) Exomphalos major.
b) Malrotation is invariably associated with an exomphalos. Commonly associated problems include congenital heart deformities, and Beckwith–Wiedermann syndrome (exomphalos, macroglossia, gigantism and hypoglycaemia.
psd

179 a) The physical sign shows a loss of red-reflex above caused by a curtain of retina hanging over a visual axis.
b) The patient has a retinal detachment.
c) This should be urgently referred for surgery and it must be remembered that there may be retinal weaknesses in the other eye which can be treated in such a fashion so as to prevent an outright detachment.
od

180 Horner syndrome. There is a narrow palpebral fissure, miosis, enophthalmus of the left eye and absence of facial sweating caused by injury to the cervical sympathetic chain of the first and second thoracic segment.
pd

181 a) Enlargement of the ¾ lumbar intervertebral foramen with scalloping of the back of the body.
b) A dumb-bell neurofibroma.
c) The lesion is well below the cord—which ends at L_1—and will be compressing the cauda equina. The sacral roots will be most severely affected, so in addition to back pain there will be bilateral sciatica, difficulty with micturition, numbness over the posterior aspect of the lower limbs ('saddle anaesthesia') and loss of the ankle jerks.
cn

182 a), b) and d).
gm

183 a) Systemic sclerosis (scleroderma).
b) Proteinuria.
rd

184 a) Myxovirus parotitis.
b) The virus is diesseminated by infected saliva and gains access through the respiratory passages. Virus is also found in urine, but there is no evidence that this is important in the spread of mumps.
c) About one third of all attacks are subclinical.
id

185 a) Peutz–Jegher's syndrome.
b) Intestinal polyps—usually benign adenomas although malignant change may occur.
c) This is transmitted as an autosomal dominant characteristic.
om

186 d) and e) Calcified aortic knuckle is commonly seen in the X-rays of old people who may have associated atheroma.
gm

187 a) Irregular long ragged stricture of

deep urethra.
b) Carcinoma of urethra.
ur

188 a) There is a corneal foreign-body just below and to the left of the pupil and it must be removed.
b) This is best done by anaesthetizing the eye and an attempt should be made first to sweep it off with some cotton wool wrapped around an orange stick. If this fails it should be removed with a disposable needle or referred for specialist treatment.
od

189 A thoraco-lumbar myelo-meningocele with Arnold–Chiari malformation and lack of sphincter control (incontinence). There is marked neck retraction, the brainstem and cerebellum are displaced downwards into the cervical canal. The meningocele is covered with skin and a vascular membrane containing nerve tissue.
pd

190 Faecalith.

191 a) Tuberculosis.
b) Normal lower moiety. Tuberculosis may completely spare one moiety of the kidney.
ur

192 a) A small, well-defined round shadow in the fourth right interspace.
b) A rheumatoid nodule.
rh

193 Concentric left-ventricular hypertrophy due to benign hypertension.
cpa

194 a) 'Main-en-lorgnette' due to destructive absorption of phalanges.
b) It is sometimes seen in rheumatoid or psoriatic arthritis.
rh

195 a) Winging of the scapulae and a lumbar lordosis suggest a muscular dystrophy. At this age the patient is unlikely to have a severe limb girdle dystrophy, and examination of the face confirmed that she had the facioscapulo–humeral variety.
b) As an autosomal dominant.
c) The disease usually runs a long, benign course, but the presence of a marked lordosis at this age is disconcerting.
cn

196 b) This is a contact entry wound, with extensively damaged underlying tissues. Flame burns and unburnt powder were found in the wound. The pink staining around the edges may be due to carbon monoxide, forming carboxyhaemaglobin.
ae

197 a) There is a level of blood in the anterior chamber. This is an hyphaema.
b) There may be other associated injuries to the globe and the patient should be referred for specialist attention.
od

198 e).
gm

199 This clinical photograph shows very nicely the occasional appearance of a step in the line of spinous processes in patients with spondylolisthesis. The superior vertebral body has slid forward in relation to that below it as a result of separation of the pars interticularis with the lamina. Put simply and somewhat crudely the

upper half of this patient is 1 cm anterior to the lower half! Step deformity described in patients with spondylolisthesis is in fact a relatively uncommon finding.
is

200 a).
ae

201 It is a teratoma partly covered with normal skin containing dental and osseous tissue. The baby is otherwise normal. There was no disability after removal of the growth.
pd

202 a) Target cells (thin hypochromic cells with central haemoglobin), helmet cells (the same type of abnormality—a bell-shaped codocyte—seen from the side), macrocytes (erythrocytes of large diameter), spherocytes (small, round, deeply staining cells) and schistocytes (irregularly fragmented cells).
b) The predominance of target cells, together with the other red cell abnormalities, makes ß thalassaemia the most probable diagnosis.
hacy

203 a) Gangrene.
b) Diabetes mellitus.
end

204 a) There is obvious limitation of movements of the right eye vertically and some enophthalmos. Further examination shows anaesthesia of the infra-orbital nerve.
b) This is a case of a blow-out fracture which should be referred for specialist attention as surgery may be necessary to alleviate the vertical diplopia which can be incapacitating.
od

205 a) Reduction in platelets as, for instance, in idiopathic thrombocytopenia. However, the reduction in platelets in early leukaemias may have a similar result.
b) In thrombocytopenia gingival bleeding and oral 'blood blisters' may occur. In early leukaemia gingival hyperplasia and bleeding may occur.
c) A common cold may produce a disconcertingly similar appearance for a short time.
om

206 b).
ae

207 The baby has lamellar ichthyosis ('collodion baby'), a disturbance of keratinisation of autosomal recessive inheritance. After a few days the superficial membrane peels off exposing a softer skin which remains scaly and itching. The condition has to be differentiated from the severest form of congenital ichthyosis ('harlequin baby') where shedding of the membrane does not occur. Affected infants do not survive.
pd

208 c).
ae

209 Mesangial (Kimmelstiel–Wilson) nodules.
Capsular drops.
Fibrin caps.
rd

210 a) Sacro-iliitis.
b) Ankylosing spondylitis, Reiter's syndrome, psoriatic arthritis, inflammatory bowel disease.
rh

211 b).
ae

212 a) Subdural effusion. In a subdural

haemorrhage, blood may track through the subdural space along the optic nerve and be visible on fundoscopy.
b) Fractured skull; meningitis.
nb

213 b).
ae

214 a) An arteriovenous malformation.
b) With 'migraine', fits and/or a subarachnoid haemorrhage.
c) Patients tend to have fits *or* haemorrhages. As resection is usually difficult or impossible, the former may best be treated medically. For those who bleed, embolization of the lesion now offers a promising alternative.
cn

215 a) 'Sciatic scoliosis', distinguished from true scoliosis by the absence of any vertebral rotation.
b) The patient tilts to the right to avoid stretching the left sciatic nerve roots.
co

216 a) There is a network of new vessels on the optic disc.
b) Proliferative retinopathy in diabetes mellitus.
c) Although asymptomatic at this stage, new vessels are fragile and may break and bleed, causing the patient to complain of symptoms such as 'floaters'. Further extensive haemorrhage into the vitreous results in severe visual loss. Subsequent vitreous organisation and fibrosis may cause traction retinal detachment.
d) Retinal photocoagulation.
esd

217 a) Variable mixtures of calcium phosphate, oxalate and organic matrix.
b) (i) Unilateral.
(ii) Alkaline.
c) Variable—may be symptomless, or give rise to pain, haematuria or repeated episodes of renal infection.
rd

218 c).
ae

219 a) Hirsutism.
b) Idiopathic. It is not possible to identify an adrenal or gonadal abnormality in the majoriry of patients.
c) Amenorrhoea; virilism (i.e. temporal baldness, deeping of the voice, breast atrophy, masculine habitus and clitoral abnormality).
d) Androgens, glucocorticoids, phenytoin, diazoxide.
end

220 a) Schistosmiasis.
b) Contacted irregular bladder. Strictures of the juxtavesical ureters, tortuous dilated, 'intestine-like' ureters.
c) Tuberculosis.
ur

221 d) Hysterical contraction of the hand. An analysis of the balancing forces of muscle to produce this attitude shows that it is anatomically impossible to explain by any form of nerve or tendon damage. Although it bears some resemblance to Trousseau's sign, it was confirmed to one hand only, and there was no other suggestion of tetany. It is an example of motor hysteria.
co

222 a) No.
b) The commonest are oral contraceptives, phenothiazines, tricyclic antidepressants, methyl dopa, haloperidol and reserpine.

    c) Primary hypothyroidism.
end

223 They are vocal cord nodules (singers' nodules) and occur more commonly in those occupations requiring pronounced vocalisation (teachers, singers and sargeant-majors). Most cases respond to speech therapy.
feurt

224 Venous hypertension and stasis leading to pericapillary fibrin deposition and impaired tissue oxygenation.
si

225 a) On examination the eye is slightly congested and it is seen that the lower eyelashes are abrading the front of the eye because the eyelid has rotated inwards.
b) The diagnosis is that of entropion.
c) The case should be referred for minor surgery. A useful interim step may be to pull the eyelid very gently down with a layer of adhesive transparent tape. This can be left there for days if necessary.
od

226 Keratodermia blennorrhagica in Reiter's syndrome.
rh

227 a) Right staghorn calculus, multiple small calculi in right lower pole, non-functioning right kidney. Note the normal left kidney.
b) Right vesico-ureteric reflux.
ur

228 a) Microscopic examination by polarised light after Congo Red staining.
b) Amyloid infiltration of glomerular basement membranes.
rd

229 a) Infarction of the lateral part of the medulla.
b) Traditionally, Wallenburg's lateral medullary syndrome is attributed to thrombosis of the posterior inferior cerebellar artery. In fact, it is usually due to thrombosis of the vertebral artery.
c) The main complaints are of dizziness, dysphonia and dysphagia due to damage to the vestibular and cerebellar systems and the vagus. Characteristic findings are impairment of facial sensation, a Horner's syndrome and ataxia on the side of the lesion, with loss of pain and temperature sensation on the opposite side of the body due to damage to the spinothalamic tract. The twelfth nerve, the medial lemniscus and the pyramid (which can be seen to the left of the slide) are spared.
cn

230 Abscess of the liver due to *Entamoeba histolytica*.
tmp

231 He has temporal arteritis.
b) Erythrocyte sedimentation rate, which is very elevated and a temporal artery biopsy which may reveal giant cell arteritis.
c) Blindness.
d) The patient should be treated immediately with systemic steroids which could avoid complications.
al

232 Raynaud's phenomenon. May occur in a), c), d) and e).
gm

233 Tuberculoid leprosy with damage to the ulnar nerve. This characteristic picture is referred to as the *main de predicateur*.
tmp

234 a) This is the typical appearance of a stress fracture at the junction of the upper and middle thirds of the tibia. As will be seen the fracture involves a large proportion of the cortex and is transverse/oblique.

b) Stress fractures of this type are significant in that they can readily go into a complete fracture of the bone with displacement (particularly when the crack is oblique or longitudinal) and all the other problems of tibial fracture. This is one of those sites of stress fracture, therefore, where the fracture is treated with circumspection and immobilisation may be necessary.

is

235 a) Polyp arising from the cervix or uterus.

b) The complaint is that of 'something coming down' on standing or straining.

c) Once the site from which the polyp arises has been detected, it should be removed. This polyp in fact originated from the cervix.

clgy

236 c).
bd

237 The rubella syndrome. Contact with rubella by susceptible mothers within the early weeks of pregnancy carries a high risk of congenital malformation. Active immunisation should be included in immunisation programmes.
pd

238 a) Hidradenitis suppurativa.
b) Apocrine sweat glands.
c) Inguinal regions and perineum.
si

239 Simple obesity which can produce rapid development. It has to be differentiated from the 'buffalo type' of obesity, the Cushing's syndrome (adrenocortical hyperplasia) which is of similar appearance. Here the hormonal assay is always abnormal.
pd

240 a) Atlanto-axial subluxation.
b) Rheumatoid arthritis.
rh

241 a) Increased pigmentation of the buccal mucosa which can occur in Addison's disease.

b) They may complain of fatique, anorexia and gastrointestinal upset. Occasionally they may be hypotensive, hyperglycaemic and hypothermic, with vitiligo and alopecia.

c) If the disease is not treated, coma and death may occur.
al

242 a) Acute suppurative parotitis.
b) Elderly, debilitated patients who become dehydrated especially after surgery.
c) *Staphylococcus aureus*.

243 a) Congestive type.
b) Long runs of attenuated, degenerate, muscle fibres. Some nuclei large and hyperchromatic. Some muscle fibres hypertrophic. Increased fibrosis. Scattered inflammatory cells. Mild vacuolation of centre of some muscle fibres.
cpa

244 d). The patient has angular stomatitis which tends to occur in chronic under-nourishment and multi-vitamin deficiency.
gm

245
a) Medullary carcinoma (with amyloid stroma).
b) From the parafollicular, calcitonin-secreting, C cells.
c) Adrenal phaeochromocytoma (often bilateral) and parathyroid adenoma (or hyperplasia): Sipple's syndrome, multiple endocrine neoplasia Type 2. Other associations include mucosal neuromas, intestinal ganglioneuromatosis, skeletal deformities and a marfanoid habitus (multiple endocrine neoplasia Type 2b or 3).

Apart form calcitonin, medullary carcinomas can secrete other substances including ACTH, serotonin, prostaglandins and histaminase. The ACTH-secreting tumours may be associated with Cushing's syndrome.
th

246
a) The physical sign shows a raised pinkish swelling above the temporal to the optic nerve of the right eye. The colour and shape are characteristic of a retinoblastoma.
b) The patient should be referred for urgent treatment as other tumours may be present, not only in this eye but also in the other eye. Genetic counselling may be necessary.
ot

247
a) Peutz–Jegher's syndrome—intestinal polyps associated with mucocutaneous pigmentation.
b) Complications include intussusception, recurrent gastrointestinal haemorrhage presenting with iron-deficiency anaemia and, rarely, malignant degeneration.
psd

248 c) and e).
nb

249
a) Bitot's spot. This is indicative in young children of Vitamin A deficiency.
b) No. This lesion is nasal; most are on the temporal aspect of the conjunctiva.
nd

250
a) Post-traumatic cervical meningoceles.
b) Avulsion of the cervical roots from the cord—usually in high-speed, road-traffic accidents.
c) The patient has a flaccid, areflexic, anaesthetic 'flail' arm. There will also be loss of paraspinal sensation, weakness of the rhomboids and serratus anterior, and a Horner's syndrome because the lesion is proximal to the posterior primary rami, the proximal motor and sympathetic outflows. The distal sensory fibres, though disconnected from the cord, survive because the dorsal root ganglion is distal to the lesion. Despite loss of sensation, conduction studies and the triple response (which is mediated through sensory fibres) are therefore normal. The chance of recovery is slender.
cn

251
a) Postcoital, postcontact, or intermenstrual bleeding are the most likely symptoms. If, after the menopause, it may be postmenopausal.
b) The diagnosis may be suggested by cervical cytology (i.e. malignant cells present), but biopsy is essential to confirm the diagnosis of carcinoma of the cervix.
c) Treatment depends upon the stage, but in general, it will be by radiotherapy, surgery or a combination of both.
clgy

252 Hydatid cysts. *Taenia echinococcus* is widespread in dogs. Eggs accidentally ingested by man develop into the larval, cystic stage, commonly in the liver.
tmp

253 a) The specimen shows a typical osteosarcoma arising in the lower part of the femoral shaft, abutting on the epiphyseal plate and invading the surrounding soft tissues.
b) Although no aetiological factor can be identified in the majority of cases, osteosarcomas may follow exposure to ionising radiation; in older people, the tumours sometimes arise as a complication of Paget's disease of bone. Rarely, genetic factors are involved; for example, survivors of the familial form of retinoblastoma may develop osteosarcomas outside any radiation field.
th

254 b) and c).
ud

255 a) Casal's necklace.
b) Pathognomonic of pellagra.
c) It is treated with 500 mg nicotinamide daily.
nd

256 a) Pneumatosis intestinalis with detailed loops of intestine.
b) Necrotizing enterocolitis.
c) Nasogastric suction, parenteral nutrition and broad-spectrum antibiotics. Surgery is reserved for impending or frank intestinal perforation.
psd

257 a) Scurvy (vitamin C deficiency).
b) Elderly male patients suffering from self-neglect.
c) A significant proportion of patients with scurvy are extreme 'food fadists' who may be quite young. There is no element of self-neglect in the ordinary sense of the term in these patients.
om

258 An infra-orbital oedema, a gaping mouth due to nasal obstruction, hypertrophic tonsils and a geographical tongue. The child is suffering from perennial rhinitis.
pd

259 a) Pilonidal sinus.
b) Granulation tissue.
c) Free hairs from the skin above the sinus.

260 a) Swelling of the optic disc; hyperaemia; haemorrhage.
b) Papilloedema or papillitis. In papilloedema the blind spot is enlarged; in papillitis visual acuity is severely affected.
esd

261 The girl has idiopathic thrombocytopenic purpura of the recurrent type. This illness is triggered off by viral infections or sensitizing agents like drugs leading to increased platelet destruction and haemorrhage. Recovery followed splenectomy.
pd

262 a) Beta-cell adenoma of the pancreatic islets of Langerhans. Hyperinsulinism. (The tumour may also be called an 'insulinoma.')
b) Tumours of the islets may be associated with:
(i) the Zollinger–Ellison syndrome—intractable peptic ulceration with hypergastrinaemia;
(ii) glucagonoma syndrome—necrolytic migratory erythema, anaemia, stomatitis, diabetes, venous thrombosis, weight loss,

diarrhoea and mental disturbances;
(iii) the somatostatinoma syndrome—achlorhydria tolerance curve;
(iv) the Verner–Morrison syndrome or 'pancreatic cholera'—watery diarrhoea with achlorhydria, hypokalaemia and acidosis (WDHA syndrome). Islet-cell tumours can also produce a variety of other hormones, including ACTH (with Cushing's syndrome), ADH, serotonin, parathormone and prostaglandins.
th

263 a) Multiple fistulae in ano; 'watering-can perineum'.
b) Crohn's disease.

264 b) This is trenchfoot of both feet, caused by prolonged wearing of soaking boots in temperatures just above freezing.
ae

265 Brushfield's spots; speckling of the iris by stromal fibres around the iris near the limbus. It occurs with Down's syndrome and tends to disappear with age.
pd

266 Congenital toxoplasmosis.
tmp

267 a) Osteolytic metastases of left lesser trochanter.
b) Re-calcification.
c) Hypernephroma.
ur

268 a) This is a speckled leukoplakia.
b) In lesions of this type there is almost always a candidal involvement, although it is not known whether this is a true aetiological factor or whether superinfection occurs after the initial formation of the lesion. Tobacco smoking is strongly implicated in the production of these lesions.
c) Speckled leukoplakias and those shown histologically to have candidal infiltration have a reputation for a relatively high incidence of malignant transformation.
om

269 a) Prominence of the subcutaneous border of the tibia on both sides due to wasting of the anterior tibial group of muscles.
b) Wasting, weakness and areflexia suggest a gradual destruction of lower motor neurones. Such profound abnormalities are unlikely to be due to polyneuritis when the arms are normal and sensation is intact. A cauda equina lesion would usually produce pain in the back and legs, saddle anaesthesia and loss of sphincter control. The age and speed of onset, and the general appearance are not in keeping with peroneal atrophy. Motor neurone disease, however, occasionally presents as a slowly progressive paraplegia with loss of reflexes and gross wasting. There may be little or no fasciculation, and the wasting may be concealed by dependent oedema. In this instance the arms were involved in 18 months, and the diagnosis was confirmed at autopsy.
cn

270 c) This is a small laceration of the jejunum 5 cm from Treitz' angle, after a closed trauma. Repair and recovery.
chtr 1

271 A sequence of normal neutrophil granulocytes including a myeloblast, with several nucleoli

and marked cytoplasmic basophilia; a promyelocyte (with a single vacuole) retaining nucleoli but with basophilia less conspicuous and confined to the cytoplasmic rim and with a scattering of azurophilic granules; a myelocyte with oval nucleus, minimal nucleolar traces and mixed azurophil and neutrophil granules; a metamyelocyte with U-shaped nucleus and neutrophilic granularity of cytoplasm; and two stab cells, each with a densely pachychromatic twisted rod-shaped nucleus and fine neutrophil granularity.
hacy

272 a) A salivary gland tumour—most probably a pleomorphic adenoma.
b) Yes. In spite of the slow growth of the lesion, it could be one of the more aggressive forms of salivary neoplasm.
c) Fairly radical excision—salivery gland neoplasma are quite unpredictable in their behaviour.
om

273 a) Ingrowing toenail (onychocryptosis).
b) Incorrect cutting of toenails and tight footwear.
c) Avulsion of toenail, wedge resection of nail bed, complete ablation of nail bed.

274 Synechia vulvae (adhesion of the labia minora). The introitus is covered by a thin, translucent membrane which can initially be easily removed by stretching. Left untreated it may lead to ascending urinary infection and later with menarche to haematocolpos.
pd

275 b) This is cellulitis affecting the right forearm and arm. It resolves completely with antibiotics and rest.
ae

276 a) Myelination of the optic disc and retina. Affected nerve fibres partially obscure the retinal vessels and edge of the optic disc, characteristically giving rise to a shiny white lesion with feathery margins.
b) This condition occurs spontaneously in about 1 per cent of the population and more frequently in cases on neurofibromatosis (von Recklinghausen's disease).
c) It is usually asymptomatic and requires no treatment.
esd

277 b) This is a pilonidal abscess, resulting from infection of a pilonidal sinus.
ae

278 a) Left renal artery stenosis with post-stenotic dilatation.
b) Underlying cause is atheroma.
ur

279 a) Wasting of the legs and the distal part of the thighs ('inverted champagne bottle legs'), high arched feet and ulceration of the toes.
b) Wasting of the hand muscles, areflexia, a positive family history and possibly fasciculation, loss of vibration sense, hypertrophy of nerves and ataxia.
c) Peroneal muscular atrophy—a condition which may be due to a demyelinating or an axonal neuropathy or to distal spinal muscular atrophy. It is closely related to familial hypertrophic polyneuritis and to the Roussy Levy hereditary ataxia.
cn

280 b).
ae

281 The most significant pre-disposing factor is maternal infection with condylomata acuminata (genital warts), and if such lesions are active around the time of delivery an elective Caesarian section should be considered.
feurt

282 a) Apart from two probable lymphocytes or lymphoplasmacytoid cells (the small nucleated cells with coarsely staining chromatin and somewhat 'clockface' marking) the remaining cells are all early granulocyte precursors; they show varying degrees of cytoplasmic basophilia; Auer rods are present in two myeloblasts and in one of two promyelocytes with azurophil granules; there are two early myelocytespresent, one showing degenerative changes with breakdown of cytoplasmic membrane and a large pale nucleolus.
b) The diagnosis is acute myeloblastic leukaemia.
hacy

283 Megacolon due to chronic Chagas' disease. The responsible organism is *Trypanosoma cruzi*.
tmp

284 a) The right temporal lobe is swollen and inflamed. To a lesser extent the rest of the brain is also injected, and there is a cerebellar pressure cone. The picture is that of herpes simplex encephalitis.
b) Fever, headache, impairment of consciousness, fits and/or hemiparesis.
c) The EEG often shows a characteristic periodic slow wave discharge. Serological studies may ultimately confirm the diagnosis, but for immediate confirmation a brain biopsy is required.
cn

285 a) A carcinoid tumour, featuring the typical eosinophilic basal granulation of the cells.
b) From the argentaffin cells of Kulchitsky which are members of APUD series of paracrine cells. APUD is an acronym derived from the common biochemical properties of the cells: amine-precursor uptake and decarboxylation.
c) Carcinoid tumours, particularly those with bulky metastases in the liver, may be associated with the 'carcinoid syndrome': bouts of flushing with mottled cyanosis, bronchospasm, diarrhoea, abdominal pain and borborygmi, and fluctuations of blood pressure. A pellagra-like syndrome sometimes develops and the occurrence of scleroderma-like lesions has also been reported.

Carcinoid heart disease is characterised by the deposition of hyaline fibrous tissue on the value cusps, the mural endocardium and the intima of the great veins. The chordae tendineae become thickened. The pulmonary valve becomes stenotic and the tricuspid valve is usually fixed and the incompetent.
th

286 Leprosy.
ud

287 Paget's disease of the upper femur. Pathological fracture of the upper femoral shaft.
rh

288 A ball thrombus arising in the left auricular appendage. The thrombus commonly forms in association with

chronic mitral-valve disease.
cpa

289 b) This is an infected sebaceous cyst. It can be differenciated from a carbuncle by the history of a pre-existing swelling in the area.
ae

290 Keratoconus. Milder cases require visual correction with a contact lens, but severe cases may need a corneal transplant.
al

291 a) Microcephaly.
b) Half are recessive. The recurrence risk is 1 in 8.
c) A normal, small brain.
cg

292 a) Here the osteophytes are sufficiently large to make the introduction of the fibroscope difficult.
chtr 2

293 Lepromatous leprosy.
ud

294 a) Rhagades. A chronic form of angular stomatitis.
b) It is seen in infants with congenital syphilis, but usually due to riboflavin deficiency in older subjects.
nd

295 b).
ae

296 b), d) and e).
rd

297 a) The physical signs shows a tense fluctuant mass caused by an abscess of the lacrimal sac.
b) Stagnation of tears, because of a blocked naso-lacrimal duct which is a chronic condition giving a running eye, has become acutely infected.
c) Such cases require antibiotics and, almost certainly at this stage, incision to drain the abscess with subsequent surgery to restore the patency of the tear passages on this side.
od

298 a) Broncho pulmonary dysplasia.
b) Mechanical ventilation following treatment for hyaline membrane disease; high F_1O_2.
nb

299 a) A group of six promyelocytes, showing variable fine-to-coarse azurophil granularity largely filling the cytoplasm, and with conspicuous multiple Auer rods visible in several cells. The nuclei are generally oval or round but with a tendency to indentation, more striking in one cell.
b) The diagnosis is acute promyelocytic leukaemia.
hacy

300 a) Hyperparathyroidism.
b) Bone cyst and subperiosteal erosions.
c) Raised calcium; low phosphate; raised alkaline phosphatase; raised parathyroid hormone.
d) Pseudogout, due to precipitation of calcium pyrophosphate crystals.
end

301 a) He has a central dysphasia and perseveration. The flow of words is free, but the patient is unable to express ideas in properly constructed sentences or, by reading what he has written, to perceive the repetition and errors. A patient with an expressive dysphasia would have made numerous amendments or abandoned the letter.

    b) In patients who are right-handed the lesion would be in the left temporo-perietal region.
    c) If the disability appeared suddenly the lesion is probably vascular. If it developed slowly it is more likely to be neoplastic.
    cn

302 a) Corneal abrasions may be caused by trauma or a foreign body.
    ae

303 a) Further exploration, as seen here, exposes the small bowel (D), the stomach (E) and the colon (F). The left lobe of the liver (G) is visible through the diaphragmatic rupture (arrows).
    chtr 2

304 a) Anal atresia.
    b) Vater syndrome.
    c) No.
    cg

305 a) Extensive consolidation of the right middle and basal lobes.
    b) Impaired respiratory effort and depressed cough reflex in the postoperative period lead to retention of pulmonary secretions and pulmonary atelectasis. Superadded infection leads to pneumonic consolidation.
    si

306 Post-kala-azar dermal leishmaniasis (PKDL). This syndrome is a sequel to visceral leishmaniasis due to *Leishmania donovani* following treatment. The dermal lesions contain amastigotes in large numbers.

307 c).
    ae

308 Bilateral adrenal calcification. This occurs a few weeks after adrenal haemorrhage and may remain as a permanent radiological curiosity.
    nb

309 b) Penetrating injuries to the perineum carry a high risk of damage to the anal canal, rectum, urethra and bladder. A careful examination under general anaesthesia should be undertaken. In all cases, digital rectal examination should be carried out. Blood on the examining finger suggests a tear, even if the latter cannot be felt.
    ae

310 Salicylate-associated rhinitis, which usually comprises rhinitis, nasal polyps, sinusitis and asthma—all of which are exacerbated by aspirin and other NSAIDs.
    al

311 Onchocerciasis. The condition of this patient is sometimes called 'leopard skin' and is almost pathogenetic of late *Onchocerca volvulus* infection.
    tmp

312 Cutaneous larva migrans or 'creeping eruption' due to infective larvae of various species of animal hookworms.
    tmp

313 a) Williams syndrome.
    b) Hypercalcaemia.
    c) Supravalvular aortic stenosis.
    cg

314 a) Paget's disease of the nipple.
    b) The epidermis is infiltrated with large, palely-staining, pleomorphic carcinoma cells ('Paget's cells'). The cells often contain intracytoplasmic mucin.
    c) In the overwhelming majority of cases, Paget's disease of the nipple is associated with carcinoma in the subjacent

breast, although the tumour is impalpable in about 50 per cent of the patients. Treatment should be planned on the assumption that a mammary carcinoma is present.

d) Extra-mammary Paget's disease occurs in the skin of the vulva, the perianal region, the groin and the axilla; very rarely in other sites.

th

315 c) This is pseudo-pneumothorax. The patient has a tension gastrothorax following a rupture of the diaphragm.

chtr 1

316 a) Tetracyclines.
b) Tetracyclines do not cause hypoplasia of tooth substances. These changes may be due to the condition for which the antibiotic was administered.
c) From interuterine life to approximately 11 years of age—it is possible to produce staining after this age but it is unlikely to prove a cosmetic problem.

om

317 a) Dilated bladder; dilated proximal ureter; narrow distal stream.
b) Urethral valves.

nb

318 Vernal catarrh.
ud

319 Ascariasis. Examination of stools will reveal numerous, characteristically shaped eggs of *Ascaris vermicularis*.
tmp

320 a) Peripheral retinal angioma with a prominently dilated and tortuous feeding artery and draining vein.
b) Cerebello-retinal haemangioblastomatosis (von Hippel–Lindau syndrome).
c) Increased production of erythropoietin caused by a tumour of the kidney.

esd

321 b) and d). The patient has a left-sided ptosis. Causes include congenital simple ptosis, third-nerve palsy, vascular lesions, tumours, Horner's syndrome, multiple sclerosis, myasthenia gravis and traumatic. Posterior cerebral infarction causes visual problems but not ptosis.

st

322 a) Apart from two normoblasts with very dense nuclei and a probable megakaryocyte nuclear fragment with an associated scattering of platelets, the nucleated cells are all of the granulocyte series. They include a myeloblast, a promyelocyte, a poorly granular myelocyte and stab cell, three neutrophil polymorphs, and no fewer than five basophils of various stages of maturity.
b) The probable diagnosis is chronic myeloid leukaemia.
c) Cytochemical staining would show a low leucocyte alkaline phosphatase score, and cytogenetic studies would reveal the Ph1 chromosome (a 9;22 translocation).

hacy

323 *Trichuris trichiura* infection.
tmp

324 b) This a prepatellar bursitis which has become infected. There is gross cellulitis in the surrounding tissue.

ae

325 c) This is empyema necessitatis. An untreated pyothorax can spread through the chest wall and appear under the skin.
chtr 1

326 The patient had treated coeliac disease, and this biopsy was obtained 6 hours after a gluten challenge. The normal intestinal villi are absent, the mucosa is flattened and there is hyperplasia of the crypts. The surface mucosa is cuboidal, and there is lymphocytic infiltration.
al

327 c) Fundoscopy sometimes reveals obstructed retinal vessels with foci of ischaemia.
chtr 1

328 Henoch–Schönlein purpura.
al

329 c) Some shoulder dislocations compress or even rupture the axillary vessels.
ae

330 a) There are several typical asbestos bodies.
b) Pleural plaques, diffuse pleural fibrosis, pulmonary fibrosis (pneumoconiosis, asbestosis) malignant mesothelioma, pulmonary carcinoma (particularly adenocarcinoma).

An increased incidence of cancer of the oesophagus, colon and rectum, larynx, kidney, oro-pharynx and perhaps stomach has been reported also.
th

331 Rheumatic heart disease.
cpa

332 Periosteal frills along the phalanges and metacarpals due to hypertrophic pulmonary osteoarthropathy.
rh

333 b) The muscle belly lies more distally on the arm.
ae

334 Chronic infection with *Schistosoma mansoni*. Inflammatory reaction around the eggs causes periportal fibrosis of the liver.
tmp

335 a) Multiple papillary transitional-cell carcinomas of the bladder.
b) Urothelial tumours occur as an occupational hazard in workers exposed to certain chemicals, especially α-naphthylamine, ß-naphthylamine and benzidine. An increased incidence of bladder cancers has been found in workers in the aniline dye, rubber and cable industries, and amoung workers in the retort houses of gas works. Cigarettes smoking and analgesic abuse are predisposing factors.
th

336 a) The right vocal cord has been infiltrated along its length by a keratinising squamous cell carcinoma.
b) This disease is invariably associated with smoking, and may be preceded by an area of leukoplakia. A small number of these patients have or will develop a bronchial carcinoma. Hoarseness is usually the presenting feature, and any patient with unresolving hoarseness of greater than 3 weeks duration should be referred for laryngoscopy.
feurt

337 Paragonomiasis. The adult flukes are commonly embedded in the lung tissue in which they deposit their eggs.
tmp

338 a) A Galeazzi fracture-dislocation.
ae

339 b) This procedure involves taking a radial artery blood gas sample. It provides useful data in salicylate poisoning.
ae

340 This field shows two neutrophils (one stab cell and one polymorph), a normal lymphocyte and four 'hairy cells', showing the typical eccentric nucleus with moderately coarse 'spongy' chromatin, the pale slate-blue cytoplasm and the fine surface projections or hairs. A rod-shaped negatively-staining inclusion in one of the hairy cells may represent a ribosome—lamella complex. The diagnosis is hairy-cell leukaemia. Hairy cells characteristically show a strong tartrate-resistant acid phosphate positivity.
hacy

341 Still's disease.
ud

342 b).
ae

343 a) Carbuncle.
b) Diabetic patients.
c) Staphylococci.

344 a) Calcified ova of schistosoma haematobium.
b) The schistosome eggs are passed in the urine, After hatching out, the larvae (miracidia) undergo further development in fresh-water snails and emerge as actively motile cercariae. The cercariae penetrate the human epidermis and eventually migrate to the perivesical venous plexus and the rectal veins.
th

345 Asthma itself causes growth retardation, buut the major cause in his case is long-term oral steroid treatment, evident from his Cushingoid facial features.
al

346 b) Immediate odynophagia is followed by deep emphysema along the entire posterior oesophageal wall.
chtr 2

347 a) Hydatidiform mole.
b) Assessment of HCG levels, especially in dilution will confirm the diagnosis (apart from histology).
c) The risk for the patient is that of choriocarcinoma, and all women who have a hydatidiform mole are advised to avoid becoming pregnant for at least one year, preferably two.
clgy

348 Aphthous ulceration. The cause is unknown, though trauma, infection and occasionally allergy are probable factors.
al

349 a), b), c) and d).
ud

350 b) An occipital bedsore. An alopecic necrotic area developed on the back of the head.
chtr 1

351 a) Renal tuberculosis.
b) Haematogenous spread usually from a primary focus in the lung.

352 b).
ae

353 a).
ae

354 Pyorrhoea (periodontitis).
nd

355 a) Acrodermatitis enteropatheica.
b) It responds to 100 mg zinc sulphate daily.

nd

356 a) There are two neutrophil metamyelocytes and a single lymphocyte; all other nucleated cells are plasma cells, many with dense nuclei and deeply basophilic cytoplasm reflecting high RNA content and active protein synthesis, and often showing a paler perinuclear 'hof' around the region of the Golgi apparatus. Other plasma cells have more lightly staining nuclei and paler cytoplasm and there is a quadrinucleate cell with partially disrupted cytoplasm.
b) This pattern of variability in size and staining characteristics is not uncommon in multiple myeloma, despite the clonal origin of the neoplastic plasma cells.

hacy

357 Toxoplasmosis. When this disease is found in association with a systemic illness, the patient may have a high fever, lymphadenopathy and perhaps a focal maculopapular rash.

ud

358 a) The tumour is composed of a mixture of epithelial tubules and cartilaginous (chondroid) tissue.
b) Pleomorphic adenoma ('mixed tumour').
c) In other major and minor salivary glands, in the lacrimal gland, in the skin, and rarely in the lung and breast.

th

359 a) Thyrotoxicosis (Graves' disease).
b) A diffuse goitre (over which a vascular bruit could be heard) and exophthalmos.

al

360 a) Seminoma.
b) The tumour is very radiosensitive. With modern methods of treatment, a cure rate of about 90 per cent is to be expected.
c) In the ovary (where it is called dysgerminoma); also in certain other (extragonadal) sites, particularly the anterior mediastinum, and in the pineal and suprasellar regions.

th

361 a) A Bennett's fracture.

ae

362 a) Diabetic gangrene.
b) Peripheral neuropathy, microangiopathy, atheromatous disease of major limb vessels and increased susceptibility to infection.

363 c) Three mallet finger deformities in the hand of a patient with rheumatoid arthritis. Tendons are particularly liable to rupture from trivial actions.

ae

364 a) Thymoma; predominantly epithelial, but featuring a moderate number of lymphocytes.
b) Chiefly myasthenia gravis, red-cell agenesis (especially with spindle-cell thymomas) and hypogammaglobulinaemia. Other rarer associations include mucocutaneous candidiasis, polymyositis granulomatous myocarditis, systemic lupus erythematosus, pemphigus vulgaris, autoimmune haemolytic anaemia and Sjögren's syndrome.

th

365 a) Hartnup disease.
b) Due to a defect in absorption of tryptophan.

c) It responds to 100—200 mg nicotinamide daily.
nd

366 Cysticercosis. These are the larval stages of *Taenia solium* normally found in the pig. The adult tapeworm is the usual stage found in man.
tmp

367 Ocular toxocariasis.
ud

368 d) and e). The typical claw-hand deformity is due to a lesion of ulnar nerve with associated wasting of the small muscles of the hand.
st

369 b).
ae

370 b) Callus formation brings a series of pseudarthroses.
chtr 1

371 a) Ludwig's angina.
b) Anaerobic bacteria.
c) Upper respiratory tract obstruction.

372 Yaws. Small outbreaks of yaws have recently occurred and one must be on the look-out for this condition despite the fact that the prevalence of this infection diminished dramatically after the yaws eradication campaign, of the 1950s.
tmp

373 Retinal tear causing focal retinal detachment, which has secondarily caused vitreous hemorrhage and a multitude of floaters presenting in the patient's visual field.
ud

374 c).
ae

375 b) This should be assumed unless proven otherwise by radiography.
ae

376 a) Staghorn calculi.
b) Calcium, magnesium and ammonium phosphate.

377 The picture shows spastic right hemiplegia. Lack of early physiotherapy and rehabilitation may result in a patient developing such spastic postures of the hemiplegic limbs. Frozen shoulder is a frequent complication of a recent stroke, but is not shown in this picture.
st

378 Intraocular larva which needs to be surgically removed from the patient's eye.
ud

379 a) There is a pleomorphic picture, with conspicuous eosinophil polymorphs and some neutrophils, lymphocytes with dark nuclei and minimal cytoplasm, centrocytes with lighter nuclei and somewhat larger size, occasional still larger centroblasts and immunoblasts, together with a few plasma cells and some monocyte—macrophages. There is a single large Reed–Sternberg cell with twisted or overlapping double nucleus and large dark violaceous nucleoli in each figure.
b) The appearance is strongly suggestive of Hodgkin's disease, probably of the mixed cellularity variant.
hacy

380 a).
ae

381 Infection with *Schistosoma haematobium*. Fibrosis around eggs in the bladder wall leads to ureteric obstruction.
tmp

382 CT showing a left convexed meningioma. This patient presented with unsteadiness, falls and confusional episodes. He was diagnosed as a case of recurrent transient cerebral ischaemic attacks but later on he developed contra-lateral upper motor neurone signs with dysphasia, hemiplegia and urinary incontinence.
st

383 a) Bartholin's gland abscess.
b) *Bacteroides* species and anaerobic streptococci.

384 Fatty infiltration, or cardiac adiposity. Extensive adipose tissue extends amongst atrophic myocardial fibres.
cpa

385 Only occasionally is this congenital but this patient has received radiotherapy to the larynx and this is the commonest cause of telangiectasia in this area. Radiotherapy reactions affecting the larynx are diverse and include mucositis, laryngitis sicca, oedema of the larynx and adhesion formation.
feurt

386 a) Pseudomembranous colitis.
b) *Clostridium difficile*.

387 b) Steering wheel syndrome, with fracture of sternum and cardiac contusion.
chtr 2

388 Opposing granulomas (1) lie over the vocal processes (2) of both arytenoid cartilages. Such granulomas classically occur following long-term intubation.
feurt

389 Subphrenic abscess.

390 a) A massive or saddle thrombotic embolus suddenly occluding the bifurcation of the pulmonary artery.
b) A deep vein thrombosis. In this case it had detached itself from a thrombosis in the left calf of the patient.
cpa

391 a) There are three very large cells (<40um diameter) with a normal-sized nucleus but extensive cytoplasm which shows a mixed granular, fibrillary and onion skin pattern of lipid inclusion material. These are Gaucher cells. The field also shows a scattering of lymphocytes, with minimal cytoplasm, a metamyelocyte and a possible monocyte.
b) The condition is Gaucher's disease, a rare familial disorder in which defective activity of the catabolic enzyme ß-glucocerebrosidase leads to the accumulation of glucocerebroside in cells of the monocyte–macrophage system.
hacy

392 A probable massive subcutaneous emphysema due to airways rupture; the hands are steadying the neck in the absence of a definite diagnosis.
chtr 2

393 a) Branchial cyst.
b) Cervical sinus, a second branchial arch derivative.
si

394 a) Osteitis pubis.
b) Widening of the symphysis pubis and rarefaction of the adjacent pubic bones.
si

395 a) There is a slight fluid reaction, but no haemopericardium.
chtr 2

396 Regressed retinoblastoma in the fellow eye.
ud

397 b) This was seen at autopsy seven days after the accident. Death ensued due to multiple haemorrhagic injuries and to a crush syndrome.
chtr 2

398 d) Sub-hyaloid haemorrhage is a classical feature of subarachnoid haemorrhage but is not seen very commonly.
st

399 a) Facial cellulitis.
b) Septic cavernous sinus thrombophlebitis.
si

400 Saliva is seen encroaching upon the arytenoid cartilages (2) and this sign is present in post-cricoid or upper oesophageal neoplasms or foreign bodies, or in neuromuscular disorders which affect the swallowing mechanism.
feurt

Index

Figures refer to question numbers

Achilles tendon rupture, 380
Acrodermatitis enteropathica, 355
Acromegaly, 12, 162
– enlarged pituitary fossa, 3
Addison's disease, 98, 241
Adenoids (nasopharyngeal tonsil enlargement), 36
Adolescent kyphoscoliosis (Scheuermann's disease), 69
Adson's test, 122
Adrenal gland calcification, 308
Adreno-genital syndrome, 6
Albright's syndrome, 48
Amaurosis fugax, 177
Anal atresia, 304
Angular cheilitis, 114
Angular stomatitis, 244, 294
Ankle, rupture of lateral ligament, 352
Anopheles, 34
Anterior fossa of skull fracture, 25
Aortic aneurysm, 125
Aortic knuckle calcification, 186
Aortic valve, 72
Aphthous ulceration, 348
Arteriovenous malformation, 214
Arthritis, septic, 295
Arthropathy, 44
Asbestos body, 330
Ascariasis, 319
Asthma, short stature in, 345
Atlanto-axial subluxation, 240
Atrial appendages, 72
Atrial septal defect, 397
Autoimmune (Hasimoto's) thyroiditis, 82

Ball thrombus of auricular appendage, 288
Bartholin's abscess, 63, 383
Basophil, 322
Basophilia, 8
Bedsore, occipital, 350
Behçet's disease, 93
Bennett's fracture, 361

Bitot's spot, 249
Black eyes, bilateral, 143
Blow-out fracture, 204
Bladder
– dilated, 317
– 'fir-tree', 43
– transitional cell carcinoma, 335
Blue sclerae, 145
Bone
– giant-cell carcinoma, 169
– secondary deposit, 128
Borrelia duttoni, 166
Borrelia vincenti, 32
Branchial cyst, 393
Breech delivery with extended legs, 84
Bronchopulmonary dysplasia, 298
Bullous myringitis, 5
Burns, 206, 208
Brushfield's spots, 265
Burst abdomen, 121

Calcaneal apophysitis, Sever's, 55
Calcinosis circumscripta, 1
Cancrum oris (noma; infective gangrene of mouth), 32
Candidiasis, acute pseudomembranous (thrush), 110, 119, 159
Carbuncle, 343
Carcinoid tumour, 285
Carcinoma, 182
Cardiac contusion, 387
Cardiomyopathy, congestive type, 243
Casal's necklace, 255
Cataract, 76
Cellulitis, 275
Central dysphasia and perseveration, 301
Centroblast, 379
Centrocytes, 379
Cephalhaematoma, bilateral, 111
Cerebello-retinal-haemangioblastomatosis (von Hippel-Lindau syndrome), 320
Cerebral fat embolism, 280
Cerebral ischaemic attack, transient, 382
Cerebrovascular disease, ocular

abnormalities, 153
Cervical carcinoma, 251
Cervical polyp, 235
Chagas' disease, 283
Cheiralgia paraesthetica, 172
Chickenpox virus pneumonia, 146
Chloroquine, 136
Chondrocalcinosis, 116
Chondromalacia patellae, 94
Claw-hand deformity, 368
Cleft palate, 70
Cleidocranial dysplasia, 167
Coeliac disease, 326
"Collodion baby" (lamellar ichthyosis), 207
Condylomata acuminata (genital warts), 281
Congested eye, 31
Conjunctiva
– lymphoma, 15
– melanosis, 123
– sarcoidosis, 15
Contact allergic dermatitis, nickel-induced, 51
Contralateral visual neglect (topagnosia), 13
Cornea
– abrasions, 302
– foreign body, 188
Coronary artery occlusion, 116
Cutaneous larva migrans, 312
Cysticercosis, 366
Cystic fibrosis, 19
Cystic hygroma (lymphangioma), 86

Deep vein thrombosis, 200
Déjérine myopathy (facioscapulohumeral dystrophy), 21, 195
Dengue haemorrhagic fever, 71
Dermatitis herpetiformis, 65
Diabetes mellitus
– gangrene, 203, 362
– hypopigmentation, 173
– infant of diabetic mother, 20
– proliferative retinopathy, 216
Diaphragm
– hernia, 109
– rupture, 127, 303
Dislocated lens (ectopia lentis), 132

Down's syndrome, 52
Dracunculus medinensis (Guinea worm), 107
Dyschondroplasia (Ollier's disease), 57

Ear injury, 81
Ectopia lentis (dislocated lens), 132
Eczema herpeticum, 155
Emphysema, subcutaneous, 392
Empyema necessitatis, 325
Endothelial cell, 104
Entropion, 225
Epithelial cell (podocyte), 104
Erythema marginatum (rheumatic erythema), 33
Erythroblast, 156
Erythrocyte (red blood cell), 9, 104, 156
Erythroid series, 85, 156
Espundia, 139
Exomphalos major, 178
Extensor tendon damage, 374
Extradural haematoma, 95

Facial cellulitis, 399
Facial palsy, 61
Facioscapulohumeral dystrophy (Déjérine myopathy), 21, 195
Faecalith, 190
Femur, fractured neck, 375
Fish bone impaction, 89
Fistula-in-ano, 263
Flexor digitorum profundus/ sublimis injury, 369
Fluorosis, 58
Fusobacterium fusiformis, 32

Galactorrhoea, 222
Galeazzi fracture-dislocation, 338
Gangrene, 203, 362
Gas gangrene, 102
Gastro-oesophageal retrograde prolapse, 150
Gaucher's disease, 391
Genital warts (condylomata acuminata), 281
Genu recurvatum, 78
Giant-cell tumour of bone, 169

Giant hairy naevus, 62, 168
Glaucoma, 99, 103
Glomus jugulare tumour, 29, 74
Glossitis, median, 126
Gout, tophaceous, 198
Granuloma, laryngeal, 388
Graves' disease (thyrotoxicosis), 359
Guinea worm (*Dracunculus medinensis*), 107

Hairy cells, 340
Hand deformities, 68
Hartnup disease, 365
Hasimoto's (autoimmune) thyroiditis, 82
Heart, right, perforation by pacemaker electrode, 395
Helmet cells, 202
Hemiplegia, spastic, 377
Henoch-Schönlein purpura, 328
Herpes hominis type 1, 4
Herpes simplex encephalitis, 284
Herpes zoster, 148, 163
Herpetic vulvovaginitis, 170
Hidradenitis suppurativa, 238
Hirsutism, 219
Hodgkin's disease, 379
Horner syndrome, 180
Hydatid cyst, 252
Hydatidiform mole, 347
Hydrocephalus, 87, 142
Hydronephrosis, 11
Hypernephroma, osteolytic metastases, 267
Hyperparathyroidism, 80, 300
Hypertension
– malignant, 164
– renal lesions, 160, 164
Hypertrophic pulmonary osteoarthropathy, 332
Hyphaema, 197
Hypopyon, 53
Hypothyroidism, infantile, 129
Hysterical contracture of hand, 221

Idiopathic thrombocytopenia, 205
Imperforate hymen, 2
Incisional hernia, 91
Infantile spinal muscular atrophy (Werdnig-Hoffman disease), 113
Infective gangrene of mouth (cancrum oris; noma), 32
Ingrowing toe nail (onychocryptosis), 273
Insulinoma (beta-cell adenoma of islets of Langerhans), 262

Jejunal laceration, 270

Keloid scar, 137
Keratoconus, 290
Keratoderma blennorrhagica, 226
Kidney
– amyloid infiltration of glomerular basement membrane, 228
– cyst, 64
– horse-shoe, 96
– hypertensive lesions, 160
– malignant tumour, pelvic urothelial origin, 296
– multicystic disease, 83
– – adult type, 96
– multiple calculi, 227
– non-functioning, 227
– staghorn calculus, 217, 227, 376
– tuberculosis, 191, 351
Kimmelstiel-Wilson (mesangial) nodules, 209
Knee joint
– hypermobility with hyperextension (genu recurvatum), 78
– protective spasm of hamstring muscles, 23
– rupture of synovial membrane, 14

Lacrimal sac abscess, 297
Lamellar ichthyosis ("collodion baby"), 207
Larva, intraocular, 378
Laryngeal juvenile papillomatosis, 281
Lateral rectus palsy, 73
Laurence-Moon-Biedl syndrome, 9
Left ventricle
– concentric hypertrophy, 193
– rupture of wall, 134
Leishmaniasis
– mucocutaneous, 139
– post-kala-azar dermal, 306

Leprosy, 112, 124
- lepromatous, 293
- scleritis, 254
- tuberculoid, 135, 233
- uveitis syndrome, 286
Leukaemia
- acute promelocytic, 299
- chronic lymphatic, 213
- chronic myeloid, 322
- hairy cell, 340
- myeloblastic, 283
Leukoplakia, speckled, 268
Liver
- abscess, 230
- hydatid cysts, 252
Loaiasis, 60
Long tendon of biceps rupture, 333
Long thoracic nerve lesion, 182
Lower motor neurone facial palsy, 61, 74
Ludwig's angina, 371
Lymphangitis, acute, 38
Lymphangioma (cystic hygroma), 86
Lymphocytes, 85, 282, 356
Lymphoma, 42
Lymphoplasmacytoid cells, 282
Lymphosarcoma, 147

"Main-en-lorgnette", 194
Malar bone fracture, 100
Malaria, 34
Malignant hypertension, 164
Mallet finger, 363
Mallory-Weiss syndrome, 140
Marfan's syndrome, 132
Measles, 67
Medulla, infarction of, 229
Megacolon, 283
Megaloblast, 85
Megaloblastic anaemia, 85
Meningocele, post-traumatic cervical, 250
Mesangial cell, 104
Mesangial (Kimmelstiel-Wilson) nodule, 209
Metamyelocyte, 85, 271, 356
Microcephaly, 291
Minnigerode's sign, 346
Monilial vulvovaginitis, 22
Morquio-Brailsford disease, 40

Motor neurone disease, 269
Multiple sclerosis, bladder abnormalities, 43
Myeloblast, 271, 282, 322
Myelocyte, 85, 271, 282, 322
Myelo-meningocele, thoraco-lumbar, 189
Myocardium
- fatty infiltration, 384
- infarction, 116
Myositis ossificans progressiva, 10
Myxoedema
- hypopigmentation, 173
- localised, 59
Myxovirus parotitis, 184

Nail-bed injury, 353
Nasal polyp, allergic, 19
Nasopharyngeal tonsil enlargement (adenoids), 36
Necrotizing enterocolitis, 256
Necrotizing retinochoroiditis, 141
Nephrotic syndrome, 171, 228
Neural tube defect, 157
Neurofibroma, dumb-bell, 181
Neurofibromatosis, 88, 101
Neuromuscular disorders, 395
Noma (cancrum oris; infective gangrene of mouth), 32
Normoblast, 322

Obesity, simple, 239
Odynophagia, 346
Oesophagus
- atresia, 79
- stenosis, 151
- upper, neoplasm, 400
- vertebral osteophyte impression, 292
Onchocerciasis, 90, 311
Onchocryptosis (ingrowing toe nail), 273
Optic disc myelination, 276
Osteitis pubis, 394
Osteodystrophy, renal, 58
Osteogenesis imperfecta, 145
Osteoid osteoma, 128
Osteomyelitis, 248
Osteoporosis circumscripta, 50

Osteosarcoma, 253

Paget's disease of bone, 80, 287
Paget's disease of nipple, 314
Paget's sarcoma of humerus, 27
Papillitis, 260
Papilloedema, 260
Paragonomiasis, 337
Parkinsonism, drug-induced, 38
Paronychia, 47
Parotid gland, pleomorphic adenoma (mixed tumour), 358
Parotitis
– acute suppurative, 242
– myxovirus, 184
Patellar fracture, 307
Pectus excavatum, 97
Pellagra, 255
Pericardium, secondary carcinoma, 46
Perineal penetrating wound, 309
Periodontitis (pyorrhoea), 354
Perivasculitis, 349
Pernicious anaemia, hypopigmentation, 173
Peroneal muscular atrophy, 279
Peutz-Jegher's syndrome, 185, 247
Pilonidal abscess, 277
Pilonidal sinus, 259
Plasmodium falciparum, 17
Plasmodium malariae, 171
Plasmodium vivax, 75
Platelet reduction, 205
Pneumatosis intestinalis, 256
Podocyte (epithelial cell), 104
Polydactyly, 9
Polymorphs, 322, 340
– eosinophil, 379
– neutrophil, 379
Post-cricoid neoplasm, 398
Prepatellar bursitis, 324
Primary acquired refractory sideroblastic anaemia, 156
Proerythroblast, 8, 156
Proliferative retinopathy, 216
Promyelocyte, 271, 282, 299, 322
Prostate carcinoma, secondaries, 58
Protein-energy malnutrition, chronic, 54
Proteinuria, 44

Pseudoarthroses of ribs, 370
Pseudocyst, post-traumatic, of pancreas, 154
Pseudomembranous colitis, 386
Pseudopneumothorax, 315
Ptosis, 321
Pulmonary artery embolus, 390
Pulmonary consolidation, 305
Pulmonary valve, 72
Pulmonary veins, right/left, 72
Pupil, unilateral fixed dilated, 342
Purpura, recurrent idiopathic thrombocytopenia, 261
Pyelonephritis, 138
Pyorrhoea (periodontitis), 354
Pyostomatitis gangrenosum, 133

Ranula, 49
Raynaud's phenomenon, 232
Rectum
– prolapse, 161
– villus tumour (adenoma), 30
Red blood cells, 9, 104, 156
Reed-Sternberg cell, 379
Reiter's syndrome, keratoderma blennorrhagica, 226
Renal artery stenosis, 278
Replacement arthroplasty, staphylococcal infection, 144
Retina
– detachment, 179, 373
– myelination, 276
– peripheral angioma, 320
– tear, 373
Retinal artery block, 108, 177
Retinal vessels, fat globules in, 327
Retinitis, reactive, 357
Retinitis pigmentosa, 9
Retinoblastoma, 246, 396
Retinochoroiditis, necrotizing, 141
Rhagades, 294
Rheumatic erythema (erythema marginatum), 33
Rheumatic heart disease, 331
Rheumatoid arthritis, 254
Rheumatoid nodule, 192
Rhinitis
– perennial, 258
– salicylate-associated, 310
Ringed sideroblast, 156

Rubella syndrome, 237
Rubeosis iridis, 165

Sacro-iliitis, 210
Salivary gland tumour, 272
Sarcoidosis, perivasculitis, 349
Scalded skin syndrome (toxic epidermal necrolysis), 77
Scheurmann's disease (adolescent kyphoscoliosis), 69
Schistocytes, 202
Schistosomiasis, 220
– calcified ova, 344
– *Schistosoma haematobium* infection, 381
– *Schistosoma mansoni* infection, 334
Sciatic scoliosis, 215
Scleroderma (systemic sclerosis), 183
Scoliosis, sciatic, 215
Scurvy, 257
Sebaceous cyst, infected, 289
Sebaceous glands, labial, with black domed secretion, 39
Sella turcica enlargement, 162
Seminoma, 360
Septic arthritis, 295
Serratus magnus paralysis, 182
Shotgun wound of chest, 196
Shoulder dislocation, 329
Sickle cell anaemia, 24
Singers' nodules (vocal cord nodules), 223
Snapping (subluxing) peroneal tendons, 174
Speckled leukoplakia, 268
Spherocytes, 202
Spondyolisthesis, 199
Sprengel's shoulder, 176
Stab cell, 271, 340
Stab wound, suicidal, 218
Staghorn calculi, 217, 227, 376
Steering wheel syndrome, 387
Sternal fracture, 387
Still's disease, 341
Stress fracture, 234
Subdural effusion, 212
Subhyaloid haemorrhage, 398
Subphrenic abscess, 389

Sucking cushions, 26
Sugar baby, 41
Superior vena cava, 72
Synechia vulvae, 274
Syphilis
– oral, 118
– perivasculitis, 349
Systemic lupus erythamatosus, **44**, 149
– vasculitis, 349
Systemic sclerosis (scleroderma), 183

Tapir mouth, 21
Target cells, 202
Telangiectasis, 385
Temporal arteritis, 231
Tenosynovitis, acute crepitating, 7
Teratoma, 201
Tetanus, 211
Tetracyclines, 316
– thalassaemia, 202
Thanatophoric dysplasia, 158
Third nerve palsy, 148, 153
Thrush (acute pseudomembranous candidiasis), 110, 119, 159
Thymoma, 364
Thyroid gland, medullary carcinoma, 245
Thyrotoxicosis (Graves' disease), 359
Tibia
– osteomyelitis, 248
– stress fracture, 234
Tonic neck reflex, 28
Topagnosia (contralateral visual neglect), 13
Toxic epidermal necrolysis (scalded skin syndrome), 77
Toxocariasis, ocular, 367
Toxoplasmosis, 357
– congenital, 266
Traumatic asphyxia, 66
Trenchfoot, 264
Trichuriasis, 45, 323
Trisomy, 18, 37
Trypanosoma gambiense, 175
Trypanosoma rhodesiense, 175
Tuberculosis
– cold abscess, 92

– dactylitis, 105
– perivasculitis, 349
– renal, 191, 351
Turner's syndrome, 131

Ulnar nerve palsy, 368
Ureter, dilated proximal, 317
Urethra
– carcinoma, 117, 187
– carbuncle, 117
– papilloma, 117
– prolapse, 117
– tear, 18
– valves, 317
Uterus, prolapse, 130, 161

Vater syndrome, 304
Venous hypertension, 224
Ventricular tachycardia, 56
Vernal catarrh, 318
Vesico-ureteric reflux, 43, 227

Vocal cord
– carcinoma, 336
– nodules (Singers' nodules), 223
– palsy, left, 120
von Hippel-Lindau syndrome (cerebello-retinal haemangioblastoma), 320
Vulva
– carcinoma, 106
– condylomata, 106
Vulvovaginitis, herpetic, 170

Wallenburg's lateral medullary syndrome, 229
Werdnig-Hoffman disease (infantile spinal muscular atrophy), 113
Wucheria bancrofti, 152
Williams syndrome, 313

Yaws, 372